DOPING IN SPORT AND FITNESS

RESEARCH IN THE SOCIOLOGY OF SPORT   VOLUME 16

DOPING IN SPORT AND FITNESS

EDITED BY

APRIL HENNING

University of Stirling, UK

And

JESPER ANDREASSON

Linnaeus University, Sweden

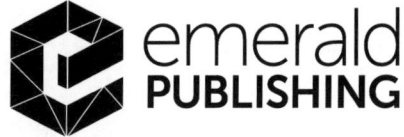

emerald
PUBLISHING

United Kingdom – North America – Japan
India – Malaysia – China

Emerald Publishing Limited
Howard House, Wagon Lane, Bingley BD16 1WA, UK

First edition 2023

Reprints and permissions service
Contact: permissions@emeraldinsight.com

British Library Cataloguing in Publication Data
A catalogue record for this book is available from the British Library

ISBN: 978-1-80117-158-8 (Print)
ISBN: 978-1-80117-157-1 (Online)
ISBN: 978-1-80117-159-5 (Epub)

ISSN: 1476-2854 (Series)

Printed and bound by CPI Group (UK) Ltd, Croydon, CR0 4YY

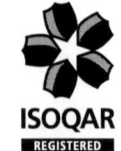

ISOQAR certified
Management System,
awarded to Emerald
for adherence to
Environmental
standard
ISO 14001:2004.

ISOQAR
REGISTERED
Certificate Number 1985
ISO 14001

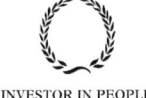

INVESTOR IN PEOPLE

CONTENTS

PART 3 DOPING ARENAS AND COMMUNITIES

PART 4 GENDERING DOPING

ABOUT THE AUTHORS

Jesper Andreasson has a PhD in Sociology and is Professor of Sport Science in the Department of Sport Science at Linnaeus University, Sweden. He has extensive experience of working with ethnography and different internet methods. Andreasson has published widely within the areas of doping, gym/fitness culture, carnalizing sociology and gender theory. He oversees a PhD programme in Sport Science and teaches at the graduate and postgraduate levels, mainly in the areas of research methods, sport science and social theory.

Geoff Bates is a Research Associate at the Institute for Policy Research, University of Bath. His research focuses on identifying and using evidence to inform the development and implementation of services, interventions and policy, and in understanding decision-making and health and social behaviours. With his background in health psychology and public health, Geoff's research applies behavioural and implementation science perspectives to a range of health and social care topics.

Cornelia Blank is Professor and Deputy Head of the Institute for Sports Medicine, Alpine Medicine and Health Tourism at the Private University for Health Sciences and Health Technology (UMIT Tirol) in Hall in Tirol, Austria. She is an international published and cited researcher with experiences in several international and doping-related projects. With a background in health sciences and psychology, her research focuses on prevention and health promotion in and by means of sport. Topics include the perception of doping prevention measures from an athlete's and athlete support personnel perspective. She is furthermore interested in developing and evaluating current doping prevention strategies integrating the athletes' and ASP perspectives.

Andrew Bloodworth is a Senior Lecturer in the School of Sport and Exercise Sciences, Swansea University. His teaching and research is in the field of sports ethics, more specifically the ethics of anti-doping policy. Andrew is also Chair of the College Research Ethics Committee.

Luke Cox is a post-doctoral research fellow at KU Leuven, where he is programme coordinator for the world's first Interdisciplinary Centre for Ethics, Regulation and Integrity in Sport (iCERIS). His PhD examined doping within recreational sport, focusing on ethical aspects of player responses to performance and image enhancing drugs in the context of anti-doping policy. Luke has previously published on doping within Welsh Rugby Union and ethical aspects of the Therapeutic Use Exemptions Policy.

Lovely Dasgupta, PhD, Associate Professor, Law and Director NUJS Centre for Sports Law and Policy, has been teaching and researching in the field of Sports Law since 2003. Her specific interest is doping, sports and third world approach. She has published three books on issues relating to sports law. Her latest book, published by Routledge, is titled *Doping in Non-Olympic Sports-Challenging the Legitimacy of WADA?*

Matthew Dunn, PhD, is a Senior Lecturer in Public Health in the School of Health and Social Development, and a member of the Institute for Health Transformation, at Deakin University, Australia. His research interests include the use of, as well as harms and benefits associated with, licit and illicit substances. His primary research interest is in the field of human enhancement drugs, including anabolic-androgenic steroids.

Bertrand Fincoeur holds a PhD in Criminology from KU Leuven. He is a Senior Lecturer in Sports Sociology and Sports Management at the Institute of Sports Sciences from the University of Lausanne. He is also Senior Lecturer at the College of Humanities from the Swiss Federal Institute of Technology (Lausanne). His research areas primarily cover sports ethics and integrity.

Katharina Gatterer is a senior scientist in doping and anti-doping at the Private University for Health Sciences and Health Technology (UMIT Tirol). With a pedagogical background (teacher training) and a PhD in Sports Medicine, Health Tourism and Leisure Science, her research focuses on adolescent athletes and current anti-doping education and its perception from an athlete's point of view, as well as current doping prevention strategies and its evaluation.

April Henning has a PhD in Sociology and is Lecturer in Sport Studies at the University of Stirling. Henning has published widely on image and performance enhancing drugs in relation to sport and fitness, policy and gender. She is a Director of the International Network of Doping Research. She teaches on undergraduate and postgraduate degree programmes in sport studies, mainly on substance use, social theory and gender.

Helen Jefferson Lenskyj is a Professor Emerita at the University of Toronto, Canada, where she taught Sociology. Her work as a researcher and activist on gender and sport issues began in the 1980s, and she has published eight books critiquing the Olympic industry, as well as five books on gender and sport. Her most recent publication is *The Olympic Games: A Critical Approach* (Emerald, 2020). She completed her PhD at the University of Toronto in 1983 and was a Professor from 1986 until retiring in 2007. Her website is www.helenlenskyj.ca.

Charlotte Mclean is a Visiting Research Fellow with the Public Health Institute at Liverpool John Moores University, where she recently completed her PhD exploring women's use of anabolic-androgenic steroids and growth hormone within bodybuilding culture.

Mike McNamee is Professor of Ethics at KU Leuven, Belgium, and Professor of Applied Ethics, at Swansea University, UK. He has dual backgrounds and qualifications in Philosophy and in Sports Sciences. He has published several books including *Sports, Virtues and Vices* (Routledge, 2008) and *Sport, Medicine, Ethics* (Routledge, 2016), *Bioethics, Genetics, and Sport* (Routledge, 2018). He is the Founding Editor of the international journal *Sport, Ethics and Philosophy* (2007–2017), and Co-Editor of Routledge's 'Sport Ethics' book series (1998–). He is Chair of WADAs Ethics Expert Group.

Jim McVeigh holds the post of Professor in Substance Use and Associated Behaviours at Manchester Metropolitan University. He has worked within the field of substance use for 30 years initially as a Nurse at The Maryland Centre working with people who inject drugs, before moving into academia and building an international reputation within the field of human enhancement drugs, in particular, the use of anabolic steroids and associated drugs. In 2019 he co-edited the Routledge book *Human Enhancement Drugs* and in 2020, he founded the Anabolic Steroid United Kingdom Network and leads the National Institute for Health Research (NIHR) funded research 'Image and Performance Enhancing Drug Use in the United Kingdom'.

Jessica Rullo holds an MSc in Sports Sciences from the University of Lausanne. She graduated and has worked as a Research Assistant on a project on drug use and sports in prison.

Sarah Teetzel is a Professor in the Faculty of Kinesiology and Recreation Management at the University of Manitoba in Winnipeg, Canada. Her research focuses on applied ethical issues in sport with emphasis on gender inclusion and doping.

Honor D. Townshend is a final-year PhD student, Visiting Lecturer and Researcher at University of Hertfordshire, UK. Her research predominantly revolves around gendered identities and IPED use, but other research areas have included: dark web and IPED marketplaces.

Luke A. Turnock has a PhD in Sociology for his research into IPED use among lifting cultures in UK gyms and is a Senior Lecturer in Criminology at the University of Lincoln, UK. He is author of the book *Supplying Steroids Online*, exploring the cultural and market contexts of IPED access and supply on digital fitness forums.

Mair Underwood is an Anthropologist of the body, and Lecturer in the School of Social Science at the University of Queensland, Australia. She specializes in human bodies and their modification, and has spent the last five years exploring online bodybuilding communities. Much of her research has focussed on image and performance enhancing drug use. She is particularly interested in the social lives of enhancement drugs, drug communities as risk and enabling environments, and harm reduction as practised by people who use drugs.

Gemma Anne Yarwood is a Senior Lecturer and Interdisciplinary Researcher studying social care, health and social justice across the life-course with a focus on substance use and associated behaviours. A key focus of Gemma's work is on 'The Body as a Project': body modification, enhancement and social constructs. She has written many publications, including: journal articles; website content; book chapters and reports for various organizations, local authorities and national charities.

INTRODUCTION: UNBINDING DOPING CONTEXTS

April Henning and Jesper Andreasson

ABSTRACT

This chapter introduces the main aims and ambition with the anthology, which is to bring together research from diverse perspectives on doping and Image and Performance Enhancing Drug (IPED) use. The chapter highlights existing but often backgrounded links between sport and fitness doping research and present a re-reading of the cultural history of doping through which simplistic divisions, such as that between sport and fitness, are deconstructed. Further, by unbinding the hegemonic divide between sports doping and fitness doping, new insights (and themes) concerning anti-doping, health and risk, new emerging doping spaces and the gendering of this field of research are brought to the fore. These themes are then used as point of departure when introducing the different chapters and scholars that contribute to the volume at hand.

Keywords: Sport and fitness; doping history; anti-doping; health; doping spaces; gender

Historically, doping and how this practice and phenomenon has been understood has largely been a question of socio-cultural contexts, perspectives and structures (Andreasson & Henning, 2021a). Indeed, users, policymakers, researchers, media stakeholders and others have all taken somewhat different stands towards doping. Their situatedness in varying contexts impacts how they make meaning of doping use and their views on how that use should be handled. In sport, doping has largely been debated in terms of governance and different anti-doping incentives. Among policymakers and health professionals in different countries, developing strategies to prevent people from engaging in doping use and reduce harm if they do so have been the priority. Though situated meaning-making can provide significant insights into particular doping contexts and perspectives, they

Doping in Sport and Fitness
Research in the Sociology of Sport, Volume 16, 1–14
ISSN: 1476-2854/doi:10.1108/S1476-285420220000016001

may also serve to background more general trends, missing insights that are relevant across contexts and the people operating in them.

This anthology is titled *Doping in Sport and Fitness*. We chose to include both sport and fitness in order to direct attention to one of the clearest contextual separations found in the field of doping research: doping in formally governed competitions in elite sports known as *sports doping* and doping as a public health issue – that is, as a social problem predominantly connected to gym and fitness settings, also called *fitness doping*. There are clear overlaps in terms of how issues such as anti-doping, health, risk, gender and more are addressed in these contexts. However, this cultural and contextual divide has been drawn, if not sedimented, in research and fuelled for decades both by the scholarly debate and in public discourse. Therefore, sports researchers have tended to pay the most attention to doping in particular sports (such as cycling, weightlifting, American football etc.), the work and significance of the World Anti-Doping Agency (WADA) and issues of fair-play, as well as how anti-doping is implemented and understood by professional athletes (Dimeo & Møller, 2018; Henning & Dimeo, 2022). In media and public discourse, sports dopers have been condemned for their (immoral) actions and may continue to be stigmatized by a rules violation even after serving their punishments for doping offences. To this end, anti-doping in sport can be ruthless.

In contrast, somewhat different lenses have often been used in the realm of fitness doping. Zooming in on the development of gym and fitness culture, doping has been debated as semi-legitimized, bound to subcultural and often masculine spaces, but still with some level of cultural acceptance within the broader fitness industry (Andreasson & Johansson, 2020; Christiansen, 2020; Klein, 1993; Locks & Richardsson, 2012; Monaghan, 2001). In this realm, researchers have focused on how individuals – mostly men – engage in doping practices to form bodies and lifestyles. This has included specific topics such as how doping communities and ethnopharmacological cultures develop over time, within spaces like gyms or online communities, and as a subcultural practice (Bilgrei, 2018; Henning & Andreasson, 2021; Underwood, 2017).

In the wake of this hegemonic divide between sport and fitness, doping experiences and doping as a phenomenon have sometimes been reduced to a matter of context. This divide has had a huge impact on how doping has been addressed. But times are changing. Since the turn of the century, this field of research has expanded significantly and the focus has broadened. Doping has increasingly been recognized as a public health issue affecting sport, fitness and society (Bates et al., 2019; McVeigh & Begley, 2017). And while previously understood as a more or less solely male phenomenon, the interest in women's use of Image and Performance Enhancing Drugs (IPEDs) has grown (Andreasson & Henning, 2021b; Germain et al., 2020; Havnes et al., 2020; Henning & Andreasson, 2021; Sverkersson et al., 2020). Further, it has been recognized that there is substantial variation among and between use populations in terms of motives, effects and, more broadly, how the drugs are understood in different cultural contexts (Thualagant, 2012; Turnock, 2021; Van Hout & Kean, 2015). This has led to acknowledgement of the need to explore and analyze alternative narratives of doping (Mulrooney et al., 2019; Salinas et al., 2019). Indeed, variability has not only been called for in terms of user experiences but also in terms of the diversity of drugs themselves, including the role of poly drug use and how this can be met and dealt with in diverse contexts, as well as its impact on users' health and lifestyles (Henning & Andreasson, 2021b). Feeding on this scholarly zeitgeist, this anthology hopes to further contribute a broadening of the debate on doping in sport, fitness and elsewhere.

ANTHOLOGY AIMS

A central thought steering this volume is that rigid differentiations between doping contexts and perspectives can be misleading. Eager to zoom in and find a focal point, we as researchers sometimes tend to overlook or background commonalities and potential overlaps, favouring strict categories such as sport and fitness, men and women, online and offline. We may also downplay or even ignore the agency and mobility of bodies and lifestyles, which rarely, if ever, operate in one context exclusively. Elite athletes in sport, for example, do not start out as elite athletes. Rather, they go through a process of training that includes various sport-specific skills and drills beginning in a recreational sport context, and there are probably relatively few top-level athletes who do not combine their sport activities with gym workouts to further boost their performance, image or well-being. Hence, the lines between even the highest performing sports stars and everyday gym-goers are less clear in some ways than has been appreciated in the academic literature.

For this anthology, we are proud to have gathered both established and emerging scholars and colleagues in the field of doping research to illustrate that doping experiences, contexts and perspectives are seldom solely a question of either/or – something that can be culturally/contextually pinpointed in time. Challenging the notion of contextual rigidity, *Doping in Sport and Fitness* aims to bring together diverse perspectives and disciplinary research on doping and IPED use and lay a mosaic in which the contributions together bring the debate and field of research forward. In the shadow of the hegemonic sport and fitness divide in this field, we have structured the contributing chapters around four themes: (1) anti-doping; (2) health and risks; (3) doping arenas and spaces; and (4) the gendering of doping and IPED use. We will use these themes as point of departure in our discussion. Rather than using them as ways of dividing up the broader doping topic, we use them as a cross-cutting organizational tool. The themes here function to illustrate, understand and address doping and IPED use in contemporary society. They apply across contexts and other categorizations common in doping research, in effort to spotlight the areas of commonality between and among research topics previously understood as totally separate. Taken together, this volume will allow for a more complex picture and understanding of substance use patterns, behaviours and responses, pointing towards future developments in this field of research.

For us to meet our aim of breaking down some of the persistent divisions related to doping, it is necessary to reconsider how this phenomenon has developed historically. In doing so, we will show the interconnections between various contexts and highlight some of the more general trends. This overview will be necessarily brief, and others have published more extensively on the history of doping (see Andreasson & Henning, 2021a; Andreasson & Johansson, 2014; Dimeo, 2007; Gleaves, 2014; Henning & Dimeo, 2022). Still, this re-framing of the sport and fitness doping history, in which commonalities and overlaps between and across contexts are emphasized, serves as a suitable foundation for this anthology. We have chosen to frame our discussion around different historical phases. Following this, we will pick up our themes and introduce the contributing colleagues in the next section.

RE-READING DOPING HISTORY

Though people's efforts to boost performance using different means stretch back to ancient cultures, a more contemporary discussion on sports and fitness doping connects to the early twentieth century. During this time, various stimulants were introduced to the consumer market and became available without prescription (Courtwright, 2009). Initially, the use of cocaine, amphetamine and other drugs was largely unrelated to sport and physical culture. These were often used medicinally or even recreationally. However, as there were no rules against their use, it is hardly surprising that they soon bled into performance cultures of the time (Andreasson & Henning, 2021a; Rasmussen, 2008). In the 1950s, these and other forms of drugs also started to appear on the bodybuilding and gym scenes, including early synthetic forms of testosterone, though use of animal testosterone extracts had been tried earlier (Yesalis & Bahrke, 2005). Consequently, during large parts of the early twentieth century, roughly up until the 1960s, stimulants and synthesized testosterone in sport and fitness contexts were met by curiosity and a lust for experimentation. This mirrored social use and views of these substances at the time. The drugs were debated roughly in terms of their potential usefulness for enhancing or restoring human capacities in different social and cultural spheres of society (increasing workplace productivity, improving soldiers' stamina, treatment for frigidity, and more). Gradually, this rhetoric changed. Concerns about the negative effects of doping substances were raised in the broader social context, with similar concerns within sport following closely behind. At this point, the idea of some form of organized anti-doping began to gain ground (Dimeo, 2007).

In the mid-1960s, the question of doping became an issue on the sport agenda. The International Olympic Committee (IOC) set up a Medical Commission in 1967 with remit for developing anti-doping, including drawing on and developing the appropriate scientific methods and tools (Henne, 2014). Sports officials knew athletes were using steroids at this point, yet the Medical Commission was reluctant to prohibit them without a way of enforcing such a rule, namely in the form of a scientific test. Reliable tests for stimulants were used for anti-doping in competitions by then, but a similar test for steroids took several more years to develop. Once this became available, the IOC formally prohibited steroids in 1974 and began full testing at the 1976 Olympics. The anti-doping movement in organized sport was also boosted by a more general concern about drugs in society and the initiation of the 'war on drugs' in the United States and elsewhere in the 1960s and 1970s. In bodybuilding and gym culture, however, a somewhat different atmosphere prevailed. Here, the effects of steroids became visible on the bodies of gym-goers – mostly bodybuilders – and there was a move towards extreme muscle mass and definition (Locks & Richardson, 2012). This became evident via the body of Arnold Schwarzenegger, world famous bodybuilder of the 1970s who remains a beacon of bodybuilding culture. Schwarzenegger used steroids as part of his training to achieve the ideal gym look of the era, which made him a movie star (Andreasson & Johansson, 2020; Schwarzenegger & Petre, 2012). As in the era of organized sports before anti-doping, there were no prominent reasons for bodybuilders to not engage in doping practices presented in public discourse or by policymakers. Steroids and other IPEDs were legal in most countries, and in contrast to the sport context, their use was largely situated as part of the medicalization of society, instead of a concern related to the war on drugs. It was also near the end of the 1970s and into the 1980s that women began entering gyms in greater numbers (Fair, 1999), beginning the re-gendering of this culture.

Whereas the 1970s were marked by rudimentary anti-doping work and cultural acceptance of doping, we can see how the views of doping and IPED use began shifting in both sports and fitness during the 1980s and early 1990s. Within bodybuilding, the use of steroids was gradually problematized as it was linked to ideas about fragile men and masculinities, insecurities and health issues (see Klein, 1993). Testosterone-fuelled bodies were thus painted in a more negative light, and reports on steroid abuse and eating disorders were published. Different autobiographical publications focusing on the dark sides of IPED use also reached the public (see Fussell, 1991). This was also connected to different drug scandals in sports, such as the infamous Canadian sprinter Ben Johnson and his 1988 positive test for steroids at the Summer Olympics that highlighted the issue of doping in sports for spectators around the world. The aftermath of the Johnson scandal saw investigations into doping in several countries and national level policies prohibiting or further restricting IPEDs (Henning & Dimeo, 2022). In parallel with these scandals and policy shifts, there remained an ongoing interest in the impact of doping on the body that echoed interest from earlier decades. Dedicated international bodybuilders exceeded their genetic maximum and broke records for muscle mass, symmetry and vascularity, while elite sports athletes continued to break world records. To a certain extent, the dark sides of use (obsessive behaviours, psychological impacts etc.), existing prohibitions and harsh judgements of doping could co-exist with a cultural attraction to the extreme and to the idea of spectacular – and potentially doped – bodies (Andreasson & Johansson, 2019).

The 1990s constituted a pivotal era in the history of doping. During this time, several events coincided to change the face of IPED use across contexts. For example, natural bodybuilding, done without the use of drugs, emerged around the time when steroids became more heavily regulated in some countries (Liokaftos, 2019). This also related to the broader health and fitness focus of the fitness revolution, a transformation in which a previously exclusive masculine basement culture gradually became a more gender inclusive fitness culture for the masses (Andreasson & Johansson, 2014). These updated ideas of fitness were much more commercialized and 'clean' than the previous iterations of bodybuilding gyms that tended to be exclusive masculine and homosocial spaces (Sassatelli, 2010). The wave of women becoming more engaged in fitness pursuits occurred alongside changes in women's bodybuilding, as the sport itself opened up new competition disciplines that encouraged less muscular forms and prioritized what were considered to be more traditional and accurate feminine forms (Andreasson & Johansson, 2020). This wave of change was situated alongside the theoretical developments of feminist theory in the 1990s. Academics and scholars such as Judith Butler and Donna Haraway helped to fuel the intellectual debate on the gendering of bodies. In general, we can see an increasing fascination on how people with modern body techniques may stretch the limits of what is humanly possible to reshape bodies, and to the reach or challenge the bodily ideals of the time.

Sports also undertook a clean sweep of doping in this period, not least through the development of international anti-doping policies, often led by the IOC. A watershed moment came in 1998 when French border guards found IPED substances and paraphernalia in a search of a car belonging to the Festina cycling team. Though it is likely that cycling officials had some idea of the doping occurring in cycling, French police oversaw the investigation. The investigation expanded to include and then implicate several other teams set to compete in that year's Tour de France (Dimeo, 2014). The ensuing scandal and pressure from media and national governments led to the IOC convening a 1999 meeting in Lausanne, Switzerland, to strategize a path forward. The result was the agreement to establish the WADA, the body that would be charged with policymaking and harmonization of global anti-doping efforts. Across sport and fitness in the 1990s, there was a strong push towards the idea of clean and doping-free contexts. Previously secluded and subcultural spaces were opened and ideals of health and inclusion were brought to the fore in the debate. These changes did not mean that the use of doping decreased. Rather they suggest that the social, cultural and demographic landscape of doping was about to change.

Entering the twenty-first century, the demographics of doping and IPED use appear to be evolving further. Doping is still commonly associated with bodybuilding and elite sports, especially as high-profile scandals continue to haunt events like the Olympics (McLaren, 2016). At the same time, scandals have not prevented the spread of doping among recreational sports athletes (cf. Henning & Dimeo, 2015; Seifarth et al., 2019). Similarly, fitness doping is adapting to demographic changes within the fitness industry (Andreasson & Johansson, 2020). New groups of users, including women and other more routine gym-goers, have opened new markets and new online spaces for doping (Bates & McVeigh, 2016; Hanley Santos & Coomber, 2017). The market and distribution for IPEDs have also followed a roughly similar route as the overall development of the doping landscape. Between the 1970s and 1990s, the IPED market tended to follow a more social and less commercially driven model (van de Ven & Mulrooney, 2017). In this system, experienced users or coaches 'helped out' and mentored newbies on how to use IPEDs. The enforcement of anti-doping policies in sport and laws in some countries has diminished the level of sociability among both users and suppliers as a way to protect against discovery of their activities. As such, the emergence of the online doping space is unsurprising. This new virtual meeting place and trade route has fostered an ever-growing doping market and the development of online doping eco-systems and communities (Fincoeur et al., 2015; van de Ven & Mulrooney, 2017). What we see today is the initiation of a new phase in the historical development of doping and IPED use. Increasingly, critical debates on the effectiveness of various drug control systems in both sport and fitness and the medical curiosities found in the early twentieth century also seem to be reappearing in discussions on human enhancement drugs and ideas about safer or less harmful doping.

In this section, we have illustrated that though the sport and fitness contexts may not always move in lockstep, there is a historical link in approaches and responses. This is exemplified not only through how anti-doping has been implemented but also how questions concerning health, gender and performance manifest. This points to future doping and anti-doping developments potentially becoming even more intertwined than in the past, an idea this volume will investigate further throughout.

THEMES AND CHAPTERS

For much of the twentieth century, sports and fitness doping could be understood as a rational choice for individuals to make. The drugs that many anti-doping policies would eventually prohibit were originally introduced to the public as technologies for improving and enhancing minds, bodies and lifestyles. Such ideas have, of course, lingered, despite the emphasis on health risks and anti-doping heavily promoted by policymakers and other stakeholders. Even after different policies and laws prohibiting their use were implemented, opportunities for use have continued and the range of use populations has grown. Though any number of examples or illustrations might work to describe the global doping milieu, we would like to draw on the idea of nesting dolls. Nesting dolls are a set of dolls that fit one inside the other in descending order of size. A complete set may look like the dolls separated and lined up next to each other as individual dolls, or in their nested state, it may appear as a single doll, the largest obscuring the others. Each doll plays a part in creating the whole in either state, as it would be incomplete if any were to be missing. Similarly, doping is an issue composed of multiple layers. It is possible to take the topic apart and focus on a single layer – say, specific policy strategies or the experiences of a single user group – as much research in this area does. Individually, these provide in-depth looks at discreet pieces of puzzle and improve our understanding of these important component parts. We are fortunate here to have a range of topics covered in a single place, allowing us to see how the topics and themes nest together to form a whole. Even as this picture will be necessarily incomplete, it offers a way to understand how these themes are inextricably linked and how each discreet piece fits within the higher order themes we have used here.

The blurring of doping in sport and fitness also spotlights other themes that have come to form our understandings of the doping phenomenon, such as the development of both anti-doping and new doping arenas and spaces, as well as how IPED use is understood in relation health and gender. These four themes – or layers to our doll – are inextricably linked to one another and seemingly cut across the history of fitness and sport doping. As such, we have chosen to use them as a way of framing this volume's contents. However, these themes are not intended as a way to once and for all systematize this field of research and establish new divides. Instead, the themes serve as an analytical and organizational point of departure. They will help us arrange the contributed chapters for clarity and to dig more deeply into this phenomenon, helping to widen and develop our understanding. Surely, the themes are constructs and there will be overlaps between themes. In the concluding chapter, we will foreground the interconnections between each theme to bring the picture together.

Part I: Anti-Doping Approaches

In this introductory chapter, we have provided an overview of the topic area, the aims of this volume and given an updated historical outline of doping and anti-doping in sport. This historical foundation foreshadowed some of the contemporary debates around IPEDs and doping, as well as some of the considerations key to painting a fuller picture of doping and anti-doping. One of the first considerations relates to the rules and approaches to addressing doping, which often take the form of anti-doping. Doping, and the way it is defined legally and by many researchers, is directly related to questions of governance and how it is regulated through anti-doping (or anti-drug in some contexts) policies. Rather than more 'common sense' understandings of doping as using a substance to enhance performance, doping under WADA's Code, the central policy document for Olympic and member sports, is defined as a violation of its rules. As these policies are the foundation of both individual experience, public perception and research in this field, our first theme includes multiple perspectives on anti-doping law and governance.

In Chapter 1, Lovely Dasgupta considers the implications of the WADA Code for athletes, particularly those from developing countries, from a legal perspective. Exploring the relationship between athletes' rights and sports law within the anti-doping narrative, Dasgupta's chapter argues for revising existing anti-doping legal procedures to improve their impact on athletes' rights. Also taking a critical approach, in Chapter 2 Helen Lenskyj focuses on who has power in anti-doping and how that power translates into rights and responsibilities for both athletes and sport-governing bodies. Lenskyj shows several instances in which athletes have received varying outcomes under the WADA Code, calling into question

WADA's ability to ensure equitable treatment. Katharina Gatterer and Cornelia Blank further interrogate the role of policy in Chapter 3, focusing on prevention strategies and how research on this topic may be interpreted and coherently implemented to stop doping before it starts. Overall, this theme presents a critical discussion on anti-doping policy, governance and the implications for both doping users and athletes in general.

Part II: Health and Risks

Policies, as argued in the literature (Henning et al., 2021; Henning & Andreasson, 2020), produce socio-legal environments in which doping cultures form. Beyond determining what is legal to use, possess or sell, these policies can impact how individuals learn about and acquire IPEDs and what resources for ensuring safer use they have available to them. In sport, for example, prohibitions against a range of substances may limit athletes' access to medical supervision or possibly lead to a more systematic approach to reduce use-related risks. Similarly, fitness doping may be enabled by national policies that either legalize or criminalize various aspects of IPED acquisition and use. Despite the distinctions between athletes and gym-goers being potentially less clear cut than commonly thought (Andreasson & Henning, 2021a), health and risk related to substance use are primary concerns for all people who engage in IPED use. To this end, under the theme of *health and risks*, we have gathered three chapters. In Chapter 4, Jim McVeigh, Geoff Bates and Gemma Anne Yarwood depart from the increasing use and widening of anabolic steroid user groups to explore whether doping should be understood as a public health issue or not. In doing so, this chapter addresses recent developments within doping demography and contributes to the evidence base on doping and health, as well as offering criteria for debating public health and anabolic steroids. Following this, Matthew Dunn investigates healthcare professionals' experiences with IPED (also known as PIED) con- sumers and the experiences of IPED consumers with healthcare professionals in Chapter 5. Through reviewing the literature on this topic, the chapter provides insights into the interactions between health professionals and users of IPEDs. Further, it illustrates some of the barriers to and facilitators for consumers in accessing healthcare, regardless of contextual situatedness. Finally, this theme includes Chapter 6 by Mair Underwood. Focusing on how a particular drug, Trenbolone, is understood by users, this chapter initiates a discussion on the physical, psychological, social and sexual harms that may follow with use of Trenbolone and how it is debated among users in the context of an online forum. This chapter provides significant insights into drug particularities and how use is legitimized, despite potential harms.

Part III: Doping Arenas and Communities

As described above, IPED use is no longer confined to the worlds of elite sport or extreme bodybuilding, or even to either sport or fitness. Rather, doping has expanded into new spaces and places, giving rise to new communities of users that may bear little resemblance to their predecessors in terms of motivation, use behaviours and trajectories. These emergent forms of doping highlight the overlaps between groups who use IPEDs, as well as between groups who use substances more generally. In Chapter 7, Bertrand Fincoeur and Jessica Rullo explore IPED use in prison settings in Belgium, showing how prison use is both similar to and distinctive from other forms of prison-based substance use, as well as from doping in sport and fitness. Further they show how steroid use is viewed by inmates and prison staff in comparison with other recreational substances in a prison setting. Turning to another emergent site for doping research, Luke Turnock and Honor Townsend look at doping fitness forums and address how social communities of users develop in the context of online communication in Chapter 8. This chapter also discusses how harm reduction behaviour can develop in relation to the particularity of the online doping context (also reconnecting to the previous *health and risk* theme). In doing so, this chapter provides implicit insights into how online doping spaces may be formed, partly independently from offline doping contexts. Rather than looking to new spaces, Luke Cox, Andrew Bloodworth and Mike McNamee in Chapter 10 focused on a population with potentially growing engagement with doping: recreational athletes. Chapter 10 considers the updates to the 2021 WADA Code and the ethical and practical implications for recreational athletes now explicitly covered by the Code.

Part IV: Gendering Doping

Given the historical links between masculinity and muscles, broader questions of gender and how gender is done with regards to IPEDs have gone largely unanswered. This is despite women's history of engagement with such substances, from the unwittingly doped East German women athletes to the steroid-enhanced built bodies on stages in bodybuilding competitions. To understand how and why men have and continue to dominate the popular and research IPED focus, April Henning and Jesper Andreasson elaborate the concept of cultural manspreading. In Chapter 11, this concept captures how men continue to take up more than their equitable share of fitness space, leading to women and their voices and experiences being pushed out or to the side both in online and offline sport and fitness spaces. Next, in Chapter 12, Charlie McLean invites us to join an autoethnographic journey into the world of women's bodybuilding and the role IPEDs play in the pursuit of female muscularity. This chapter not only problematizes the decision-making around doping and how it is influenced by cultural norms, peer influence and personal experiences but also reflects on the personal and professional challenges that comes with autoethnographic research. In Chapter 13, Sarah Teetzel weaves together an exploration of gender by looking at the development of sex and anti-doping testing and the impacts these have had on sport and athletes. It also considers the implications of such tests for intersex and transgender athletes.

Following these contributed chapters, in the final chapter, we bring together the central arguments within and across the themes that have structured the book. In doing so, we highlight the main outcomes and implications and present possible future directions and debates within this field.

KEY READINGS

(1) Andreasson, J., & Henning, A. D. (2021). *Performance cultures and doped bodies. Challenging categories, gender norms and policy responses.* Common Ground.

This book initiates the debate on why doping as a practice and social phenomenon has been approached as a question of context. It argues that stark categorizations (e.g. sport/fitness; masculine/feminine; health/risk) have continued to ignore lived experiences and aims to widen our understanding of doping, both empirically and through introducing new conceptual tools for analysis.

(2) Henning, A., & Dimeo, P. (2022). *Doping: A sporting history.* Reaktion Books.

This book provides a cultural history of doping within sport, putting contemporary understandings of doping into historical perspective. This book shows how current understandings of doping as something evil or as an expression of a sport crisis is a rather new way of thinking. It highlights the historical variability on doping and how it for large parts in history has been debated in terms of experimentation and innovation, unhindered by talk of cheating or health risks.

(3) Germain, J., Leavey, C., Van Hout, M. C., & McVeigh, J. (2020). 2,4-Dinitrophenol: It's not just for men. *International Journal of Drug Policy.* Article 102,987. https://doi.org/10.1016/j.drugpo.2020.102987

While the scholarly debate has often focused on men and their use of steroids, this chapter provides significant insights on women's use of the organic compound 2,4-dinitrophenol (DNP). The article discusses women's diverse motivations for using DNP and differences in experiences, dosing regimens, willingness to take risks and more. In doing so, the article provides interesting insights concerning how women navigate male-dominated protocols without gender sensitive treatment pathways.

(4) Fussell, S. (1991). *Muscles. The confession of an unlikely bodybuilder.* Scribners.

This autobiography chronicles how the author gradually became part of a bodybuilding subculture and engaged in drug use practices. It shows not only how the bodybuilding lifestyle and the associated drugs impact social life, body and identity but also how disengagement from this culture may manifest. Written in the 1990s, this book shows the particularity of changing doping perspectives of the time.

(5) Salinas, M., Floodgate, W., & Ralphs, R. (2019). Poly drug use and poly drug markets amongst image and performance enhancing drug users: Implications for harm reduction interventions and drug policy. *International*

Journal of Drug Policy, 67(2019), 43–51.

Departing from the fact that the use of IPEDs has increased in recent decades and transcended the elite sport context to include recreational sport athletes and fitness enthusiasts, this chapter focuses on steroid use in body-building gyms. It demonstrates the intersectionality across IPEDs, diverted medication, and both illicit and licit substance use. The chapter contributes to our understanding of changing doping demographics and this necessitates a review of current dominating harm reduction advice for IPED users and policy developments.

REFERENCES

Andreasson, J., & Henning, A. D. (2021a). *Performance cultures and doped bodies: Challenging categories, gender norms and policy responses.* Common Ground.

Andreasson, J., & Henning, A. D. (2021b). Challenging hegemony through narrative: Centering women's experiences and establishing a sis-science culture through a women-only doping forum. *Communication & Sport.* https://doi.org/10.1177/21674795211000657

Andreasson, J., & Johansson, T. (2014). *The global gym. Gender, health and pedagogies.* Palgrave Macmillan.

Andreasson, J., & Johansson, T. (2019). *Extreme sports, extreme bodies. Gender, identities & bodies in motion.* Palgrave Macmillan.

Andreasson, J., & Johansson, T. (2020). *Fitness doping. Trajectories, gender, body ideals and health.* Palgrave Macmillan.

Bates, G., Begley, E., Tod, D., Jones, L., Leavey, C., & McVeigh, J. (2019). A systematic review investigating the behaviour change strategies in interventions to prevent misuse of anabolic steroids. *Journal of Health Psychology, 24*(11), 1595–1612.

Bates, G., & McVeigh, J. (2016). *Image and performance enhancing drugs: 2015 survey results.* Liverpool John Moores University.

Bilgrei, O. R. (2018). Broscience: Creating trust in online drug communities. *New Media & Society, 20*(8), 2712–2727.

Christiansen, A. V. (2020). *Gym culture, identity and performance-enhancing drugs: Tracing a typology of steroid use.* Routledge.

Courtwright, D. T. (2009). *Forces of habit: Drugs and the making of the modern world.* Harvard University.

Dimeo, P. (2007). *A history of drug use in sport 1876–1976. Beyond good and evil.* Routledge.

Dimeo, P. (2014). Why Lance Armstrong? Historical context and key turning points in the 'cleaning up' of professional cycling. *International Journal of the History of Sport, 31*(8), 951–968.

Dimeo, P., & Møller, V. (2018). *The anti-doping crisis in sport: Causes, consequences, solutions.* Routledge.

Fair, J. D. (1999). *Muscletown USA: Bob Hoffman and the manly culture of York Barbell.* The Pennsylvania State University Press.

Fincoeur, B., van de Ven, K., & Mulrooney, K. J. D. (2015). The symbiotic evolution of anti-doping and supply chains of doping substances: How criminal networks may benefit from anti-doping policy. *Trends in Organized Crime, 18*(3), 229–250. https://doi.org/10.1007/s12117-014-9235-7

Fussell, S. (1991). *Muscles. The confession of an unlikely bodybuilder.* Scribners.

Germain, J., Leavey, C., Van Hout, M. C., & McVeigh, J. (2020). 2, 4 Dinitrophenol: It's not just for men. *International Journal of Drug Policy.* Article 102987. https://doi.org/10.1016/j.drugpo.2020.102987

Gleaves, J. (2014). A global history of doping in sport: Drugs, nationalism and politics. *International Journal of the History of Sport, 31*(8), 815–819.

Hanley Santos, G., & Coomber, R. (2017). The risk environment of anabolic–androgenic steroid users in the UK: Examining motivations, practices and accounts of use. *International Journal of Drug Policy, 40*, 35–43. https://doi.org/10.1016/j.drugpo.2016.11.005

Havnes, I. A., Jørstad, M. L., Innerdal, I., & Bjørnebekk, A. (2020). Anabolic-androgenic steroid use among women: A qualitative study on experiences of masculinizing, gonadal and sexual effects. *International Journal of Drug Policy*. Article 102876. https://doi.org/10.1016/j.drugpo.2020. 102876

Henne, K. (2014). The emergence of moral technopreneurialism in sport: Techniques in anti-doping regulation, 1966–1976. *International Journal of the History of Sport, 31*(8), 884–901.

Henning, A., & Andreasson, J. (2020). Preventing, producing, or reducing harm? Fitness doping risk and enabling environments. *Drugs: Education, Prevention and Policy*. https://doi.org/10.1080/ 09687637.2020.1865273

Henning, A., & Andreasson, J. (2021). "Yay, another lady starting a log!": Women's fitness doping and the gendered space of an online doping forum. *Communication & Sport, 9*(6), 988–1007. https:// doi.org/10.1177/2167479519896326

Henning, A., & Andreasson, J. (2021b). New frontiers in IPEDs and polydrug use: Knowledge gaps and new perspectives. *Performance Enhancement & Health, 9*(3), 100206. https://doi.org/10. 1016/j.peh.2021.100206

Henning, A., McLean, K., Andreasson, J., & Dimeo, P. (2021). Risk and enabling environments in sport: Systematic doping as harm reduction. *International Journal of Drug Policy, 91*, 102897. https://doi.org/10.1016/j.drugpo.2020.102897

Henning, A., & Dimeo, P. (2015). Questions of fairness and anti-doping in US cycling: The contrasting experiences of professionals and amateurs. *Drugs: Education, Prevention & Policy, 22*(5), 400–409.

Henning, A., & Dimeo, P. (2022). *Doping: A sporting history*. Reaktion Books.

Klein, A. (1993). *Little big men: Bodybuilding, subculture and gender construction*. State University of New York Press.

Liokaftos, D. (2019). Natural bodybuilding: An account of its emergence and development as competition sport. *International Review for the Sociology of Sport, 54*(6), 753–770.

Locks, A., & Richardson, N. (Eds.). (2012). *Critical readings in bodybuilding*. Routledge.

McLaren, R. (2016). *Independent Investigation Report: Part 1*. WADA. https://www.wada-ama.org/en/ resources/mclaren-independent-investigation-report-part-i

McVeigh, J., & Begley, E. (2017). Anabolic steroids in the UK: An increasing issue for public health. *Drugs: Education, Prevention & Policy, 24*(3), 278–285.

Monaghan, L. F. (2001). *Bodybuilding, drugs and risk: Health, risk and society*. Routledge.

Mulrooney, K. J., van de Ven, K., McVeigh, J., & Collins, R. (2019). Commentary: Steroid madness: Has the dark side of anabolic-androgenic steroids (AAS) been over-stated? *Performance Enhancement & Health, 6*(3–4), 98–102. https://doi.org/10.1016/j.peh.2019.03.001

Rasmussen, N. (2008). America's first amphetamine epidemic 1929–1971: A quantitative and qualitative retrospective with implications for the present. *American Journal of Public Health, 98*(6), 974–985. https://doi.org/10.2105/AJPH.2007.110593

Salinas, M., Floodgate, W., & Ralphs, R. (2019). Polydrug use and polydrug markets amongst image and performance enhancing drug users: Implications for harm reduction interventions and drug policy. *International Journal of Drug Policy, 67*, 43–51.

Sassatelli, R. (2010). *Fitness culture: Gyms and the commercialisation of discipline and fun*. Palgrave Macmillan.

Schwarzenegger, A., & Petre, P. (2012). *Total recall: My unbelievably true-life story*. Simon & Schuster.

Seifarth, S., Dietz, P., Disch, A. C., Engelhardt, M., & Zwingenberger, S. (2019). The prevalence of legal performance-enhancing substance use and potential cognitive and or physical doping in German recreational triathletes, assessed via the randomised response technique. *Sports, 7*(12), 241. https://doi.org/10.3390/sports7120241

Sverkersson, E., Andreasson, J., & Johansson, T. (2020). 'Sis science' and fitness doping: Ethnopharmacology, gender and risk. *Social Sciences, 9*(4), 55. https://doi.org/10.3390/socsci9040055

Thualagant, N. (2012). The conceptualization of fitness doping and its limitations. *Sport in Society: Cultures, Commerce, Media, Politics, 15*(3), 409–419. https://doi.org/10.1080/17430437.2012. 653209

Turnock, L. (2021). *Supplying steroids online. The cultural and market contexts of enhancement drug supply on one of the world's largest fitness & bodybuilding forums.* Plymouth Policy Research Press.

Underwood, M. (2017). Exploring the social lives of image and performance enhancing drugs: An online ethnography of the Zyzz fandom of recreational bodybuilders. *International Journal of Drug Policy, 39,* 78–85.

van de Ven, K., & Mulrooney, K. J. D. (2017). Social suppliers: Exploring the cultural contours of the performance and image enhancing drug (PIED) market among bodybuilders in the Netherlands and Belgium. *International Journal of Drug Policy, 40,* 6–15. https://doi.org/10.1016/j.drugpo.2016.07.009

Van Hout, M.-C., & Kean, J. (2015). An exploratory study of image and performance enhancementdrug use in a male British South Asian community. *International Journal of Drug Policy, 26*(9), 860–867. http://doi.org/10.1016/j.drugpo.2015.03.002

Yesalis, C. E., & Bahrke, M. S. (2005). Anabolic steroid and stimulant use in North American sport between 1850 and 1980. *Sport in History, 25*(3), 434–451.

PART 1

ANTI-DOPING POLICY

Chapter 1

ATHLETES, LAW AND THE WORLD ANTI-DOPING CODE: A PERSPECTIVE

Lovely Dasgupta

ABSTRACT

This chapter explores the relationship between athletes and sports law within the anti-doping narrative. The World Anti-Doping Code is the most important reference to understand this relationship. Athletes are constantly pressured to meet standards beyond reasonable expectations. This chapter explores the anti-doping narrative from the athletes' perspective, mapping out the inherent legal hurdles impeding delivery of equitable outcomes for the athletes. Such hurdles are the result of lack of bargaining power by the athletes. This chapter critically evaluates the existing literature on the anti-doping narrative and identifies the gaps in the structures affecting the athletes, Sports Governing Bodies and the World Anti-Doping Agency (WADA). This chapter then focuses on the usurpation of athlete's rights through the instrumentality of the WADA Code that appears to predominantly promote and protect the interests of the governing class against those it governs. It is one of the first to analyze the existing anti-doping narrative and its impact on athlete's right within the 2021 WADA Code, which has not introduced any fundamental changes to the existing anti-doping narrative. The chapter argues for a more equitable treatment of the athletes while enforcing the 2021 Code, and for revising the existing anti-doping measures vis-à-vis athletes and opens possible areas of future research.

Keywords: Athletes; doping; sports law; anti-doping; compliance; WADA code

Doping in Sport and Fitness
Research in the Sociology of Sport, Volume 16, 17–33
Copyright © 2023 by Emerald Publishing Limited
All rights of reproduction in any form reserved
ISSN: 1476-2854/doi:10.1108/S1476-285420220000016002

INTRODUCTION

On 17 May 2021, the Office of the National Drug Control Policy (ONDCP) of the United States updated Congress about reforms within the World Anti-Doping Agency (WADA). This report highlighted the existing conflicts within the anti-doping programme. After the Russian doping scandal, the issue of reforms has plagued WADA and there are ongoing efforts to reform and fundamentally change WADA. The ONDCP report is an example of such attempts in overhauling WADA. In the broad scheme of things, as proposed by ONDCP, athletes have an important role to play. However, as the Russian doping scandal established, the stake of athletes gets subverted due to the vested interests of sports administrators, including those within national governments. This does not, however, discount the fact that elite athletes do also tend to manipulate the system to evade detection under the WADA Code. Given the complexities involved, the WADA Code has been revised time and again to balance these different interests. Unfortunately, this balance is not always achieved, as the Code itself tends to waver between just and unjust outcomes. The athletes participating in international competitions are literally barred from accessing domestic legal forums. Their only recourse is to find justice within the system constructed by the WADA Code. This system is aided and supported by the International Olympic Committee (IOC) as well as the different International Federations (IFs).

WADA is understandably reluctant to bring in reforms and truly becoming an autonomous and independent body. Widespread reforms have the danger of upsetting the status quo and ruffling many stakeholders. The greater the transparency, the greater the accountability. Avoiding increased transparency and accountability vis-à-vis WADA also ensures that the IFs and IOC are equally reluctant to bring in fundamental reforms. The ongoing crisis within sports due to COVID-19 underlines that the interests of the sports administrators and organizers supersede that of the athletes. In hosting the Olympics in 2021, commercial interests of IOC superseded those of the athlete's interests. Consequently the concerns about health of athletes were brushed aside in run up to the Games. The reference to the Olympics is relevant, as it exemplifies the dominance of IOC in sports administration. WADA is administratively dominated by the IOC. Hence each and every stance of the IOC on issues relating to sports governance impacts the athletes. Thus, the anti-doping narrative is shaped by the IOC's stance vis-à-vis WADA. It means that within this IOC dominated anti-doping narrative the athletes cannot take an effective stance on the issue. The situation is worse for athletes from developing and least developed countries, as they are sandwiched between their dreams and reality. Further, their access to better health infrastructure is compromised due to socio-economic pressures. And, as the current pandemic reveals through the inequity in vaccine distribution, it similarly impacts the sports scene and adds to the current inequities in which the athletes are stuck.

There is a vast literature on the rights of the athletes within the context of the anti-doping narrative. However, the 2021 Code is yet to receive extensive attention in terms of athletes' rights. The predicament of the athletes under the

2021 Code thus needs to be analyzed. For purposes of this chapter, the law in the title does not indicate municipal law or international law. Rather, the law in the title refers to the regulations and codes framed under the aegis of the IOC. As already referred to above, the IOC is the supreme sports administrator. And WADA Code is part of the several rules and regulation that the IOC has approved and is binding for athletes. Hence the inevitable question that comes up is the extent to which the 2021 Code is equitable. The concern for equity is the primary focus of this chapter, since, of all the stakeholders, the athletes have the weakest bargaining power. Equity in the context of anti-doping regulation entails accessibility to information, to legal aid and to justice. Further, the anti-doping narrative is equally impacted by the personal experiences of the athletes. Accordingly, the perspective of a developed country athlete is far different from that of a developing country athlete. Hence, the Code needs to be dynamic enough to accommodate different perspectives. Accordingly, it needs to be understood the extent to which the Code is dynamic.

This chapter is aimed at undertaking a holistic analysis of the 2021 Code. It is written against the background of the ONDCP report. The question of equity thus predominates the narrative. The chapter begins by explaining the existing anti-doping programme and structures within. The explanation is aimed at mapping the framework that governs athletes. The second part highlights the challenges faced by the athletes in being Code compliant, and also discusses the challenges thrown up by the 2021 Code. The third part collates the various debates on the existing anti-doping programme to analyze the question of equity within the 2021 Code. Finally, this part will also highlight the conflicts that exist between the various stakeholders. As noted above, it is these conflicts that skew the anti-doping programme against the athletes, who may get caught within its ambiguities. Finally, the chapter will discuss possible refinements that should to be introduced. Such refinements need to be tested against the standards of equity. The chapter contends that incorporation of equity will ensure greater inclusivity and dynamism within the WADA Code.

THE ANTI-DOPING NARRATIVE AND STRUCTURES

The current anti-doping programme comprises three pillars of the Code: the International Standards and Technical documents and Models of Best Practice and Guidelines. Of these, it is the Code that spells out the guidelines that are binding on all stakeholders, particularly athletes. The standards and the model guidelines are supplementary documents that assist in fine-tuning the system. However, athletes are expected to be informed about these supplementary documents as well. The Code spells out the structures and framework that are crucial for anti-doping regulation. These structures play the most important role in deciding the fate of athletes, as well as defining the roles and responsibilities of the other stakeholders. Accordingly the roles of national sport governing bodies, national governments, the IFs and the IOC are clearly defined. It also identifies the role that WADA has to play. The entire framework is designed to have effective control of athletes, as punitive sanctions and other consequences that an anti-doping rule violation attracts are all geared towards this objective. In other words, the entire anti-doping narrative is focused on athletes and their roles and responsibilities, as it is the athletes that provide the causa causans in all anti-doping actions.

Athletes are also needed to establish the legitimacy of the anti-doping narrative. The history of the anti-doping programme reveals that it was developed to make sports viable commercially, and that could be only done by selling an ideal of clean sports (Johnson, 2016). The best way to achieve this ideal was to vilify the taking of performance enhancing drugs (PEDs) (Abbott, 2012). Hence, commercial interest coupled with the mission of strengthening the IOC led to the codification of anti-doping measures (Barney, 2002). Once athletes were put up on pedestals as icons, there was no scope for mistakes. The gradual rise of the anti-doping movement was premised on this portrayal of a model athlete. The addition of the moral justification to the existing anti-doping narrative was used to legitimize the entire process (Beamish & Ritchie, 2006). The more purified the idea of sports became, the more burdensome the role of the athletes became. The various scandals involving doped athletes, however, did not deter the advocates of purity in sports from pursuing a stringent anti-doping programme (Bertling, 2007). Consequently, each revision of the Code and the associated documents upped the ante for athletes. The level of compliance becomes more skewed after each revision.

The 2021 Code is the latest in the series and has further raised the bar of compliance for athletes. Thus the 2021 Code recognizes a wider basket of incidents that will amount to anti-doping rule violations (ADRVs). Accordingly, the 2021 Code has laid down the following 11 scenarios that amount to ADRVs.

(1) Presence of prohibited substance in the samples of the athlete (Article 2.1).
(2) Use or attempted use of a prohibited substance or method (Article 2.2).
(3) Refusal/Evasion/Failure to submit to sample collection (Article 2.3).
(4) Whereabouts Failure (Article 2.4).
(5) Tampering or attempted tampering with any part of the doping control (Article 2.5).
(6) Possession of any of the prohibited substance or method (Article 2.6).
(7) Trafficking or attempted trafficking in prohibited substance or method (Article 2.7).
(8) Administration or attempted administration (either in-competition or out of competition) of prohibited substance or method (Article 2.8).
(9) Complicity or attempted complicity in the form of assisting, encouraging, aiding, abetting, conspiring, covering up an ADRV etc. (Article 2.9).
(10) Prohibited Association (Article 2.10).
(11) Acts amounting to discouragement from, or retaliation for, reporting to authorities (Article 2.11).

The addition of the new Article 2.11 reinforces the carrot and stick approach of the WADA Code vis-à-vis athletes. This chapter aims to protect the whistle-blower but also puts pressure on the athletes to turn against the system. The onus is on the athletes to cooperate and reveal all kinds of secret doping programmes. The problem is that athletes are lowest in the pecking order of bargaining power (Beamish, 2011). Hence it might be difficult for them to blow the whistle against their coaches, national federations or even national governments. It also underlies the point stated above that athletes hold the key to detecting secret doping programmes. The Lance Armstrong scandal as well as the Russian doping scandal are examples of secret and sophisticated doping programs. It also establishes that WADA is entirely dependent on the cooperation of the athletes to make the anti-doping programme a success. Importantly, it is the athletes who can help WADA gain legitimacy as the ultimate anti-doping regulator. From the athlete's perspective, there are hardly any fundamental changes brought in by the 2021 Code. For instance, the Prohibited List and the criteria for a substance being included on it remain the same, barring a few cosmetic touch ups. Similarly, the purpose and scope of the WADA programme, as spelled out in the Code, remains the same. Thus, doping-free sport continues to be the only fundamental right that the Code aims to protect. The 2021 Code declares deterrence as one of the primary objective of the programme and, as argued above, gives greater emphasis to stringency. This stringency is evident from the fact that the health of athletes has been given the place of utmost importance in the 2021 Code. Accordingly, the fundamental rationale of the 2021 Code has been amended. Through this amendment, protection of health of the athletes has been cited as one of the rationale of the Code. Further, the definition of spirit of sport has been rephrased citing health as the most important value. This ties up with using health risk as one of the criteria for preparing the Prohibited List.

A key change brought in by the 2021 Code is the specific recognition of athletes' rights, brought in through an amendment to the fundamental rationale of WADA Code. As per Article 20.7.7, WADA undertakes the responsibility:

> ...to submit to the WADA Executive Committee for approval, upon the recommendation of the WADA Athletes Committee the Athletes' Anti-Doping Rights Act which compiles in one place those Athletes' rights which are specifically identified in the Code and International Standards, and other agreed upon principles of best practice with respect to the overall protection of Athletes' rights in the context of anti-doping.

The Athletes' Anti-Doping Rights Act (the Act) documents the code of best practices that anti-doping organizations are expected to follow. The Act embodies the recommendations of the athletes, but has no legally binding effect and does not supersede the WADA Code. It therefore lays down the desirable standards to protect athletes' rights while implementing the anti-doping programme. Accordingly, the Act is divided into two parts, the one that the Code recognizes and the other that the athletes recommend. The athletes' recommendations include a corruption-free anti-doping system, participation in decision-making processes and governance, and access to legal aid. These are fairly reasonable recommendations on the part of the athletes, though not realistically implemented by the IFs, WADA or the IOC.

Another significant change is the shifting of the burden of proof. As per the amendment to Article 3.2.3, the anti-doping organization has the burden of proving that deviations from international standards did not cause the adverse analytical finding/whereabouts failure/anti-doping rule violation in each of the cases of departure from: the International Standard for Testing and Investigations (related to Sample collection or Sample handling); the International Standard for Results Management or International Standard for Testing and Investigations (related to an Adverse Passport Finding); the International Standard for Results Management (related to the requirement to provide notice to the Athlete of the B Sample opening); the International Standard for Results Management (related to Athlete notification). The newly added comment to Article 3.2.3 elaborates further that, '…An Anti-Doping Organization would meet its burden to establish that such departure did not cause the Adverse Analytical Finding by showing that, for example, the B Sample opening and analysis were observed by an independent witness and no irregularities were observed'. It further clarifies that, 'Departures from an International Standard or other rule…may result in compliance proceedings by WADA but are not a defense in an anti-doping rule violation proceeding and are not relevant on the issue of whether the Athlete committed an anti-doping rule violation'.

The shifting of burden, however, does not appear to have had any impact on the overall philosophy and structure of the Code and its implementation process. On the other hand, stringency of the rules vis-à-vis athletes has increased. Thus, the 2021 Code has expanded the monitoring system in order to include newer substance to the Prohibited List. The comment to Article 4.5 accordingly explains, 'In order to improve the efficiency of the monitoring program, once a new substance is added to the published monitoring program, laboratories may re-process data and Samples previously analyzed in order to determine the absence or presence of any new substance'.

The 2021 Code has amended Article 6 to introduce changes in the principles applicable to sample analysis. Article 6.1 has been broadened to permit analysis of samples in non-WADA accredited laboratories. The same is permitted to prove anti-doping rule violations through indirect means as given under Article 3.2. Article 6.1.1 accordingly declares that, 'As provided in Article 3.2, facts related to antidoping rule violations may be established by any reliable means. This would include, for example, reliable laboratory or other forensic testing conducted outside of WADA-accredited or approved laboratories'. This increases the discretion of the anti-doping organization in terms of sample testing and renders athletes more vulnerable. Similarly, Article 6.8 has been introduced to grant unbridled rights to WADA to take possession of samples/data from a lab or an anti-doping organization. No prior notice is needed to be given to the lab or the anti-doping organization. Further, the lab or the anti-doping organization is duty-bound to cooperate with WADA on the issue. This is clear from the explanation to Article 6.8:

> Resistance or refusal to WADA taking physical possession of Samples or data could constitute Tampering, Complicity or an act of non-compliance as provided in the International Standard

for Code Compliance by Signatories, and could also constitute a violation of the International Standard for Laboratories. Where necessary, the laboratory and/or the Anti-Doping Organization shall assist WADA in ensuring that the seized Sample or data are not delayed in exiting the applicable country.

The 2021 Code has introduced a change at the level of fair hearings under Article 8. The amendment advises the anti-doping agency to provide 'a fair hearing within a reasonable time by a fair, impartial and Operationally Independent hearing panel in compliance with the WADA International Standard for Results Management'. Further, the 2021 Code defines the concept of operational independence. Effectively, it means that none of the officials/employees/members of the anti-doping organizations are to be part of the hearing panel. This is to ensure the hearing panel will operate without any influence or interference from the investigating team. Further, the anti-doping organization shall not have any say in the constitution or operation of the hearing panel. Importantly though, the amendment does not specify the consequences of defaulting on the requirement of operational independence. A related change that the 2021 Code introduces is with respect to single hearing. While the 2015 Code did have the same provision under Article 8.5, the 2021 Code has introduced an explanation. The explanation to Article 8.5 gives the rationale for the provision on single hearing, noting it is justified where, 'the combined cost of holding a hearing in the first instance at the international or national level, then rehearing the case de novo before CAS can be very substantial'. Hence, if all the concerned parties agree that the Court of Arbitration for Sport (CAS) will be the best for deciding the matter, a single hearing suffices. The anti-doping organization is allowed to 'participate in the CAS hearing as an observer'. The viability of single hearing, however, skews the narrative for the athletes from developing countries, as they are economically disadvantaged and, hence, effective accessibility to CAS is a farfetched dream.

On the whole, the 2021 Code has rendered lip service to the question of equity and fairness in so far as athletes are concerned. Though changes in terms of concern for health of athletes and their rights have been specifically incorporated, this does not deviate attention from the fact that the 2021 Code mostly fine tunes the existing structures. Further, the fundamental principle of strict liability that forms the core of the anti-doping programme is retained in all its glory. Hence, irrespective of the changes introduced, the 2021 Code appears to be more like an old wine in a new bottle. Consequently, the jurisprudence developed over the years by CAS will continue to be relevant and, importantly, will be helpful in dealing with the challenges that athletes face while negotiating the WADA Code.

Athletes will continue to face greater challenges while negotiating the 2021 Code. This is evident from the amendments introduced in Article 10 of the WADA Code. For instance, Article 10.2.4 is a new addition in the 2021 Code. As per Article 10.2.4.1, a substance abuse unrelated to sports performance attracts a sanction of three months. This essentially widens the jurisdiction of the Code and renders the athlete more vulnerable. One is not justifying substance abuse and it definitely merits interference. However, the problem is interference via the Code, which has made the health of athletes its most important rationale. Such a justification cannot take away from the fact that 2021 Code, like its previous versions, is attempting to further the agenda of doping-free sport. In contrast, substance abuse is largely unrelated to performance enhancement. Hence its separate inclusion is another attempt by WADA to morally police athlete. In this context, there might be a view point that the reduced duration of sanction for substance abuse may not deter the athlete. On the contrary, the athletes might just risk the chance of getting caught due to reduced period of sanction. Substance abuse primarily has nothing to do with performance enhancement, hence using health argument to monitor its abuse is further encroachment. WADA through such expansion is taking on the role of Pseudo State. This creates a dangerous precedent since WADA can use the health pretext to regulate each and every aspect of an athlete's life. It is clearly an intervention in the athlete's private space. This interference is absolute since the defence based on No-Fault/Negligence or No-Significant Fault/Negligence is not available in cases of substance abuse. As such, the 2021 Code furthers the agenda of WADA, the IFs and anti-doping organizations to restrict the autonomy of the athletes. The extent of this control over the choices of the athletes is further expanded as one reads through the remaining Article 10.2.4.1. It is specified therein that the sanction period of three months can be brought down to one month. The prerequisite being the successful completion of 'Substance of Abuse treatment program approved by the Anti-Doping Organization with Results Management responsibility'. The athlete, accordingly, has no choice but to comply with this directive; More so because the scope of Article 10.2.4.1 is aimed at out-of-competition substance abuse. In addition, the burden is on the athlete to prove successful completion of the said programme. Finally, the amendment to Article 10.2.4.2 deals with in-competition substance abuse. Herein too, the burden is placed on the athlete to prove that the said abuse was unrelated to sport. In that case, the same shall not be treated as intentional and will not attract the sanction of four years.

ATHLETE'S DILEMMA AND LEGAL BOUNCERS WITHIN THE CODE

As noted above, the 2021 Code brings in newer challenges for athletes. At the same time, it does retain the status quo ante vis-à-vis athletes. Thus, the key areas that troubled athletes in the earlier versions of the Code continue to haunt them under the 2021 Code. To begin with, the 2021 Code continues to apply the strict liability rule. The strict liability principle is based on the assumption that all are guilty unless proven innocent. In USA Shooting & Q./Union Internationale de Tir (UIT) (CAS 94/129), CAS held that 'in principle the high objectives and practical necessities of the fight against doping amply justify the application of a strict liability standard'. This declaration by CAS reflects the current philosophy of the WADA Code. The comment to Article 2.1.1 reiterates the point thus 'An anti-doping rule violation is committed under this Article without regard to an

Athlete's Fault. This rule has been referred to in various CAS decisions as "Strict Liability"'.

In the UIT case (as described above), CAS noted with concern that the absence of the strict liability rule will make it nearly impossible for the sports federations to prove anti-doping rule violations. CAS urged that 'a requirement of intent would invite costly litigation that may well cripple federations-particularly those run on modest budgets-in their fight against doping'. Further, CAS vehemently declared in the UIT case that the fact that strict liability is unfair in a few cases does not make it problematic since the rule balances the interests of the entire athletic community against the interests of a few individuals. As per CAS, the strict liability rule on the whole 'appears to be a laudable policy objective not to repair an accidental unfairness to an individual by creating an intentional unfairness to the whole body of other competitors'.

The underlying objective of advancing the strict liability principle is to establish a level playing field for all athletes. This is reiterated within the fundamental rationale for the WADA Code. Amongst other things, the spirit of sport includes ethics, fair play and honesty. It further reiterates 'Doping is fundamentally contrary to the spirit of sport'.

In Q v UIT (1994), CAS dismissed the concerns that the strict liability principle was unreasonable or that it is 'contrary to natural justice, because it does not permit the accused to establish moral innocence'. Further the CAS rejected all the arguments that the strict liability principle 'is an excessive restraint of trade'. A similar line of argument has been used by others to justify the strict liability principle as the core of the Code. du Toit (2011) thus argues that 'In cases such as anti-doping rule violations it will be very difficult if not impossible to [prove] that the defendant had acted with fault or negligence'. (p. 164).

In Gasser v Stinson and Another (1988), Judge Scott reiterated the virtue of the strict liability principle. As per the judge, if an athlete or his/her support staff denies doping, it will be as good as a cause los, as it will be nearly impossible for the anti-doping organizations to prove doping in such a case. The underlying point being that the inclusion of proof of intent would, as per Scott, nullify the efficacy of the anti-doping programme. Thus, Scott summarized the virtue of the strict liability regime by declaring that, 'if a defence of moral innocence were open, the floodgates would be opened and the [Sport Governing Body's] attempts to prevent drug-taking by athletes would be rendered futile'.

A similar stance has been taken by Sebastian Coe (2004), while writing for the Telegraph: 'strict liability – under which athletes have to be solely and legally responsible for what they consume – must remain supreme. . ... we cannot, without blinding reason and cause, move one millimeter from strict liability – if we do, the battle to save sport is lost'. Coe is currently the president of World Athletics (formerly the International Associations of Athletic Federations [IAAF]). It would appear that given the overwhelming support for the principle of strict liability, it is entrenched within the anti-doping narrative. In IOC v. Xinyi Chen (Arbitration CAS anti-doping Division (OG Rio) AD 16/005), CAS underlined that 'Even if the Panel is willing to give the Athlete credit for being a young, honest person and her Coach credit for developing her outstanding performance results using exclusively fair and accepted training methods, such facts neither eliminate nor diminish the Athlete's duty under the IOC ADR to ensure that no Prohibited Substance enters her body, and in case of an Adverse Analytical Finding, her duty to explain the source of the Prohibited Substance'.

Another legal bouncer that athletes continue to face is the difficulty in proving flaws within the sample testing process. Modahl v British Athletic Federation Limited ([1999] UKHL 37) is a classic pre-WADA case that highlights the difficulties of challenging the sample testing processes or the test itself. The case primarily involved allegations based on the breach of contract by the UK Athletics/British Athletics (formerly called the British Athletic Federation [BAF]). However, the origin of the said claim was the outcome of the dispute surrounding the lab test. Based on the sample test, BAF suspended Modhal, claiming an anti-doping rule violation. Subsequently, Modhal filed an appeal and was able to successfully get an acquittal from the charges of doping. The independent tribunal had doubts about the authenticity of the lab tests. On being reinstated Modhal filed suit against BAF, claiming compensation for breach of contract. She argued 'that her suspension and the initiation of disciplinary proceedings were in breach of the contract between her and the BAF....She claims damages for the financial loss she suffered because for nearly a year she was unable to compete in international athletics'.

Another legal provision within the Code that is a matter of contention is the therapeutic use exemption (TUE). TUEs provide an escape route to athletes from getting caught in the whirlwind of anti-doping rule violations. In effect, the role of TUEs within the Code is to allow athletes to use a prohibited substance/method in very limited situations. The TUE is granted in a situation where the athlete can treat his/her medical condition without enhancing performance (Brown, 2016). As per Article 4.2 of the International Standard Therapeutic Use Exemptions (ISTUE, 2021):

> An Athlete may be granted a TUE if (and only if) he/she can show, on the balance of probabilities, that each of the following conditions is met: a) The Prohibited Substance or Prohibited Method in question is needed to treat a diagnosed medical condition supported by relevant clinical evidence. b) The Therapeutic Use of the Prohibited Substance or Prohibited Method will not, on the balance of probabilities, produce any additional enhancement of performance beyond what might be anticipated by a return to the Athlete's normal state of health following the treatment of the medical condition. c) The Prohibited Substance or Prohibited Method is an indicated treatment for the medical condition, and there is no reasonable permitted Therapeutic alternative. d) The necessity for the Use of the Prohibited Substance or Prohibited Method is not a consequence, wholly or in part, of the prior Use (without a TUE) of a substance or method which was prohibited at the time of such Use.

Further, in the comment section to the said Article it has been clarified that:

> The WADA documents titled "TUE Physician Guidelines," posted on WADA's website, should be used to assist in the application of these criteria in relation to particular medical conditions. The granting of a TUE is based solely on consideration of the conditions set out in Article 4.2. It does not consider whether the Prohibited Substance or Prohibited Method is the most clinically appropriate or safe, or whether its Use is legal in all jurisdictions...

The proof pertaining to the medical condition of the athlete is a *sine qua non* for being eligible of applying for TUE. Further, the athlete must prove that the current treatment protocol is the only option and there are no alternatives available. In addition, the athlete must prove that the granting of the TUE will not enhance performance or violate the spirit of sport. The sole object of the granting of TUEs is to bring the athlete to a normal state. The rationale behind TUEs is problematic considering that it contradicts the philosophy of the existing anti-doping regime. As mentioned, the anti-doping regime is premised upon the argument that doping is cheating. Hence, to permit exemption on the ground of medical reasons undermines the justification for prohibiting substances/methods. The argument that use within the ambit of a TUE is meant to bring the athlete's health to normal state is not acceptable. For example, an athlete born with a medical condition would never have had a normal state minus that condition. Hence to treat that medical condition with banned substance/methods is adding to the performance, since the normal state was that with the medical condition.

The other problem in the argument justifying TUEs for raising the athlete's health condition to normal level is the word 'normal' itself. For instance, in Dutee Chand v. Athletics Federation of India (AFI) and International Association of Athletics Federations (IAAF) (2014), the problem of defining the word normal or natural was highlighted and the legality of the Hyperandrogenism Regulations of the World Athletics was challenged. Chand contested that the high testosterone level in some female athletes resulting from genetic formation was normal and inherent to the biology of the concerned athlete. Accordingly, the same was comparable to the other inborn and unusual traits like height, lung capacity, foot size or visual acuity that some athletes have. The athlete argued that 'athletes who achieve sporting success are usually those who fall outside normal parameters... Male athletes with testosterone levels falling above the upper limit of the "normal" range of male testosterone are permitted to compete without having to satisfy any medical criteria or to undergo any medical examination or treatment as a precondition to eligibility. Female athletes – unlike their male counterparts – must therefore satisfy an additional eligibility criterion before they are permitted to compete. The differential treatment between male and female athletes constitutes discrimination...' (pp. 24–25).

In the context of TUEs, these arguments surrounding the word 'normal' thus make sense. And the problematic use of the word normal is further underlined by the explanation given in the comment section of the ISTUE 2021 viz. 'An Athlete's normal state of health will need to be determined on an individual basis. A normal state of health for a specific Athlete is their state of health but for the medical condition for which the Athlete is seeking a TUE'.

As mentioned above, in case of an athlete suffering from an ailment, it will be difficult to assess his/her normal state. For example, if an athlete is born with an incurable condition and must take medication for life, how does one assess their normal condition? Mulhall sums up the problem with the word *normal* by stating that:

...an athlete who suffers a reduction of natural testosterone due to testicular cancer would be allowed to use that substance from an external source to return to a state of 'normal' health. Does 'normal' mean normal for that athlete or within the range of normal for males of the human race? It may be that there is no reliable record of 'normal' for a particular athlete prior to the athlete's illness. Further, 'normal'; hormonal levels in each individual vary over time. So the only available criterion may be the range of "normal" for all (male) humans who have been tested. In that circumstance the athlete would only have to ensure his enhanced testosterone levels are within the 'normal' range, and he could be near or at the top of that range without violating the Code. On the other hand, an athlete who has not suffered from a testosterone-reducing disease is not permitted to increase 'low-normal' levels of his testosterone to at or near the top of the normal range. (Mulhall, 2006)

The word *normal* thus stratifies physiological hierarchies and this creates problems for athletes from developing and poor countries.

Kayser et al. (2007) argue that, 'depending on their nationality and sports speciality, athletes may differ enormously with regard to their access to care, supervision, and a high quality medical and technological environment'. The impediment thus created by the resource crunch can impede the athletes from successfully pleading a TUE. The existing structures, too, add to the dilemma of the athletes by creating legal impediments. Thus Article 6.8 of the ISTUE 2021 states that 'Any costs incurred by the Athlete in making the TUE application and in supplementing it as required by the TUEC are the responsibility of the Athlete'. Notwithstanding the explanation added to the ISTUE 2021, the process of determining what is normal remains as contentious as ever. Consequently, an athlete will remain mired in a dilemma as to the manner or the method of proving the normal state and the need for TUE. This would burden the athletes with financial costs.

There is another problem in addition to those pertaining to the rationale of TUEs that was highlighted when a group of hackers called Fancy Bear leaked the confidential data of several athletes. From 13 September, 2016, to 3 October, 2016, they hacked the WADA database and leaked athletes' confidential data, including TUE data. Some of the high-profile athletes like Olympic gold medallist Simon Biles and tennis superstar Serena Williams were victims of this hacking. One thing that the leaked information revealed was the ease with which the elite athletes were successful in getting TUEs. And though there was nothing untoward about the process by which they got a TUE, it does appear to be unfair. The hackers also wanted to convey and prove that the TUE process was being abused by those who have better accessibility. The scope of alleged abuse by the powerful arises due to the nature of the TUE process itself. The TUE applications of all athletes are vetted and sanctioned/rejected by the concerned National/ International Federation. The role that WADA plays is only to review the decisions of the National/International Federations or event organizers such as the IOC. Thus, the role of WADA is limited and continues to be so under the 2021 ISTUE. The problem with such a decentralized process is that it can possibly lead to bias. The report from the Cycling Independent Reform Commission (CIRC) (2015) supports the existence of such a possibility. The CIRC found evidence of abuse of the TUE process based on the statements of riders who went on record to admit the ease of getting TUEs. Accordingly, CIRC noted that '90% of TUEs were used for performance-enhancing purposes'. Hence, for the athletes it is a system that can work as a double-edged sword. Genuine cases might get rejected and cheats might succeed in getting TUEs.

A final point on the legal bumps that the athletes continue to face under the 2021 Code is in the area of sanctions for anti-doping rule violations. Though the 2021 Code has added to the existing bouquet of sanctions, it has not changed the underlying philosophy associated with sanctions. This is evident from the comment to Article 10, as given in the 2021 Code:

> Harmonization of sanctions has been one of the most discussed and debated areas of anti-doping. Harmonization means that the same rules and criteria are applied to assess the unique facts of each case. Arguments against requiring harmonization of sanctions are based on differences between sports including, for example, the following: in some sports the Athletes are professionals making a sizable income from the sport and in others the Athletes are true amateurs; in those sports where an Athlete's career is short, a standard period of Ineligibility has a much more significant effect on the Athlete than in sports where careers are traditionally much longer. A primary argument in favor of harmonization is that it is simply not right that two Athletes from the same country who test positive for the same Prohibited Substance under similar circumstances should receive different sanctions only because they participate in different sports. In addition, too much flexibility in sanctioning has often been viewed as an unacceptable opportunity for some sporting organizations to be more lenient with dopers. The lack of harmonization of sanctions has also frequently been the source of conflicts between International Federations and National Anti-Doping Organizations.

Thus, the jurisprudence developed by CAS with respect to the imposition of sanctions or its reduction/elimination will continue to apply and athletes will continue to face the same rigour as under the earlier versions of the Code. For instance, in World Anti-Doping Agency (WADA) v. Sri Lanka Anti-Doping Agency (SLADA) and Don Dinuda Dilshani Abeysekara (CAS 2015/A/4273), it was held that '[t]he need for an athlete to establish how a prohibited substance entered his or her system is a condition precedent to a finding of absence of fault or no significant fault'. It was further reiterated that the 'World Anti-Doping Code is intended to harmonise sanctions in such a way that is equally applicable to athletes young and old, amateur or professional'.

In this case, the age of the athlete, who was a minor, was not considered convincing grounds to reduce the sanction period. In Nikola Radjen v. Fédération Internationale de Natation (FINA) (CAS 2015/A/4200), it was held that 'Cheating is a key element of the notion of "intent" as contained in the World Anti-Doping Code (WADA Code). By using a Prohibited Substance, an athlete wishes to obtain an advantage in comparison to other athletes'. CAS went on to hold that an 'athlete... who pleads for the application of No Significant Fault or Negligence... based on the fact that at the time he consumed the Prohibited Substance he was suffering from depressions, caused by his father's death, has to provide... evidence of medical diagnosis for such disease, or testimony of an expert...'

CAS accordingly refused to entertain the argument of the athlete that the anti-doping rule violation was the outcome of depression. CAS noted that the athlete 'knew that he used a Prohibited Substance and he did it deliberately'.

In Niksa Dobud v. Fédération Internationale de Natation (FINA) (CAS 2015/A/4163), CAS declared that the proof of '[c]omfortable satisfaction is less than beyond reasonable doubt and more than on a balance of probabilities. The less probable the matter sought to be proved to that standard, the more cogent must be the evidence to prove it'. CAS further declared that the 'regulations governing test evasion do not require the governing body to establish why an athlete may have evaded a test; only that he had in fact done so'. CAS rejected the reasons given by the athlete for evading the tests. In doing so, CAS noted that '[t]he Panel is acutely conscious of the grave consequences to the Appellant of dismissal of the Appeal, especially in an Olympic year'.

In the World Anti-Doping Agency (WADA) v. Africa Zone V Regional Anti-Doping Organization and Anti-Doping Agency of Kenya (ADAK) and Athletics Kenya (AK) and Sharon Ndinda Muli (CAS 2017/A/5157), CAS underlined the rigour of the anti-doping system for the athletes. Explaining this, CAS declared that:

> ...[i]n order to establish... how a prohibited substance entered an athlete's body, it is not sufficient for the athlete merely to protest their innocence... an athlete must adduce concrete evidence to demonstrate that a particular supplement, medication or other product that the athlete took contained the substance in question.

Further, CAS clarified the burden of proof to be discharged by the athletes under the Code by reiterating that the 'standard of proof of balance of probabilities requires an athlete to convince the CAS panel that the occurrence of the circumstances on which the athlete relies is more probable than their non-occurrence'. CAS applied this assessment to the given scenario and rejected the athlete's defense against the finding of anti-doping rule violation. As per CAS, the athlete 'did not prove on the balance of probability how the prohibited substance entered her body or the origin of the prohibited substance'.

Similarly, in Filip Radojevic v. Fédération Internationale de Natation (FINA) (CAS 2018/A/5581), CAS noted that '[t]he prescription of a medicinal product by an athlete's doctor does not excuse said athlete from investigating to their fullest extent that the medication at stake does not contain prohibited substances. Athletes cannot rely on the advice of their support personnel'. CAS reiterated that 'The concept of no significant fault or negligence requires more of an athlete than a conscious bona fide use of a prescribed medication. Athletes are required to seek information actively and to take precautions in order to avoid any ingestion of a prohibited substance'. It was emphasized that '[a]n athlete must demonstrate the same level of diligence with regard to all substances included in the World Anti-Doping Agency Prohibited List irrespective of their capability of enhancing performances'.

And thus goes the dilemma of the athletes facing the legal bouncers of the Code. The athletes' predicament vis-à-vis the Code is evident from the decision of the CAS in Shayna Jack v. Swimming Australia and Australian Sports Anti-Doping Authority (CAS A1/2020). Herein, the Sole arbitrator, deciding the matter for CAS, was completely convinced that the ADRV was not intentional. The Sole arbitrator in the judgement emphatically noted that the athlete was clearly an honest person and the sole arbitrator clearly believed the evidence given by the athlete. Based on this reasoning, the Sole arbitrator justified the conclusion so arrived at by declaring that:

> The Applicant did not come across to the Sole Arbitrator as someone who would intentionally cheat by deliberately taking a Prohibited Substance. She did not come across as a person who engaged in conduct that she knew constituted an ADRV or that she intentionally engaged in conduct which she knew to bring with it a significant risk that it may result in an ADRV. She did not present as a person who manifestly disregarded the risk that her conduct might result in an ADRV. On the contrary, the evidence she gave, and the way she presented herself, convinced the Sole Arbitrator that she was a person who conscientiously sought, at all times, to comply with the anti-doping policies...

This finding saved the athlete from being banned for four years and instead was sanctioned for two years. This is so because the 2015 Code made a distinction between intentional and unintentional violation of the Code. This continues to be the positon under the 2021 Code. As per Article 10.2.3 of the 2021 Code, 'intentional' is meant to identify those 'Athletes or other Persons who engage in conduct which they knew constituted an anti-doping rule violation or knew that there was a significant risk that the conduct might constitute or result in an anti-doping rule violation and manifestly disregarded that risk...'

In effect, this emphasis on intention to determine the length of the sanction to be imposed is to treat the cheats differently from the innocent. Accordingly, the relief of additional defences like No-Significant fault/Negligence or No-Fault/ Negligence is available only to the innocent. Herein lies the dilemma for the athletes. Despite proving lack of intent to cheat, the athletes are not spared the sanction. They must further prove 'how the Prohibited Substance entered the Athlete's system'. The definition of No-Fault/Negligence and No-Significant Fault/Negligence insists on this requirement. Accordingly in the above case, CAS held that:

> The Applicant has not established how ligandrol entered her system... There is simply no evidence before the Sole Arbitrator upon which it could be concluded, on the balance of probabilities, that any of these speculative possibilities was in fact the reason for the presence of the Prohibited Substance in her system.

CONCLUSION: THE WAY FORWARD

The more things change the more they remain the same, and the developments within the anti-doping programme prove this. The WADA Code's revision and the ongoing demand and suggestion for reform will not change the fundamentals; it is the fundamentals that shapes and legitimizes the entire edifice of the anti-doping structures. WADA will lose its teeth and bite without the strict lia-bility principle. The athlete will get far more leeway in deciding upon the system that they would like to follow. The harmonization of sanctions across the varied sports is another feature that adds to the might of the WADA Code. Importantly, though, the recognition of the Code as the primary document to determine all anti-doping measures gives it strength. The WADA Code thus overrides all domestic legislation, in so far as international sports are concerned. Further, absence of recognition by the IFs/IOC – which requires compliance with the Code – nullifies all legitimate sporting activity. Hence, WADA Code compliance is a must for being included within the sports hierarchy. Accordingly, athletes are cornered in their attempt to prove their innocence within the framework of the Code. Hence, while various suggestions are made to reform WADA, its core principles are neither revisited nor questioned. Mere reference to athletes' right within the Code and adding explanation does not ensure equity for them. For if athletes must be ensured fairness and justice, then equity should not only be textual but also substantive. The only way of achieving this is by protecting the independence of WADA. An independent WADA should be mandated with powers to take on the most powerful IFs as well as the IOC. WADA should formally recognize the rights of athletes to have access to legal aid, formalized through adoption of a separate document comprising the International Standard for Access to Legal Aid. Finally, the Code needs to be revisited again to be fairer towards the athletes who have not intentionally committed anti-doping rule violations. On the whole, the perspective of the athletes needs to be built within the Code and not outside it for equitable outcomes.

KEY READINGS

(1) David, P. (2017). *A guide to the World Anti-Doping Code: The fight for the spirit of sport*. Cambridge University Press

This book reviews the Code and explains the role of CAS in evolving the jurisprudence that conditions the interpretation of the WADA Code. It analyzes the anti-doping regime as it evolved from the pre-WADA days, up to the 2015 Code. It is an important read to understand the nuances of the Code.

(2) Rabin, O., & Pitsiladis, Y. (Eds.). (2017). *Acute topics in anti-doping*. Karger Medical and Scientific Publishers.

This book looks at the problem of doping among athletes from a holistic perspective. The various contributors bring in their unique perspective to the debate on doping in sports.

(3) Healey, D., & Haas, U. (Eds.). (2016). *Doping in sport and the law*. Bloomsbury Publishing.

This book contains an in-depth analysis of the crisis that doping in sports has caused. It provides a thorough analysis of the interaction that policy and varied concepts of law such as tort, corporate governance, employment law and human rights law have when it comes to international doping regulation within sports.

(4) Dimeo, P., & Møller, V. (2018). *The anti-doping crisis in sport causes, consequences, solutions.* Routledge.

This book critically reviews the role of WADA in handling the crisis of doping in sports. It highlights the deficient handling of doping cases by WADA, leading to dubious convictions as well as human right violations.

(5) Dasgupta, L. (2019). *The World Anti-Doping Code: Fit for purpose?* Routledge.

This book is the first of its kind to revisit the WADA Code following the Russia doping scandal. It primarily argues for a more equitable anti-doping system that co-opts the perspective of developing country athletes.

REFERENCES

Abbott, K. (2012). The 1904 Olympic marathon may have been the strangest ever. Smithsonian.com. https://www.smithsonianmag.com/history/the-1904-olympic-marathon-may-have-been-the-strangest-ever-14910747/Athens 1896https://www.olympic.org/athens-1896

Barney, R. K. (2002). An Olympian dilemma: Protection of Olympic symbols. *Journal of Olympic History*, *10*(3), 7–9. http://library.la84.org/SportsLibrary/JOH/JOHv10n3/JOHv10n3f.pdf

Beamish, R. (2011). *Steroids: A new look at performance enhancing drugs.* Praeger.

Beamish, R., & Ritchie, I. (2006). *Fastest, highest, strongest: A critique of high-performance sports.* Routledge.

Bertling, C. (2007). The loss of profit? The rise of professionalism in the Olympic movement and the consequences for national sport systems. *Journal of Olympic History*, *15*(2), 52.

Brown, A. (2016). Fancy Bears hack: 107 athletes; 23 countries; 25 sports. http://www.sportsintegrityinitiative.com/fancy-bears-hack-107-athletes-23-countries-25-sports/

Coe, S. (2004). We cannot move from strict liability rule. *The Telegraph.* https://www.telegraph.co.uk/sport/othersports/drugsinsport/2373729/We-cannot-move-fromstrict-liability-rule.html

du Toit, N. (2011). Strict liability and sports doping - What constitutes a doping violations and what is the effect thereof on the team? *International Sports Law Journal*, 3–4.

Johnson, M. (2016). *Spitting in the soup: Inside the dirty game of doping in sports.* VeloPress.

Kayser, B., Mauron, A., & Miah, A. (2007). Current anti-doping policy: A critical appraisal. *BMC Medical Ethics*, *8*(1), 1–10.

Mulhall, S. J. (2006). Critique of the World Anti-Doping Code. *Advocate (Vancouver)*, *64*, 29.

Chapter 2

RIGHTS, RESPONSIBILITIES AND POWER IN SPORT ANTI-DOPING: THE COURT OF ARBITRATION FOR SPORT

Helen Jefferson Lenskyj

ABSTRACT

The chapter presents a critical analysis of the functions of the Court of Arbitration for Sport (CAS), identifying how athletes who appeal to CAS for resolution of doping disputes face the problems of 'stacked decks' and 'repeat parties'. A detailed critique of CAS's claim that it supports athletes' human rights, in the document titled 'Sport and Human Rights: Overview from a CAS Perspective', reveals the shaky ground on which the CAS authors based their argument. Detailed analyses of several recent doping cases reveal chronic problems of inconsistent and subjective awards, and, in the case of Chinese swimmer Sun Yang, issues of racist discrimination.

Keywords: Court of Arbitration for Sport; anti-doping; athletes' rights; International Olympic Committee; World Anti-Doping Agency; discrimination

High-performance athletes occupy unique positions in the labour force and in the justice system. They are not considered workers, and most do not enjoy the benefits of union organizing and collective bargaining. On the contrary, their 'employers' are sports organizations with extensive sets of rules controlling every aspect of their daily lives, with a specific focus on preventing the use of performance-enhancing drugs. If athletes are found guilty of doping, the authorities mete out what they consider appropriate penalties, all justified in the interest of protecting 'clean

Doping in Sport and Fitness
Research in the Sociology of Sport, Volume 16, 35–51
Copyright © 2023 by Emerald Publishing Limited
All rights of reproduction in any form reserved
ISSN: 1476-2854/doi:10.1108/S1476-285420220000016003

athletes' and 'clean sport'. Appeals of these often draconian punishments can only be brought to the arbitration tribunal set up by the International Olympic Committee (IOC) – the Court of Arbitration for Sport (CAS).

The IOC established CAS in 1983, prompted by the alleged need for a confidential dispute resolution process that produced 'expedient, flexible, inexpensive and informed judgments' outside of the court system (Kane, 2003, p. 2). Often characterized as a 'supreme court for world sport' (McLaren, 2010), CAS is an arbitration tribunal like any other, notwithstanding its proponents' appeals to 'sports law' and CAS jurisprudence (Straubel, 2005).

Despite proponents' claims that the sport arbitration system would be athlete-friendly, potential clients were slow to embrace CAS's services, presumably because of its close ties to the IOC. Twenty years passed before the annual number of CAS cases reached 100 (Duval & Marino, 2014). Since its inception, CAS panels have heard more doping-related appeals than any of the other major categories, including eligibility, contract, transfer, discipline, nationality and governance.

Reforms of 1994 followed a 1993 decision by the Swiss Federal Tribunal (SFT), where an athlete had appealed a CAS award. The SFT and some European courts, including the European Court of Human Rights, offer the sole recourse for appeals of CAS awards. SFT only considers procedural grounds, such as irregular designation of arbitrator/s, lack of jurisdiction, failure to respect a party's full right to be heard, or incompatibility with Swiss public policy (Martens, 2015, p. 6.3). The 1993 SFT decision noted in passing that CAS's 'organic and economic ties with the IOC' regarding finances and appointment of members could threaten its independent status (Kane, 2003, pp. 5–6).

The IOC then created what it viewed as an 'independent' body, the International Council of Arbitration for Sport (ICAS), to oversee CAS administratively and financially, although the IOC itself continued to have influence over CAS statutes and the appointment of arbitrators. Significantly, the founding president of ICAS, IOC member Judge Keba M'Baye, headed both CAS and ICAS from 1994 until his death in 2007. Italian lawyer Mino Auletta, formerly a member of the IOC's and the IAAF's Sports and Legal Commissions, held the position for three years. IOC vice president John Coates was elected ICAS president in 2010, re-elected in 2015 and again in May 2019. His expiry date as IOC member, usually set at age 70, had been conveniently extended the week before his re-election. In other words, the separation between the IOC and ICAS is far from complete.

INSIDE THE 'OLYMPIC FAMILY'

From the perspectives of the IOC, international federations, national sports organizations, and the World Anti-Doping Agency (WADA), arbitration through CAS neatly avoided what they viewed as the evils of litigation: the time and costs involved, and judges' lack of specialized sport knowledge. These key Olympic industry players objected to the 'intrusion of law into sport' and wanted 'immunity from domestic jurisdictions' (Anderson, 2000, p. 123). Presumably, the 'domestic jurisdictions' that posed the biggest threat were democracies where laws prioritized individual human rights over the 'autonomy of sport' principle that animated the Olympic industry and prompted the formation of CAS.

In the often-quoted words of veteran CAS arbitrator, Michael Beloff, 'Render unto sports the things that are sports' and to courts the things that are legal' (Beloff, 2012, p. 80). For more than two decades, the IOC and its subsidiaries have devoted extensive time and energy to ensuring that sport's autonomy and self-regulation is protected from 'outsiders' and that all disputes are kept 'within the family'. Proponents of CAS have even invoked that argument unironically: Blackshaw (2003, p. 61), for example, stated that CAS provided effective dispute resolution 'within the Family of Sport' (see also Lenskyj, 2018, Chapter 2).

HOW THE SYSTEM WORKS

CAS loosely follows the model of international arbitration tribunals. As in forced arbitration outside of sport, employees sign contracts agreeing to arbitration, not litigation, as the sole means of dispute resolution. Within high-performance sport, the longstanding Rule 61 of the Olympic Charter defines CAS's jurisdiction: any Olympic Games-related dispute 'shall be submitted *exclusively* to the Court of Arbitration for Sport in accordance with the Code of Sport-Related Arbitration' (IOC, 2020, emphasis added). Athletes' contracts and entry forms include the same restrictions on access to domestic courts.

Most CAS hearings take place in Lausanne, with provision for tele-conference or video-conference, a method routinely used in 2020–2021 because of the COVID-19 pandemic. In 1996, in a move designed to facilitate timely hearings during international competition, CAS established an Ad Hoc Division (AHD), with a 12-member team of arbitrators operating on the ground at every Olympics, as well as at other major sport mega-events and FIFA World Cups.

Most appeals are heard by a three-member panel of arbitrators, unless the parties agree to a sole arbitrator. The latter is increasingly popular, since a carefully chosen individual with arbitration experience and sport-related expertise allows parties to avoid challenges and delays. An added advantage for the athlete is the possibility of selecting a sole arbitrator who shares one's own language, cultural background and nationality. On the other hand, a panel with diverse backgrounds could arguably provide a more balanced response. For example, the first panel to hear Dutee Chand's eligibility appeal in 2014 was chaired by a relatively new arbitrator, Annabelle Bennett. A former judge in the Federal Court of Australia, she had no listed sport-related expertise, but her extensive scientific credentials may have been a factor in the panel's partial upholding of Chand's appeal, specifically, their agreement with the scientific consensus that 'there is no single determinant of sex' (CAS 2014/A/3759, S35.c), a position that dates back to the 1960s (e.g. Moore, 1968).

ARBITRATION: WINNERS AND LOSERS

In workplaces outside of sport, arbitration has been the subject of extensive critique. Lindgren (2016) identified some advantages, including privacy, confidentiality and procedural flexibility, but noted that forced arbitration, rather than mediatory procedures, may also incur more costs, delays and an adversarial approach. Moreover, arbitration awards typically affect only the parties involved, have no precedential value and therefore do not contribute to the development of law. There are chronic problems of 'repeat parties' and 'stacked decks' that threaten impartiality and fairness (Lindgren, 2016).

In CAS cases, the 'repeat parties' and 'stacked decks' problems are in full view, and, from time to time, subject to external critiques by legal scholars and investigative journalists. IOC, WADA, FIFA and the major IFs are repeat parties, as either appellants or respondents, in the majority of CAS cases, and their frequent appearances provide them with an advantage over the individual athlete or team. On the question of precedent based on CAS awards, CAS arbitrator Dirk-Reiner Martens stated that 'it should be a matter of course for arbitrators to discuss precedent in the award and, if necessary, distinguish their award from other CAS decisions' (Martens, 2015, S6:2). In practice, however, this is not a 'matter of course' (Lenskyj, 2018).

The organizations that are repeat parties have a ready supply of expensive and experienced sports law representatives at their disposal. These lawyers appear at CAS hearings on a regular basis, have easy access to unpublished awards and an 'insider' advantage because of their familiarity with the individuals and procedures involved. The average athlete has no background experience, nor can they match the financial resources and access to specialist law firms enjoyed by the multinational organizations that comprise the Olympic industry. In the case of Australian swimmer Shayna Jack, discussed below, her first CAS appeal reportedly cost her and her family $AU130k, and she resorted to GoFundMe to continue with her next appeal, following challenges from WADA and the Australian Anti-Doping Agency (ASADA) (Swimmer Shayna Jack, 2021).

The nature of legal aid provided by CAS does little towards mitigating the problem. Its legal aid guidelines require evidence of financial need on the part of the applicant and their family. If granted, the athlete may choose a pro bono counsel from the CAS list, and travel, accommodation costs for applicants, witnesses, experts and interpreters are covered. Article 21, 'Confidentiality', states that the CAS office 'must inform the other parties involved in the arbitration that legal aid has been granted to the applicant' and provide the panel with the legal aid order (TAS-CAS, 2020). How this requirement is compatible with 'confidentiality' is unclear, since the release of this information indicates that the recipient is financially disadvantaged. In these 'David and Goliath' scenarios, sports organizations have more power and resources. Yet, in an early CAS doping decision, on the issue of proving guilty intent, the arbitrators lamented that such a stringent requirement 'would invite costly litigation that may well cripple federations – particularly those run on modest budgets – in their fight against doping' (CAS 94/129, S.15). Clearly, the 'fight against doping' trumps all other parties' rights and interests.

'SPORT AND HUMAN RIGHTS: OVERVIEW FROM A CAS PERSPECTIVE'

In December 2020, presumably in response to external criticism, CAS circulated an internal document titled 'Sport and Human Rights: Overview from a CAS Perspective', authored by Estelle de la Rochefoucauld, CAS Counsel and Matthieu Reeb, successor to Francois Carrard as IOC Director General. An updated version appeared on tas-cas.org in April 2021, with additional details on the Caster Semenya case (justifying 'discrimination' to protect the 'protected class' of female athletes) and the inclusion of the Sun Yang case, discussed below (de la Rochefoucauld & Reeb, 2021, pp. 18–19). Much of the content is directly relevant to doping cases.

The overview represented what a critic might term a valiant effort to find references to 'human rights', however tangential, in IOC, WADA and various international federations' (IFs) regulations, as well as in CAS cases and SFT judgements. The human rights competence of 17 arbitrators and details of five relevant CAS seminars held over a ten-year period were provided in the final sections. A full critique of the document is beyond the scope of this discussion, which will focus only on some of its more obvious shortcomings.

In Section I, 'Human Rights in Sport Regulations', it is not clear why the authors gave CAS credit for human rights-related protections developed by FIFA, the Union of European Football Associations (UEFA), the Commonwealth Games Federation, the Formula One Group, or the UN Guiding Principles on Business and Human Rights. Certainly, athletes' human rights are currently protected, to some extent, by the policies and procedures of these selected organizations, but the links to CAS are tenuous. Perhaps the authors were making the point that these organizations already protect athletes' human rights, and therefore that appeals to CAS would represent outliers.

Also in Section I, the report's most inappropriate co-optation is the inclusion of the Universal Declaration of Players Rights of 2017, developed by the Institute for Human Rights and Business and the World Players Association (WPA). Since its inception in 2014, WPA and its leader Brendan Schwab have been vocal critics of WADA and tireless advocates for athletes' rights, in the face of the constant threats posed by anti-doping rules. In other words, if WADA, the IOC and ultimately CAS had respected athletes' human rights, there would have been little need for the numerous advocacy groups that athletes and their allies have established in the past decade, including the WPA, the Sports and Rights Alliance (SRA), Athleten Deutchland and Global Athlete. For example, in 2017, when the IOC was working on the Athletes' Declaration of Rights and Responsibilities, SRA called for 'a comprehensive human rights policy... to advance the fundamental rights of athletes – those that they inherently hold as people' (SRA, 2018).

The IOC ignored the SRA's request for dialogue and input, instead relying on a limited survey of athletes as evidence of their 'engagement' with stakeholders.

In light of the ruling on WADA's Whereabouts rule, discussed below, it is especially jarring to see, in Section II 'Selected CAS cases related to human rights issues', a reference to Article 8 of the ECHR that guarantees the individual 'respect for his private and family life, his home and his correspondence'. As an example of the 'indirect application' of this particular 'right', de la Rochefoucauld and Reeb cited the case of Mariya Savinova-Farnosova, a Russian track athlete suspended for doping, who alleged that covert recordings had been made of her private conversations and were therefore inadmissible. The sole arbitrator in that case, Hans Nater, disagreed, citing the IAAF principle that the 'courts shall balance the interest in protecting the right that was infringed [privacy] ...against the interest in establishing the truth', a principle supported by the SFT and ECHR (CAS 2016/O/4481; S4, S93). The overview quoted Nater's conclusion that 'interest in discerning the truth must prevail over the interest of the athlete' (Para 106). For this to be cited as an example of a CAS case 'related to human rights issues', despite Nater's dismissal of the privacy protection offered by Article 8, seems inconsistent, to say the least.

In Section IV, 'SFT Judgements dealing with the application of human rights by the CAS', the overview begins by citing the landmark Matuzalem appeal of 2012 (Valloni & Pachmann, 2012). This was the first time that a CAS award was overturned by the SFT on *substantive* as well as procedural grounds. SFT ruled that, by upholding FIFA's ban, CAS had violated the Swiss Private International Law guarantee of Matuzalem's personal and economic freedom, and was contrary to public policy (SFT 4A_558/211, 4.3.1). Although it could be argued that the Matuzalem decision was not one of CAS's finest hours, it nevertheless gained mention in the Overview.

Similarly, the SFT's annulment of the CAS award involving Chinese swimmer Sun Yang (discussed below) is cited in the same section of the Overview. Since SFT found clear evidence of lack of impartiality – specifically, anti-Chinese racism – on the part of the panel's chair, the situation reflected badly on CAS's screening of arbitrators – hardly an exemplar of CAS's respect for human rights.

Section V identified 17 arbitrators as having 'human rights competence'. Of these, four did not appear in the database that lists published decisions (as of June 2021), either because their decisions were unpublished or because they were very recent appointees. Four others each made only two appearances, while most of the remaining arbitrators' names appeared in between seven and 17 published cases. Longstanding arbitrator Michael Beloff was an exception, with 130 cases since 1996, and is undoubtedly a standard-bearer in terms of experience.

GLOBAL ANTI-DOPING EFFORTS

WADA was established in 1999 under the leadership of IOC vice president Richard Pound. The Word Anti-Doping Code (WADC) came into force in 2004, with CAS serving as the body responsible for the final resolution of doping disputes. For their part, CAS panels have no role in establishing anti-doping rules and policies; they merely enforce the rules on behalf of WADA by hearing appeals. As Martens warned in his 2015 guidelines for arbitrators, because CAS operates in a 'highly political' environment, arbitrators must remain 'uninfluenced by considerations of perceived sporting fairness and political governance', always remembering 'that CAS is a court of law and is called upon to apply the rules of sporting bodies, not to re-write them' (Martens, 2015, p. 6.2). In practice, largely because it is not, or does not purport to be, a precedential system, arbitrators have on occasion done the equivalent of *re-writing* rules, as discussed below. Although it has been suggested *lex sportiva* (sports law) based in CAS jurisprudence has evolved as an informal precedential system (Casini, 2011; McLaren, 2010; Mitten, 2014), as McArdle noted, '...a cynic might argue that CAS Panels use precedent when doing so reinforces the judgment they wish to reach and ignore it when the precedents are adverse...' (McArdle, 2014, p. 33).

WADA routinely uses CAS to appeal what it considers an inadequate penalty determined by a national sports body, or to challenge an inadequate testing programme or laboratory in a non-compliant country, Russia, for example. WADA was a party in more than 120 published CAS cases between 1999 and 2020, and appellant in approximately 90% of those appeals. Parties have the option of confidentiality, and it has been estimated that published cases represent only about 30% of all awards (Spera, 2017). Because of this trend, quantitative analyses are unlikely to be accurate, but the published awards provide ample data for qualitative analysis and critique. Almost all of WADA's appeals were upheld or partially upheld, and the small number that named WADA as respondent were dismissed, giving WADA, and WADA's lawyers, specifically Ross Wenzel of Kellerhals Carrard law firm, a high success rate.

THE POTENTIAL FOR CONFLICT OF INTEREST

The problems of 'role-switching' and 'repeat parties', and the subsequent potential for conflict of interest, have been identified by critics of forced arbitration (Comsti, 2014; Lindgren, 2016). Switzerland offers sports organizations a large number of specialized law firms whose counsel are repeat parties in a significant number of CAS cases. Conveniently, it is also home to more than 65 international sports organizations. The website kellerhals-carrard.ch/en lists seven offices in Switzerland and documents the firm's extensive experience at CAS, representing the IOC, WADA, and numerous IFs and national anti-doping agencies. Significantly, its senior partner, Francois Carrard, was the IOC's Director General from 1989 to 2003, and during that period, according to CAS database, he also served as a CAS arbitrator in several appeals.

This problem of 'role-switching' was pervasive in relation to CAS proceedings, with individuals serving as arbitrator at one hearing and counsel at another, and IOC members themselves filling these roles (Lenskyj, 2018, p. 39). Of counsel listed in published cases at tas-cas.org, one person appears to have represented parties in seven CAS appeals, 1998–2004, at the same time serving as arbitrator on AHD panels at the 1996, 2000 and 2004 Olympics. Another arbitrator, whose name appeared in over 70 panels, 1998–2016, represented six parties, 1992–2006. A third arbitrator represented parties in two CAS cases, in 2006 and 2009. CAS rules permitted this kind of 'role-switching'.

ICAS has attempted to address the problem of conflict of interest. In 2004, S11 of the CAS Code restricted colleagues in the same law firm as the CAS arbitrator from representing parties in a dispute, and a 2010 revision prohibited CAS arbitrators from acting as counsel before CAS. Commenting on this, however, CAS Secretary General Mathieu Reeb claimed that ICAS would deal with infringements, and that the person's 'function... will not be called into question in the arbitration at stake' (Reeb, 2010). In other words, 'we make the rules, we break the rules'.

THE STRICT LIABILITY PRINCIPLE

On the matter of doping, CAS applies the strict liability principle, which amounts to the presumption of guilt whenever a banned substance is found, regardless of intent, negligence or involuntariness. The numerous critiques of this principle over the past 20 years have largely fallen on deaf ears (for example, Kane, 2003; McArdle, 2014; Oschutz, 2001; Pielke, 2017; Straubel, 2005). The rationale for strict liability relies on the ideal of 'fair competition' and the alleged 'unfair advantage' enjoyed by athletes who dope, regardless of intentionality, although CAS does apply the principle of proportionality in determining the penalty (see, for example, CAS 2010/A/2230; de la Rochefoucauld & Reeb, 2021). According to arguments in favour of the strict liability principle, every deterrent and penalty, however harsh, is justified to protect 'clean athletes' and 'clean sport'. What is generally unstated is the damage to the brand and the threat of sponsors' disengagement – in other words, the financial implications when doping athletes appear to be escaping detection and punishment.

Maintaining the integrity of sport demands that 'unclean' athletes face appropriate consequences: bans on future participation and deletion of their 'tainted' records. The media's public shaming of these athletes, regardless of innocence or guilt, inevitably follows (Boye et al., 2017; Greene, 2017). This is a bonus for the anti-doping 'moral crusade' because it sends a warning to the next generation of athletes as well as promoting cultural change within sports organizations – or so the theory goes. In fact, as Møller and Dimeo have clearly documented in the case of cycling, 'sport is essentially deteriorating under the current anti-doping campaign executed by an un-coordinated alliance between the WADA, law enforcement authorities, sports organizers and the media' (Møller & Dimeo, 2014, p. 260). In short, doping continues unchecked in cycling and other sports and records have become meaningless, despite ever-escalating surveillance and enforcement efforts.

Straubel's 2005 critique of CAS's approach to doping appeals identified a number of fundamental flaws. For example, he pointed to the fact that CAS treated doping violations as criminal in nature by imposing penalties on guilty parties; it failed to offer athletes the procedural protections, including the presumption of innocence and the right to appeal, that criminal cases require (Straubel, 2005, p. 1260). In one extreme example of sport exceptionalism, ASADA proposed a 2013 amendment to its 2006 rules that would remove the right to remain silent, by compelling parties to 'attend an interview with an investigator' (Australian Sports, 2013). Unsurprisingly, critics expressed their shock that a sports organization would propose subjecting athletes to 'a higher threshold ...than individuals suspected of criminal offences' (Giles & Loeliger, 2013).

CAS applies a higher standard of proof than the usual 'balance of probability' used in civil proceedings, whether or not the doping offence is criminal in nature (Oschutz, 2001, p. 696). The standard of proof – 'comfortable satisfaction' – used by arbitrators is 'greater than a mere balance of probability but less than proof beyond a reasonable doubt' (CAS 2015/A/3925). A 1998 CAS decision stated that when a 'high degree of satisfaction' has been established, the burden of proof shifts to the athlete, who may then raise intentionality to try to reduce the severity of the sanction (CAS 98/208). For a finding of NSF (no significant fault or negligence) or NF (no fault or negligence), the athlete has to demonstrate, on balance of probabilities, that the doping was not intentional. A change to WADC in 2009 introduced *aggravating circumstances*, including multiple violations (using or possessing performance-enhancing drugs, or tampering with samples) that warranted more severe sanctions and required the athlete to meet a higher burden of proof (WADA, 2009, p. 10.6).

WADA's annual listing of banned substances has long been controversial. The fact that it includes some that have no demonstrable positive impact on athletic performance, or that some even have a negative impact, does not affect application of the strict liability principle. In the case of Australian swimmer Shayna Jack's appeal to CAS, for example, the sole arbitrator noted that the amount of prohibited substance in her system was 'pharmacologically irrelevant'. He stated, amongst other reasons for his ruling, that 'there are very limited scientific papers...concerning the effects of taking ligandrol or of the dosages required for a performance enhancing effect especially in the case of females...' (CAS A1/2020, S100). Fortunately for Jack, the respondents were Swimming Australia and the Australian Sports Anti-Doping Authority. Had WADA been the respondent, it seems likely that their counsel would have anticipated and challenged this reasoning.

The three criteria for inclusion on the prohibited list are: potential for performance enhancement, health risk and violation of the spirit of sport (Jedlicka, 2014, pp. 438–439). Items on the list are subject to change. For example, WADA's 2018 list excluded alcohol 'after careful consideration', but recommended that international federations should establish rules to test and sanction offenders (WADA, 2018, p. 1). Cannabinoids were first listed in 2005, primarily because of their illegality in many jurisdictions and the alleged violation of 'the spirit of sport'.

WHEREABOUTS AND HUMAN RIGHTS

WADA's *Whereabouts* rule, introduced in 2004, requires elite athletes to provide WADA with their locations and availability for random testing on a daily basis. A 2015 change brought about uniform rules for all countries and sports for breaches of the *Whereabouts* rules: a standard two-year sanction, and a 'three strikes in 12-months' rule for missed tests, regardless of circumstances (WADA, 2015). Another rule change of 2015 increased the ban for doping, tampering with a sample, or helping others to dope, from two to four years, thereby guaranteeing that the athlete would miss one Olympic Games, and possibly experience the end of their career. A prominent *Whereabouts* Failure appeal to CAS in 2020–2021 involved US sprinter Christian Coleman (TAS-CAS, 2021). The CAS panel upheld the original violation finding but reduced the penalty from two years to 18 months, a change that still left him ineligible to compete in the Tokyo Olympics.

In 2010, several European sports organizations and individual players challenged the Whereabouts rule, claiming that it violated Article 8 of European Convention on Human Rights (ECHR), which protected the right to respect for private and family life. The European Court of Human Rights 2018 decision defended its legality, stating that the rule was justified on 'public interest grounds' and warning that its removal 'would be at odds with the European and international consensus' concerning the necessity for random testing in fighting 'the scourge' of doping. Furthermore, it referred to the 'protection of health' of professional athletes, and claimed that their doping would 'dangerously' encourage amateurs and 'especially young people to follow suit' (Doping control, 2018). On the issue of 'protection' of health', amateurs and youth would undoubtedly have already noticed global sports organizations' failures to achieve this goal, Russia's recent history of state-sponsored doping and USA Gymnastics' dismal failure to stop child abuse being two prime examples. Nevertheless, higher courts have been notably reluctant to criticize CAS awards; rather, as former European Court judge Helen Keller recently noted, they 'don't want to step on toes' and seem prepared to accept that CAS is 'just about compliant' with the ECHR. She also predicted the consequences; if the SFT were to be too strict vis-à-vis CAS, since its geographic location is not key, and it could be moved to Asia if necessary (Keller, 2021).

SELECTED CAS APPEALS, AND THE
CONSISTENCY PROBLEM

The Coca Tea Problem (I)

Jose Paolo Guerrero, captain of the Peruvian football team, tested positive for cocaine following the qualifying rounds of the 2018 FIFA World Cup. He claimed that contaminated tea provided by hotel staff when he requested ordinary tea was responsible for the finding of cocaine in his samples. Coca tea is a legal and traditional South American drink considered to alleviate minor health problems. Cocaine metabolites are on WADA's Prohibited List, but a modified version of the WADA Code, responding to 'stakeholder feedback', added a clause stating that cocaine and similar 'substances of abuse', used 'out-of-competition and unrelated to sport performance', would incur a suspension of only three months, to be reduced to one month if a drug rehabilitation program is completed (WADA publishes, 2020).

FIFA's provisional suspension was for 30 days, but an additional hearing increased it to one year. His appeal was successful in reducing FIFA's suspension to six months. He subsequently appealed to CAS, naming FIFA as respondent, whereupon WADA lodged an appeal to CAS, with FIFA and Guerrero as respondents. All parties agreed to let CAS consolidate the two appeals. The decision includes pages of detail debating the degree of fault for which Guerrero was responsible: should he have checked the label on the tea, was it reasonable for him to assume that sport officials had put food and beverage protocols in place at the hotel, etc.? Eventually, the panel dismissed his appeal against FIFA, partially upheld WADA's cross-appeal, and reduced the ban to 14 months (CAS2018/A/5546).

Guerrero then filed an appeal with the SFT, which it dismissed in May 2018. However, one judge froze the ban to allow him to play in the World Cup, a move to which CAS, unexpectedly, did not object. Presumably, CAS would have been well aware of the outcome if it had challenged the eight-page judgement by Swiss judge Patricia Kiss, as well as the reputational damage it would suffer in the court of public opinion. Judge Kiss pointed to the 'rare surge of solidarity' supporting his participation, including a letter signed by team captains of Peru's three major opponents – France, Denmark, and Australia. She also cited the damaging impact on his teammates if their captain was not allowed to play (Peru's Paolo Guerrero, 2018).

The Coca Tea Problem (II)

A few years later, in 2019, the coca tea issue appeared once more, this time involving Canadian show jumper Nicole Walker and Equestrian Canada as appellants and the PanAmerican Sports Organization as respondent. Walker accepted the disqualification of her individual results but challenged that of results obtained as part of team competition, thereby leading to a complex discussion of the WADA Code's definition of Team Sports vs. awards given to *teams*, as well as the PanAm rules on that issue.

The CAS panel conducted its hearing by video in May 2021. It accepted Walker's claim that she was unaware that the tea bag provided by a hotel in Lima contained coca, despite having read the Spanish label 'matte de coca'. Somewhat similar to Guerrero's defence, Walker (and Team Canada) believed that their hotel was an official PanAm hotel and that illegal food or beverage would not be provided. Walker was described as 'an intelligent, sincere and honest witness' (S255). The polygraph expert testifying on her behalf expressed 98.8% confidence that she was telling the truth, and the panel agreed that she had inadvertently and unknowingly ingested cocaine. However, the outcome remained largely unchanged: her individual disqualification carried with it the disqualification of all

Team Canada's results. Consequently, Team Canada failed to qualify for Tokyo 2020, a situation that Walker claimed was 'unfair to my teammates...Team Canada competed fairly and has earned the right to be in Tokyo' (Spencer, 2021).

It is illuminating to see the different outcomes in the Guerrero and Walker cases. Thanks to the relatively lenient Swiss judge who froze Guerroro's ban, he was allowed to play in the most significant global competition in his sport, and his team did not suffer from his absence as captain. In Walker's case, both she and her teammates were disqualified from the 2020 Olympics, in part because of different definitions of 'team sport'. Moreover, the World Cup demands world attention, given that soccer is the biggest global sport in terms of participants and fans, whereas Olympic equestrian events are of relatively low interest on all counts.

The Contaminated Blender Problem

The case of another young white woman, Australian swimmer Shayna Jack, provides further evidence of the subjective nature of CAS awards. A random test in 2019 found a banned substance, ligandrol, and Sport Integrity Australia (formerly ASADA) imposed a four-year ban. Jack denied using ligandrol, appealed to CAS, and selected Australian QC Alan Sullivan as sole arbitrator, for a hearing in September 2020. She was unable to demonstrate how the substance entered her system, but claimed that the violation was not intentional and not due to recklessness. There was no evidence of long-term use. On those grounds, she sought a finding of NSF and a reduction of the ban to two years. The sole arbitrator noted the 'speculation' offered by Jack – that her supplements were contaminated, that her housemates' previous use of a blender may be responsible or that contact with or ingestion of ligandrol came from a pool or gym.

Although Jack could not account for the adverse finding, Sullivan stated that, in his view, she was not required to do so. He interpreted the language of the relevant article more leniently than some previous awards, stating that 'the proper approach is to determine whether, on the totality of evidence, the Applicant has proven on balance of probabilities that she did not, or did not attempt to, cheat' (CAS A1/2020, S.81). The rest of the award makes his leanings very clear: Jack 'was emphatic that she did not intentionally...emphatic that she did not know...' (S.83). She described herself as 'a diligent and dedicated athlete...[who] had always had an intense disdain for intentional doping...' (S.84).

The award noted that she 'took considerable steps, at considerable expense' to find the source of the ligandrol. Finally, it stated:

> The Applicant greatly impressed the Sole Arbitrator as a witness... in cross-examination... her credibility remained completely intact. Indeed, she was one of the most impressive witness (sic) ... in more than 40 years of practice. She appeared to be completely straightforward, genuine and honest in the answers she gave... The applicant presented as an honest, decent, reliable and very plausible witness'. (S.87)

Additionally, a lineup of character witnesses supported her 'in the most glowing and praiseworthy of terms': conscientious, likeable, exceptional, fantastic and so on. Sullivan partially upheld Jack's appeal, by reducing the suspension to two years. Sport Integrity Australia and WADA may have noticed the thin ice on which he was skating. In December 2020, these two organizations lodged an appeal with CAS, but it was rejected in September 2021.

Coincidentally, the ligandrol/shared food blender defence came up again in Australia when rugby player James Segeyaro successfully appealed a ban after a failed drug test. The National Rugby League Anti-Doping Tribunal reduced his suspension to 20 months. Expert witnesses claimed that residue could be present in the blender, and one of his housemates admitted buying ligandrol (Pengilly, 2021).

Maria Sharapova

Among the high-profile athletes to appeal a doping suspension was Russian professional tennis player, Maria Sharapova, following a January 2016 doping test that had found meldonium in her sample. Meldonium was added to WADA's 2016 prohibited list, and the International Tennis Federation (ITF) imposed a two-year suspension. Sharapova's representatives explained that she had been taking Mildronate, prescribed by her doctor, for 10 years, and that her agent, responsible for all anti-doping matters, had failed to note that it had been added to the prohibited list. Sharapova sought a finding of NSF and a reduced suspension. The panel rejected the NSF argument but found less than Significant Fault and reduced the sanction to 15 months. Explaining these distinctions, the award stated that, although past doping cases 'offer guidance to a panel, all those cases are very "fact specific" and no doctrine of binding precedent applies' (CAS 2016/A/4643, S.1).

Like the 'character reference' aspect of Jack's award, the award stressed the fact that it 'was not about an athlete who cheated', there was 'no question of intent', and 'under no circumstances, therefore, can the Player be considered to be an "intentional doper"' (CAS 2016/A/4643, S.101). In fact, the panel criticized WADA and ITF for failing to notify athletes of the new prohibited substances and their brand names on the annual list.

Although this was, for the most part, a victory for Sharapova, she did not win in the court of public opinion. Most global media condemned what they saw as her failure to apologize or to show remorse, and criticized her ambition and lack of humility, character traits that are not exactly uncommon in the world of professional tennis, especially among the top male players dating back to John McEnroe.

Sun Yang

On the issue of potential bias, the high-profile appeal by Chinese swimmer Sun Yang is relevant here. These allegations involved tampering with samples, a violation that falls in the category of aggravating circumstances, as distinct from the appeals discussed above that were seeking a reduced suspension on the grounds of lack of intent. Nevertheless, the specific language used in the 2020 award to justify upholding WADA's eight-year ban on Yang together with the SFT's 2021 annulment of the award because of the chair's past racist comments make it particularly relevant to this discussion.

Although 10 Chinese-speaking arbitrators were listed on tas-cas.org, none were selected. The panel comprised Franco Frattini (Italy) as chair, and a European and a UK arbitrator. Yang's legal team included two Chinese-speaking attorneys, one French- and English-speaking Geneva-based attorney, and a London barrister (CAS 2019/A/6148). The award noted that, although his team had chosen the interpreters, there were 'apparent problems in interpreting the Athlete's testimony' and one of the Chinese-speaking attorneys had to be used until a new interpreter was in place (S.126). In spite of the acknowledged language problem, the panel saw fit to chastise Yang for asking 'an unknown and unannounced person from the public gallery ...to act as an impromptu interpreter' during the closing statement (S.358). Building on the theme of taking 'matters into his own hands', a phrase that makes four other appearances in the award, the panel chose to draw parallels between Yang's behaviour during the sample collection and his alleged lack of respect for 'the authority of others, or of established procedures' at the CAS hearing. 'He is not above the law or legal process', they warned (S.358). 'It was striking', according to S.356, that Yang did not 'express any regret as to his actions.' Rather, as stated in rather non-lawyerly language, 'he dug his heels in'. The subjective tone of these sections is itself both 'striking' and concerning.

CONCLUSION

As the preceding discussion and my earlier analysis of CAS awards (Lenskyj, 2018) have shown, it is not difficult to identify underlying systemic problems that threaten athletes' rights. Lack of consistency, transparency and fairness is unsurprising in a system that is non-precedential, and a system that offers sole arbitrators or panels selected from a closed list of over 250 lawyers who have diverse cultural backgrounds and diverse experiences in law and in sport.

The common law concept of 'a jury of one's peers' is not replicated in a CAS hearing, except, perhaps, in cases where the athlete and the sole arbitrator share some common ground: Shayna Jack and Alan Sullivan, for example. The language of Sullivan's award suggests that he had no difficulty interpreting Jack's demeanour as remorseful, and her testimony as authentic. At the other end of the spectrum, in addition to translation problems, Sun Yang faced arbitrators with whom he had little in common culturally, and a panel chair who was subsequently found to harbour anti-Chinese racist sentiments. (It is interesting to note that the panel for Yang's second hearing also comprised three European arbitrators.)

On the issue of arbitrators' subjective evaluations of athletes, a show of remorse would obviously be well received, but Sharapova did not play that game and yet the award was relatively favourable to her. Between the two extremes, we find a SFT judge in effect bending the rules to accommodate a world-class football player and his team, while a show jumper and her team are disqualified. In short, the CAS system of arbitration is not fit for purpose.

KEY READINGS

(1) Dimeo, P., & Møller, V. (2018). *The Anti-Doping Crisis in Sport*. Routledge.
  Critique of WADA's history and shortcomings, specifically ineffective testing, dubious convictions and failure to respect athletes' human rights.
(2) Duval, A., & Rigozzi, A. (2022). *Yearbook of International Sports Arbitration 2018–2020*. Asser Press.
  Review of CAS awards and other international arbitration, including doping appeals, with discussion of their significance.
(3) Lenskyj, H. (2018). *Gender, Athletes' Rights, and the Court of Arbitration for Sport*. Emerald Publishing Limited.
  Critical review of CAS cases since its inception, focusing on inconsistent awards, conflict of interest and other problematic areas, with detailed analysis of cases involving doping.
(4) Lindgren, K. (2016). International and domestic arbitration. In M. Legg (Ed.), *Resolving Civil Disputes* (pp. 209–221). LexisNexis.
  Insightful analysis of the advantages and disadvantages of arbitration when compared to litigation.
(5) McArdle, D. (2014). *Sport Dispute Resolution*. Routledge.
  Critical assessment of alternative dispute resolution procedures in sport, with a focus on CAS awards.

CAS AWARDS

tas-cas.org/jurisprudence/archive.html

CAS 94/129	USA Shooting v International Shooting Union
CAS 98/208	N. J. Y. and WADA v FINA
CAS 2010/A/2230	International Wheelchair Basketball Federation v UKAD and Simon Gibbs
CAS 2014/A/3759	Dutee Chand v IAAF and Athletics Federation of India
CAS 2015/A/3925	Traves Smikle v JADO
CAS 2016/O/4481	IAAF v All Russia Athletics Federation and Mariya Savinova-Farnosova
CAS 2016/A/4643	Maria Sharapova v ITF
CAS2018/A/5546	WADA v FIFA and Paolo Guerrero
CAS 2019/A/6148	WADA v Sun Yang and FINA
CAS 2020/A1	Shayna Jack v Sport Integrity Australia and Australia Anti-Doping Agency

SFT AWARDS

swissarbitrationdecisions.com

SFT 4A_558/2011   Matuzalem v FIFA

REFERENCES

Anderson, J. (2000). "Taking sports out of the courts": Alternative dispute resolution and The International Court of Arbitration for Sport. *Journal of Legal Aspects of Sport, 10*, 123.

Beloff, M. J. (2012). Is there a lex sportiva? In R. Siekmann & J. Soek (Eds.), *Lex Sportiva: What Is Sports Law?* (pp. 69–89). TMC Asser Press.

Blackshaw, I. (2003). The Court of Arbitration for Sport: An international forum for settling disputes effectively within the family of sport. *Entertainment and Sports Law Journal, 2*(2), 61–83.

Boye, E., Skotland, T., Østerud, B., & Nissen-Meyer, J. (2017). Doping and drug testing: Anti-doping work must be transparent and adhere to good scientific practices to ensure public trust. *EMBO Reports, 18*(3), 351–354.

Casini, L. (2011). The making of a lex sportiva by The Court of Arbitration for Sport. *German Law Journal, 12*(5), 1317–1340.

Comsti, C. (2014). A metamorphosis: How forced arbitration arrived in the workplace. *Berkeley Journal of Employment and Labor Law, 5*, 6–31.

de la Rochefoucauld, E., & Reeb, M. (2021). *Sport and Human Rights: Overview from a CAS Perspective.* tas-cas.org/fileadmin/user_upload/Human_Rights_in_sport_CAS_report_updated_16.04.2021_pdf

Duval, A., & Marino, G. (2014). Quantifying The Court of Arbitration for Sport. *Asser Sports Law.* asser.nl/SportsLaw/Blog/post/quantifying-the-court-of-arbitration-for-sport-by-antoine-duval-and-gianni-marino

Giles, A., & Loeliger, J. (2013). Australia: New powers for ASADA. *Mondaq Law.* Mondaq.com/Australia/x/248992/Sport/New+powers+for+ASAD+to+investigate+the+use+of+drugs+in+sport

Greene, P. J. (2017). When athletes are wrongly sanctioned under the World Anti-Doping Code. *Maryland Journal of International Law, 32*(1), 338–345.

IOC. (2020). The Olympic Charter. stillmed.olympic.org/media/Document%20Library/OlympicOrg/General/EN-Olympic-Charter.pdf

Jedlicka, S. (2014). The normative discourse of anti-doping policy. *International Journal of Sport Policy and Politics, 6*(3), 429–442.

Kane, D. (2003). Twenty years on: An evaluation of The Court of Arbitration for Sport. *Melbourne Journal of International Law, 4*(2), 611–635.

Keller, H. (2021). The Court of Arbitration for Sport at the European Court of Human Rights. Asser Institute. asser.nl/education-events/?id=4204

Lenskyj, H. J. (2018). *Gender, Athletes' Rights, and The Court of Arbitration for Sport.* Emerald Publishing Limited.

Lindgren, K. (2016). International and domestic arbitration. In M. Legg (Ed.), *Resolving Civil Disputes* (pp. 209–221). LexisNexis.

Martens, D.-R. (2015). The role of the arbitrator in CAS proceedings. Martens-Rechtsanwalte. martens-lawyers.com/wp-content/uploads/2015/02/Article-The-role-of-the-arbitrator-in-CAS-proceedings.pdf

McArdle, D. (2014). *Dispute Resolution in Sport: Athletes, Law and Arbitration.* Routledge.

McLaren, R. H. (2010). Twenty-five years of The Court of Arbitration for Sport: A look in the rear-view mirror. *Marquette Sports Law Review, 20*(2), 305–333.

Mitten, M. J. (2014). The Court of Arbitration for Sport and its global jurisprudence: International legal pluralism in a world without national boundaries. *Ohio State Journal on Dispute Resolution, 30*(1), 1–44.

Møller, V., & Dimeo, P. (2014). Anti-doping – The end of sport. *International Journal of Sport Policy and Politics, 6*(2), 259–272.

Moore, K. L. (1968). The sexual identity of athletes. *JAMA, 205*(11), 787–788.

Oschutz, F. (2001). Harmonization of anti-doping code through arbitration. *Marquette Sports Law Review, 12*, 675–702.

Pengilly, A. (2021). James Segeyaro has drugs ban reduced to 20 months. *WA Today*. watoday.com.au/sport/nrl/james-segeyaro-has-drugs-ban-reduced-to-20-months-20210218-p573rg.html

Peru's Paulo Guerrero Cleared. (2018, May 31). ESPN. espn.com/soccer/fifa-world-cup/story/3514197/perus-paolo-guerrero-cleared-to-play-at-world-cup-by-swiss-judge

Pielke, R. (2017, August 24). Inconsistencies between Johaug vs. Sharapova at CAS. The Least Thing Blog. leastthingblogspot.ca/2017/08/inconsistencies-between-johaug-vs.html

Reeb, M. (2010). The new code of sports-related arbitration. *TAS/CAS Bulletin*. cas.org/fileadmin/user_upload/Bulletin01112010.pdf

Spencer, D. (2021, May 4). Sport court exonerates Canadian show jumper. CBC. cbc.ca/sports/olympics/summer/nicole-walker-sports-court-olympics-1.6013513

Spera, S. (2017, January 31). Time for transparency at the Court of Arbitration for Sport. Asser International Sports Law Blog. asser.nl/SportsLaw/Blog/post/transparency-at-the-court-of-arbitration-for-sport-by-saveriospera

SRA. (2018). Athletes' rights are human rights. Sports and Rights Alliance. athletescan.com/sites/default/files/images/sra_letter_to_ioc_bach_october_2018_final.pdf

Straubel, M. (2005). Enhancing the performance of the doping court: How the Court of Arbitration for Sport can do its job better. *Loyola University Chicago Law Journal, 36*(4), 1203–1272.

Swimmer Shayna Jack Turns to Public for Donations. (2021, February 19). *The Guardian*. theguardian.com/sport/2021/feb/19/swimmer-shayna-jack-turns-to-public-for-donations-in-fight-to-clear-name

TAS-CAS. (2020). Guidelines on Legal Aid. tas-cas.org/en/add/legal-aid.html

TAS-CAS. (2021). Media release: Athletics. tas-cas.org/fileadmin/user_upload/CAS_Media_Release_7528.pdf

Valloni, L., & Pachmann, T. (2012). Switzerland: The landmark Matuzalem case and its consequences on the FIFA regulations. *Mondaq*. mondaq.com/x/184712/Sport/The+Landmark+Matuzalem+Case+And+Its+Consequences+On+The+FIFA

WADA. (2009). WADA Anti-Doping Code. WADA. wada_anti_doping_code_2009_en_0.pdf

WADA. (2015). WADA Anti-Doping Code. WADA. wada-ama.org/sites/default/files/resources/files/wada-2015-world-anti-doping-code.pdf

WADA. (2018). Summary of major modifications and explanatory notes. WADA. wada-ama.org/sites/default/files/prohibited_list_2018_summary_of_modifications_en.pdf

Chapter 3

EVIDENCE-BASED ANTI-DOPING EDUCATION: FACT OR FICTION?

Katharina Gatterer and Cornelia Blank

ABSTRACT

There are two key approaches in doping prevention research: (1) to investigate why athletes dope (i.e. risk factors) and (2) to investigate why athletes do not dope (i.e. protective factors). Both approaches aim to reduce the occurrence of doping. Even though there is a lot of evidence showing which factors protect athletes from doping, there is still the problem of putting research into practice. Currently, evidence-based prevention is lacking. In this chapter, we propose a roadmap of possible solutions in three areas: improving the translation of research findings into practice, increasing financial resources and training of human resources, and acknowledging the recipients' voice.

Keywords: Doping prevention; values-based education; International Standard for Education; risk factors; protective factors; financial resources

DOPING PREVENTION PERSPECTIVES – WHAT DOES THE EVIDENCE TELL US?

Even though doping detection measures (i.e. anti-doping testing) with the underlying purpose of deterrence might be an effective way to prevent doping, this chapter puts the spotlight on measures that might reduce doping behaviour before it occurs. Within this framework, and borrowing from the health sciences, two approaches to doping prevention research can be distinguished: (1) investigating why athletes dope (i.e. risk factors), with the long-term aim of reducing these risk factors, and (2) investigating why athletes do not dope (i.e. protective factors), with the long-term aim of enhancing these protective factors. Both approaches aim to reduce the occurrence of doping. Identifying risk factors was

Doping in Sport and Fitness
Research in the Sociology of Sport, Volume 16, 53–67
Copyright © 2023 by Emerald Publishing Limited
All rights of reproduction in any form reserved
ISSN: 1476-2854/doi:10.1108/S1476-285420220000016004

the focus of most doping prevention research in the last decade. This research was influenced by various models and theories, for example, the theory of planned behaviour (TPB) (Ajzen & Madden, 1986), deterrence theory (Paternoster, 1987), self-determination theory (Ryan & Deci, 2000), or a combination thereof (Donovan et al., 2002; Strelan & Boeckmann, 2003). Based on these theories from the fields of psychology, sociology, criminology and behavioural sciences, initial variables of interest included knowledge, attitudes, norms, motivation, beliefs and the influence of peers (Backhouse et al., 2016). In line with this, two meta-analyses summarizing variables predicting doping susceptibility, intention and behaviour found that positive attitudes towards doping, perceived social norms and subjective norms positively correlated with either doping intention or behaviour; thus, they were characterized as risk factors (e.g. Blank et al., 2016; Ntoumanis et al., 2014).

At the same time, qualitative studies based on interviews with doping athletes revealed that the reasons why those athletes dope (i.e. the risk factors) were markedly different compared to the factors listed earlier: these qualitative studies indicated that reasons to dope are usually functional, such as overcoming an illness or an injury in order to be able to compete again as soon as possible (Engelberg et al., 2015; Kirby et al., 2011); this indicates that doping is used as a coping strategy to ensure success within the sports system (Petróczi & Aidman, 2008). Following this, a study of both doped and clean athletes showed that variables defined as risk factors were not specific to doped athletes, and few of the many factors previously identified showed potential for distinguishing between doped and clean athletes (Gatterer et al., 2019). Thus, in terms of risk factors, doping was no longer only investigated at the micro-level (i.e. at the level of the individual athlete). Instead, the decision to dope was conceptualized as the product of an intentional and volitional decision-making process. The focus was extended to the macro level, to include the social context of the athlete, as well as situational factors and the sports system in other studies (Blank et al., 2016; Stewart & Smith, 2008). In this context, the comprehensive model of Stewart and Smith (2008), which aimed to explain the complexity of the doping problem, has received renewed attention. While their model had many variables in common with previous models and theories, they also included new variables pertaining to social issues (e.g. masculine sports culture) and the sporting system (Stewart & Smith, 2008). Indeed, athletes also cited some of the newly introduced factors (Engelberg et al., 2015; Kirby et al., 2011).

Overall, it seems that doping mostly stems from the environmental pressure to perform perceived by professional athletes. If the pressure becomes too great and the athletes do not have the resources to cope with it, they might choose to dope as a possible coping strategy, as outlined earlier and supported by other researchers (Petróczi & Aidman, 2008). The question remains as to what other variables may play a role in the complex decision to dope. In other words, what variables might augment resources and thus protect against doping as a coping strategy in the face of severe pressure?

Increased focus on why non-doped athletes choose not to dope is evident in anti-doping research, which has moved away from solely trying to catch dopers

(Englar-Carlson et al., 2016; Petróczi et al., 2021). Regarding protective factors, which were overlooked for a long time, a strong moral stance against cheating, an identity beyond sport, self-control and resilience against peer pressure were found to protect athletes from doping (Erickson et al., 2015). In line with this, variables that were applicable to clean athletes also included self-efficacy, sportspersonship and attitudes against doping (Gatterer et al., 2019). In addition, very recently, a 'clean athlete identity' was shown to be a strong protective factor against doping. The term 'clean athlete identity' was defined by athletes themselves, who described being clean as holding true to oneself in terms of values and morals. This clean identity is rooted in an upbringing in which significant others, such as parents and teachers, taught them to value fairness, equality and honesty, and to condemn cheating; such attitudes are then reinforced by values-based education. In addition, clean athletes are motivated by their love of sport, and are not focused only on winning (Petróczi et al., 2021). Overall, it seems that variables considered as risk factors for a very long time, and which have therefore received much attention, can rather be considered as protective factors that enhance the resources of athletes and thus allow them to remain doping-free even in the face of pressure. The associations found by Blank et al. (2016) and Ntoumanis et al. (2014), for example, still hold true, but a different perspective has emerged that is highly important for the translation of these findings into practice: changing the characteristics initially expected to be risk factors – e.g. increasing positive attitudes and positive beliefs – will not necessarily reduce doping behaviour, but might be beneficial in terms of resisting pressure. Theoretically, 'real' risk factors may have to be removed, and the pressure reduced, by changing the overall sports system. However, this is diametrically opposed to the current paradigm of professional and highly commercialized sport, and thus highly unlikely to happen.

As well as factors that could prevent athletes from doping, the age of educational target groups and the importance of young athletes have also been the focus of research. It was shown that anti-doping education is most effective when provided at a young age (Furhapter et al., 2013; Morente-Sanchez & Zabala, 2013; Vitzthum et al., 2010), as adolescence is a critical period with respect to the formation of attitudes and values (Backhouse et al., 2014; Kohlberg & Hersh, 2009). Thus, anti-doping education could exploit this development window. Early education does not necessarily need to specifically focus on doping, but rather sporting integrity in general (Petróczi et al., 2021), or the importance of values and respect (Stojanovic & Radovanocic, 2020), before moving on to the topic of doping at a later stage. In addition, and especially as young athletes are often influenced by significant others (Barkoukis et al., 2019; Hallward & Duncan, 2018; Nicholls et al., 2017), anti-doping education for coaches and parents is important. Regarding anti-doping education for parents, athletes indicated the importance of their 'clean' upbringing in helping them to stay clean (Petróczi et al., 2021). By establishing an initial sense of right and wrong, parents shape athletes' morals (Erickson et al., 2017). Especially for youth athletes, parents fulfil a wide range of roles and responsibilities, including being role models with respect to attitudes and behaviours (Fredricks & Eccles, 2004). In addition, they need to possess a range of competencies, such as understanding, applying the appropriate parenting style and managing the emotional demands of competitions. Specific parental education can help them gain more understanding, confidence and experience to better fulfil their role (Harwood & Knight, 2015). Coaches were also shown to exert a significant influence on their athletes and were found to play an important role in a number of high-profile doping incidents (Patterson & Backhouse, 2018). The World Anti-Doping Agency (WADA) has formally accepted the influence of coaches by including their roles and responsibilities in the WADA Code (WADA, 2015, Article 21.2).

EVIDENCE-BASED ANTI-DOPING EDUCATION – FACT OR FICTION?

Based on Content

Even though there is already considerable evidence as to which factors might prevent doping behaviour, the real challenge is to translate these findings into evidence-based anti-doping education. Another issue that increases the complexity of doping prevention is the gap between theory and practice, i.e. making scientific research findings more tangible and understandable for practitioners in the field of doping prevention (Backhouse et al., 2007). Values, attitudes, morals and norms have been shown to protect against doping behaviour. Thus, values-based education that catalyzes and develops these factors might be a promising approach for anti-doping education. Additionally, the 'clean athlete identity' identified as a strong protective factor against doping can be reinforced by values-based education (Petróczi et al., 2021). However, a study investigating the doping prevention programmes of National Anti-Doping Organisations (NADOs) showed that most of them do not provide values-based education. Rather, they offer information (i.e. knowledge) about doping and anti-doping (Gatterer et al., 2020), even though the WADA Code requires them to provide both information and education (WADA, 2015). According to the NADO study, the implementation of educational approaches, including values-based education, is currently unsatisfactory (Gatterer et al., 2020). In addition, a Finnish study investigating national sport organisations showed that only about one third of the organisations are carrying out top-level anti-doping activities including not only education but also testing (Finnish Center for Integrity of Sports, 2021). Further, questioning the recipients of anti-doping education, namely the athletes, about their perceptions revealed differences in access to anti-doping education depending on the overall context in which they are situated (Efverström et al., 2016b). Such differences were also obvious in another study, where the respondents felt that some athletes from countries with fewer financial resources receive anti-doping education only at events. These respondents also cited early education for all athletes as being key for clean sport (Petróczi et al., 2021).

WADA has acknowledged the importance of values-based education. Its new International Standard for Education (ISE), a mandatory global policy that came into effect in January 2021, provides Code Signatories with principles and minimum standards for education programmes (WADA, 2021a). According to the ISE, an education programme should include (1) information provision (i.e. accurate, up-to-date content on clean sport), (2) awareness raising (i.e. topics and issues related to clean sport), (3) anti-doping education (i.e. to build competencies and make informed decisions), and (4) values-based education (i.e. to develop an athlete's personal values and principles) (WADA, 2021a). Thus, even though the evidence suggests that values-based education might be key for successful doping prevention, and where key stakeholders such as WADA also acknowledge this fact, the question remains as to why implementation is still significantly lacking.

This question could be answered based on the results of scientific studies. For example, athletes themselves expressed the concern that their national federations lack responsibility and are not committed to anti-doping education (Efverström et al., 2016a). Organisations entrusted with doping prevention reported that a lack of financial and personnel resources prevented them from providing more anti-doping education (Gatterer et al., 2020; Patterson et al., 2016), which might be a barrier to meeting WADA's requirements. Even though WADA has started to focus more on prevention via education, this is not yet reflected in the distribution of monetary resources, as most of the money apportioned to prevention is still spent on doping controls; in the case of NADOs, doping control activities often take up more than half of their budgets (Kraushaar-Martensen & Moller, 2016; Westmattelmann et al., 2018). For example, in 2019, the US Anti-Doping Agency (USADA) spent $13,529,013, on testing and $2,586,827 on education and awareness (US Anti-Doping Agency, 2020). Other NADOs report similar distributions in their annual reports (e.g. UK Anti-Doping (UKAD), National Anti-Doping Agency of Germany (NADA Germany), Anti-Doping Danmark (ADD)). In addition, International Federations (IFs) spent less money on anti-doping education in 2015 than 2009 (Mountjoy et al., 2017).

Another concern is the interpretation of terms: what is actually meant by values-based education? In the early stages of values-based education research, i.e. before implementation of the ISE, the areas that should be covered by values-based education were poorly defined. Backhouse et al. (2014) investigated approaches found to be effective for doping prevention and distinguished five approaches: the knowledge-focused approach (e.g. side effects), affective-focused approach (e.g. targeting feelings of value and self-worth), social skills training (e.g. assertiveness, decision-making and resistance to peer pressure), life skills training (a multi-component approach encompassing social skills, personal skills and knowledge) and the ethic- and value-based approach (e.g. respecting the rules, fair play, honesty and integrity) (p. 53). Aside from this categorization, however, there was no further definition of values-based education; moreover, there was no explanation of how it should be delivered (i.e. methods, channels etc.). Considering this lack of examples of best practice and the cited lack of resources (also including personnel capable of developing such content), a lack of commitment might be another reason why values-based education has not yet come to fruition. Responsible organisations need to show commitment and willingness to deliver the required education. In order to do this, they need to be trained and provided with evidence-based examples and material that they can easily apply. WADA's ISE provides examples, as well as a methodological tool for developing content, lesson plans etc. These guidelines provide organisations with examples of how to plan their education, implement the four components thereof (e.g. an outreach booth for raising awareness, the 'Sport Values in Every Classroom' game for values-based education) and evaluate learning outcomes using different types of assessments. The guidelines aim to support responsible organisations at every step. Future research should aim to determine whether the guidelines have helped values-based anti-doping education move from fiction to fact.

Based on Target Group

As well as content, the target groups (i.e. athletes, athlete support personnel [ASP], parents etc.) are an important consideration. Regarding athletes, one principle of WADA's ISE is that 'an athlete's first experience with anti-doping should be through education rather than doping control' (WADA, 2021a, p. 4). This is in line with the evidence presented earlier that anti-doping education should start at a young age. However, again, it seems that bridging the gap between research and practice is a challenge. Among young, elite international athletes participating at major youth events between 2018 and 2019, one third had never received anti-doping education (Gatterer et al., 2021). This indicates the need for early anti-doping education, as also reported by several other studies (Gatterer et al., 2019; Hallward & Duncan, 2018; Stojanovic & Radovanocic, 2020). For example, Slovenia's NADO (SLOADO) published two children's books that do not focus on doping as such, but rather on sports integrity and fairness, thereby slowly introducing the topic of doping to children (Smrdu et al., 2018a, 2018b). In addition, WADA offers a programme for schools ('Sport Values in Every Classroom') for 8–12-year-olds, while a current European Union (EU) project ('I-Value') is investigating the utility of emphasizing significant values that might also, but not exclusively, act as protective factors against doping in elementary schools, starting with pupils aged six years. Based on an extensive literature review, the five values of compassion, fairness, honesty, respect and responsibility were identified, and should be covered in age-appropriate classroom interventions to not only introduce these values but also make children aware of their meaning, support them in their application and ultimately promote their transfer to contexts other than the classroom setting. Despite these examples and the importance of anti-doping education, it has not yet been globally adopted for children and adolescents (Gatterer et al., 2019; Petróczi et al., 2021).

Coaches represent another important target group for anti-doping education. They are often an important source of information for athletes (Peters et al., 2009) and are crucial to the initial decision to dope (Engelberg et al., 2015). In addition, they have a major influence on their athletes in terms of cognition, affect and behaviour (Ntoumanis et al., 2018). Worryingly, research has found that coaches showed a low level of knowledge of prohibited substances and methods (Engelberg & Moston, 2015), and of the whereabouts system (Engelberg et al., 2017). In addition, they did not view the provision of anti-doping education as part of their role (Engelberg & Moston, 2015), even though the WADA Code clearly states that the coach, as an ASP, needs to 'use his or her influence on athlete values and behavior to foster anti-doping attitudes' (WADA, 2015, Article 21.2.3, p. 114). One possible reason for this might be the marked variance in education for coaches, where anti-doping education is only received sporadically because the training of their athletes is prioritized (Patterson et al., 2016). Not surprisingly, it is universally believed by researchers that there is a need to educate coaches (Barkoukis et al., 2019; Morente-Sanchez & Zabala, 2015; Patterson et al., 2016), as they must understand the current anti-doping rules, and their responsibilities and obligations under those rules. In addition, they have the opportunity to deliver anti-doping messages to their athletes, which is apparently not happening to a sufficient degree (Engelberg & Moston, 2015).

In terms of parents, the situation is similar. Among athletes' support networks, family and friends were found to have the least doping knowledge (Mazanov et al., 2013). This is in contrast to a study conducted in Austria, where about 65% of the enrolled parents demonstrated good general doping knowledge (although these parents also showed knowledge gaps in relation to the side effects of doping) (Blank et al., 2015). However, even in-depth knowledge is futile if the parent does not believe that drug-free sport is relevant to them (Backhouse & McKenna, 2011). Given the impact that they have on their children, targeted anti-doping education for parents is of the utmost importance. This could help them recognize and accept the important role they play in shaping an athlete's attitudes and behaviours towards doping. Parents need to be equipped with sufficient knowledge about anti-doping and then educated regarding how to transmit it to their children (i.e. athletes) (Erickson et al., 2017).

Overall, the evidence shows that knowledge is an important factor in doping prevention, and that information-based education is widely implemented, at least for athletes. However, the evidence also indicates the necessity and importance of values-based education. Values, norms and morals are important factors for reducing doping, as protective factors as opposed to their initial conception as risk factors. The implementation of values-based education is obviously still in its beginning stages and has not yet been globally implemented for athletes or ASP. Possible reasons for this situation were outlined earlier and potential solutions will be presented in the next section.

TRANSLATING ANTI-DOPING EDUCATION INTO CONCRETE RESULTS – A ROADMAP OF POSSIBLE SOLUTIONS

Education is key for preventing drug use and promoting clean sport. As such, anti-doping education should support clean athletes and strengthen the concept of clean identity (Petróczi et al., 2021). However, even though anti-doping education is receiving more attention, a growing body of research is showing that anti-doping education still needs to improve in terms of quality (Gatterer et al.,

2020; Hallward & Duncan, 2018; Petróczi et al., 2021). To date, prevention programmes addressing factors shown to be important in research have not achieved significant success in terms of reducing doping behaviour. We argue that this failing is not because the wrong factors were focused on, but rather because they were simply not properly addressed. In addition, the degree of exposure of athletes and ASP to anti-doping education has not been satisfactory (Backhouse et al., 2016). In this chapter, we have outlined a number of barriers to the implementation of successful educational programmes. Based on the above, three different areas should be addressed: (1) improve the translation of research findings into practice, (2) increase financial and human resources, and (3) listen to concerns and requirements of prevention programme recipients and evaluate current initiatives.

Translating Research Findings into Practice

We cannot ameliorate the main doping risk factor – the pressure that athletes face – because that would require a change in the overall sports system. However, we can make athletes more aware of their resources and capacities by reinforcing positive values, norms and beliefs, and by educating them on other coping strategies that might be implemented through this reinforcement process. In addition to existing programmes aiming to increase the knowledge of athletes and ASP, more values-based programmes should be implemented across all countries, in accordance with the new ISE (WADA, 2021a). However, it is firstly necessary to clarify what is meant by values-based education and how it can best be developed and implemented. The new ISE guidelines might facilitate this process, by providing NADOs and IFs – as the most important providers for developing and implementing anti-doping education – with tools, examples and suggestions on 'how to do it' (WADA, 2021b). Promoting and facilitating the sharing of materials required for effective anti-doping programmes could facilitate this process and help countries and organisations with scant resources to fulfil their role, as their current ability to develop their own training materials might be limited. More than 10 years ago, Kamber (2011) proposed that larger NADOs could help smaller ones. He suggested classifying agencies such that 'A' agencies can help 'B' and 'C' agencies to develop and improve the effectiveness of their worldwide anti-doping efforts. This idea was first introduced by WADA in 2004, when they created the Regional Anti-Doping Organisation (RADO) programme to enhance anti-doping capacity in various parts of the world: 'The program supports less resourced NADOs and National Olympic Committees acting as NADOs with funding, training and ongoing anti-doping assistance' (WADA, 2021c). Next, the Institute of National Anti-Doping Organisations (iNADO), whose main task is to disseminate best practice with respect to anti-doping initiatives among their member organisations provides examples of best practice on its online platform, including recorded webinars, surveys, educative material from various members etc. (iNADO, 2021). In the same vein, WADA recently signed a 'memorandum of understanding with the Central European Anti-Doping Organisation to collaborate on anti-doping program development', starting with a project involving the Eastern Europe Regional Anti-Doping Organisation (EERADO) (WADA, 2021c). However, the platform is mostly applicable only to NADOs and RADOs, and not to other stakeholders entrusted with doping prevention measures, such as IFs. Thus, developing a new platform providing examples of best practice could be helpful, given their known positive effects. An easily accessible overview of existing evidence-based anti-doping education programmes is currently missing; this would allow NADOs and IFs to study and adopt programmes according to their needs. In particular, less-developed organisations would benefit from such an initiative, as they could implement the programmes according to the specific characteristics of their athletes. This would not only support the translation of research into practice but also allow limited resources to be deployed more efficiently.

Increasing Financial Resources and Training Human Resources

NADOs with more financial resources generally offer more advanced programmes (Gatterer et al., 2020), which justifies the call for larger budgets for anti-doping education. In order to increase the financial resources of organisations entrusted with providing anti-doping education, monetary resources could be shifted from testing to education, as also suggested elsewhere (Gatterer et al., 2020; Morente-Sanchez & Zabala, 2013). NADOs lacking financial and personnel resources (Gatterer et al., 2020) are unlikely to be able to fulfil their role of providing anti-doping education if this situation does not change. With larger budgets, they could hire more qualified personnel to create and deliver anti-doping education. Such personnel also need to be adequately trained. Teaching is only successful if the teacher is competent (didactically and in terms of content) and able to adjust to the needs of the target group (e.g. according to their age). In addition, by training those delivering the education, it is easier to regulate the content that ultimately reaches the athletes.

Acknowledging the Voice of Prevention Programme Recipients

As the ultimate goal of the World Anti-Doping Programme is to 'protect the athletes' fundamental right to participate in doping-free sport' (WADA, 2015, p. 11), the athlete, who plays the central role, should be heard. Numerous studies have indicated that anti-doping education needs to be personally relevant (e.g. Erickson et al., 2017; Hallward & Duncan, 2018; Petróczi et al., 2021). Thus, we need to ascertain what athletes think about existing prevention programmes and what they think needs to change to increase the likelihood of them participating in anti-doping programmes. This also applies to programmes for coaches and parents. Current anti-doping education programmes need to be evaluated not only in terms of efficiency (for example, by assessing the recipients' knowledge before and after programme delivery) but also in terms of their opinion about the programme itself. As indicated earlier, they must believe that the programme is personally relevant, which could be ensured by providing them with the content that they need. Athletes, coaches and parents need to be included in the evaluation process (and modification) of anti-doping programmes, as ultimately, they – and not the researcher – define the research problem.

In summary, this chapter has outlined that significant efforts have been directed towards identifying and classifying risk and protective factors to reduce doping (Blank et al., 2016; Ntoumanis et al., 2014). There are also increasing efforts to support the stakeholders entrusted with doping prevention, by translating research findings into practice or to enhance doping prevention in their target groups. As this process still has room for improvement, we made some proposals and suggestions to support this challenging work. Overall, two areas to address in the future emerged from the discussions above. Firstly, it could be worthwhile to move the focus from solely addressing 'doping' to 'integrity' issues. As described earlier, doping as a poor coping strategy is only one of many integrity issues the sports system faces (Petróczi & Aidman, 2008). By integrating anti-doping education into initiatives aimed at personal development, such education could be 'sold' more easily, especially to young athletes. Given that an appropriate mindset, as well as morals and values, contributes to a 'clean athlete identity' that ultimately protects athletes from doping (besides other negative outcomes), Petróczi et al. (2021) suggested that this might be the best approach. Education on values can and should start very early on in a person's life (Furhapter et al., 2013; Morente-Sanchez & Zabala, 2013; Vitzthum et al., 2010), and does not necessarily need to be associated with doping (Petróczi et al., 2021; Stojanovic & Radovanocic, 2020). The aforementioned I-Value project followed this approach by introducing five important values to children at the age of six years. Even though only a few of them will likely go on to be professional athletes and thus need protection from doping, all of the children developed their personalities and acquired resources to deal with pressure in their daily lives.

The second area concerns methods for scientifically approaching anti-doping education. Instead of researching risk and protective factors and applying the results to stakeholders (i.e. asking them to address these factors in their educational programmes), we could instead adapt a community-based approach similar to the EU projects RESPECT and RESPECT-P (Petróczi et al., 2021). Using this approach, the gap between research and practice will ultimately be narrowed because the 'practice' is integrated from the beginning of the process, which encompasses defining the research questions that are important to stakeholders, answering these questions with methods that they can identify with, and interpreting the results such that they have added meaning. With this approach, athletes and ASP are not only able to understand what research says but are more likely to adhere to the programmes, given their involvement in the development process. Addressing these two areas, focus and methods, might produce educative approaches for athletes and ASP that are widely accepted and used because their tenets will be clear to the recipients. Moreover, such approaches are more holistic, addressing not only doping (a term that has highly negative connotations and seemingly annoys athletes) but also integrity and personality traits that everyone needs, including outside of the world of professional sport.

KEY READINGS

(1) Petróczi, A., Heyes, A., Thrower, S. D., Martinelli, L. A., Backhouse, S. H., Boardley, I. A., & The Respect Consortium. (2021). Understanding and building clean(er) sport together: Community-based participatory research with elite athletes and anti-doping organizations from five European countries. *Psychology of Sport and Exercise, 55.* https://doi.org/10.1016/j.psychsport.2021.101932

This article investigates the protective effect of a 'clean athlete identity' on doping. Being clean in that sense is described as holding true to oneself in terms of values and morals. The authors show that a clean athlete identity is rooted in upbringing and reinforced by values-based education. They further argue that the problems of anti-doping are systemic (as identified by athletes themselves), and thus, there must be systemic solutions.

(2) Boardley, I., Chandler, M., Backhouse, S. H., & Petróczi, A. (2021). Co-creating a social science research agenda for clean sport: An international Delphi study. *International Journal of Drug Policy, 92.* https://doi.org/10.31236/osf.io/fr32a

This article provides the first social science research agenda for clean sport by using the Delphi method, including 82 anti-doping stakeholders. According to the authors, its adoption and implementation should lead to better coordination, more efficient use of funding, enhanced uptake of research findings, and more effective doping prevention education. Key topics identified for future research included examining the effectiveness of anti-doping interventions and education programmes, ASP (e.g. their role in anti-doping), and long-term studies examining the development of protective and risk factors for doping in athletes and ASP.

(3) Gatterer, K., Streicher, B., Petróczi, A., Overbye, M., Schobersberger, W., Gumpenberger, M., Weber, K., Königstein, K., & Blank, C. (2021). The status quo before the International Standard for Education: Elite adolescent athletes' perceptions of anti-doping education. *Performance Enhancement and Health, 9*(3–4). https://doi.org/10.1016/j.peh.2021.100200

This article provides an overview of the perception of adolescent athletes on the anti-doping education they received. Next to providing relevant information to athletes, anti-doping education should be multifaceted and include at least one educational approach in order to be trusted and perceived useful by the athletes. The authors conclude that via developing skills as well as knowledge for informed decision-making, Code compliance could be facilitated.

(4) Gatterer, K., Gumpenberger, M., Overbye, M., Streicher, B., Schobersberger, W., & Blank, C. (2020). An evaluation of prevention initiatives by 53 national anti-doping organizations: Achievements and limitations. *Journal of Sport and Health Science, 9*(3), 228–239. https://doi.org/10.1016/j.jshs.2019.12.002

This article evaluates prevention programmes by 53 NADOs, showing that most NADOs offer knowledge-based prevention programmes, but lack multifaceted values-based approaches. According to the authors, there is a need for concrete guidelines on how to develop and implement multifaceted, values-based education programmes.

(5) Englar-Carlson, M., Gleaves, J., Macedo, E., & Lee, H. (2016). What about the clean athletes? The need for positive psychology in anti-doping research. *Performance Enhancement & Health, 4*(3–4), 116–122. https://doi.org/10.1016/j.peh.2016.05.002

This article focuses on clean athletes and why they choose to stay clean, by concentrating on their strengths and characteristics. The authors argue that it is more effective to promote healthy behaviour ('the good') than trying to eradicate 'the bad', which is best achieved through adopting a positive psychology approach to anti-doping.

REFERENCES

Ajzen, I., & Madden, T. J. (1986). Prediction of goal-oriented behavior: Attitudes, intentions and perceived behavioral control. *Journal of Experimental Social Psychology, 22*, 453–474.

Backhouse, S., Collins, C., Defoort, Y., McNamee, M., Parkinson, A., & Sauer, M. (2014). *Study on doping prevention: A map of legal, regulatory and prevention practice provisions in EU 28*. World Anti-Doping Agency.

Backhouse, S., & McKenna, J. (2011). Doping in sport: A review of medical practitioner's knowledge, attitudes and beliefs. *International Journal of Drug Policy, 22*(3). https://doi.org/10.1016/j.drugpo.2011.03.002

Backhouse, S., McKenna, J., Robinson, S., & Atkin, A. (2007). *International literature review: Attitudes, behaviours, knowledge and education – Drugs in sport: Past, present and future*. World Anti-Doping Agency.

Backhouse, S., Whitaker, L., Patterson, L., Erickson, K., & McKenna, J. (2016). *Social psychology of doping in sport: A mixed-studies narrative synthesis*. World Anti-Doping Agency.

Barkoukis, V., Brooke, L., Ntoumanis, N., Smith, B., & Gucciardi, D. F. (2019). The role of the athletes' entourage on attitudes to doping. *Journal of Sports Sciences, 37*, 2483–2491. https://doi.org/10.1080/02640414.2019.1643648

Blank, C., Kopp, M., Niedermeier, M., Schnitzer, M., & Schobersberger, W. (2016). Predictors of doping intentions, susceptibility, and behaviour of elite athletes: A meta-analytic review. *SpringerPlus, 5*(1), 1333. https://doi.org/10.1186/s40064-016-3000-0

Blank, C., Leichtfried, V., Schaiter, R., Fürhapter, C., Müller, D., & Schobersberger, W. (2015). Doping in sports: Knowledge and attitudes among parents of Austrian junior athletes. *Scandinavian Journal of Medicine & Science in Sports, 25*, 116–124. https://doi.org/10.1111/sms.12168

Boardley, I., Chandler, M., Backhouse, S. H., & Petróczi, A. (2021). Co-creating a social science research agenda for clean sport: An international Delphi study. *International Journal of Drug Policy, 92*. https://doi.org/10.31236/osf.io/fr32a

Donovan, R. J., Egger, G., Kapernick, V., & Mendoza, J. (2002). A conceptual framework for achieving performance enhancing drug compliance in sport. *Sports Medicine, 32*(4), 269–284.

Efverström, A., Ahmadi, N., Hoff, D., & Bäckström, Å. (2016a). Anti-doping and legitimacy: An international survey of elite athletes' perceptions. *International Journal of Sport Policy and Politics, 8*(3), 491–514. https://doi.org/10.1080/19406940.2016.1170716

Efverström, A., Bäckström, Å., Ahmadi, N., & Hoff, D. (2016b). Contexts and conditions for a level playing field: Elite athletes' perspectives on anti-doping in practice. *Performance Enhancement & Health, 5*(2), 77–85. https://doi.org/10.1016/j.peh.2016.08.001

Engelberg, T., & Moston, S. (2015). Inside the locker room: A qualitative study of coaches' anti-doping knowledge, beliefs and attitudes. *Sport in Society*. https://doi.org/10.1080/17430437.2015.1096244

Engelberg, T., Moston, S., & Blank, C. (2017). Coaches' awareness of doping practices and knowledge about anti-doping control systems in elite sport. *Drugs: Education, Prevention & Policy*. https:// doi.org/10.1080/09687637.2017.1337724

Engelberg, T., Moston, S., & Skinner, J. (2015). The final frontier of anti-doping: A study of athletes who have committed doping violations. *Sport Management Review*, *18*(2), 268–279. https://doi. org/10.1016/j.smr.2014.06.005

Englar-Carlson, M., Gleaves, J., Macedo, E., & Lee, H. (2016). What about the clean athletes? The need for positive psychology in anti-doping research. *Performance Enhancement & Health*, *4*(3–4), 116–122. https://doi.org/10.1016/j.peh.2016.05.002

Erickson, K., Backhouse, S., & Carless, D. (2017). Doping in sport: Do parents matter? *Sport, Exercise, and Performance Psychology*, *6*(2). https://doi.org/10.1037/spy0000081

Erickson, K., McKenna, J., & Backhouse, S. (2015). A qualitative analysis of the factors that protect athletes against doping in sport. *Psychology of Sport and Exercise*, *16*, 149–155. https://doi.org/ 10.1016/j.psychsport.2014.03.007

Finnish Center for Integrity of Sports. (2021). Evaluation of the anti-doping activities of Finnish sports organisations. https://suek.fi/en/evaluation-of-the-anti-doping-activities-of-finnish-sports-organisations/

Fredricks, J. A., & Eccles, J. S. (2004). Parental influences on youth involvement in sports. In M. R. Weiss (Ed.), *Developmental sport and exercise psychology: A lifespan perspective* (pp. 145–164). Fitness Information Technology.

Fürhapter, C., Blank, C., Leichtfried, V., Mair-Raggautz, M., Muller, D., & Schobersberger, W. (2013). Evaluation of West-Austrian junior athletes' knowledge regarding doping in sports. *Wiener Klinische Wochenschrift*, *125*(1–2), 41–49. https://doi.org/10.1007/s00508-012-0318-7

Gatterer, K., Gumpenberger, M., Overbye, M., Streicher, B., Schobersberger, W., & Blank, C. (2020). An evaluation of prevention initiatives by 53 national anti-doping organizations: Achievements and limitations. *Journal of Sport and Health Science*, *9*(3), 228–239. https://doi.org/10.1016/j. jshs.2019.12.002

Gatterer, K., Niedermeier, M., Streicher, B., Kopp, M., Schobersberger, W., & Blank, C. (2019). An alternative approach to understanding doping behavior: A pilot study applying the Q-method to doping research. *Performance Enhancement and Health*, *6*(3–4), 139–147. https://doi.org/10. 1016/j.peh.2018.12.001

Gatterer, K., Streicher, B., Petróczi, A., Overbye, M., Schobersberger, W., Gumpenberger, M., Weber, K., Königstein, K., & Blank, C. (2021). The status quo before the International Standard for Education: Elite adolescent athletes' perceptions of anti-doping education. *Performance Enhancement and Health*, *9*(3–4). https://doi.org/10.1016/j.peh.2021.100200

Hallward, L., & Duncan, L. R. (2018). A qualitative exploration of athletes' past experiences with doping prevention education. *Journal of Applied Sport Psychology*, *31*(2), 187–202. https://doi. org/10.1080/10413200.2018.1448017

Harwood, C. G., & Knight, C. J. (2015). Parenting in youth sport: A position paper on parenting expertise. *Psychology of Sport and Exercise*, *16*(Part 1), 24–35. https://doi.org/10.1016/j. psychsport.2014.03.001

iNADO. (2021). What we do. https://www.inado.org/what-we-do/best-practices

Kamber, M. (2011). Development of the role of national anti-doping organisations in the fight against doping: From past to future. *Forensic Science International*, *213*(1–3). https://doi.org/10.1016/j. forsciint.2011.07.026

Kirby, K., Moran, A., & Guerin, S. (2011). A qualitative analysis of the experiences of elite athletes who have admitted to doping for performance enhancement. *International Journal of Sport Policy and Politics*, *3*(2), 205–224. https://doi.org/10.1080/19406940.2011.577081

Kohlberg, L., & Hersh, R. H. (2009). Moral development: A review of the theory. *Theory and Practice*, *16*(2), 53–59. https://doi.org/10.1080/00405847709542675

Kraushaar Martensen, C., & Møller, V. (2016). More money – Better anti-doping? *Drugs: Education, Prevention & Policy*, *24*(3), 1–9. https://doi.org/10.1080/09687637.2016.1266300

Mazanov, J., Backhouse, S., Connor, J., Hemphill, D., & Quirk, F. (2013). Athlete support personnel and anti-doping: Knowledge, attitudes, and ethical stance. *Scandinavian Journal of Medicine and Science in Sports*, *24*(5). https://doi.org/10.1111/sms.12084

Morente-Sanchez, J., & Zabala, M. (2013). Doping in sport: A review of elite athletes' attitudes, beliefs, and knowledge. *Sports Medicine*, *43*(6), 395–411. https://doi.org/10.1007/s40279-013-0037-x

Morente-Sanchez, J., & Zabala, M. (2015). Knowledge, attitudes and beliefs of technical staff towards doping in Spanish football. *Journal of Sports Sciences*, *12*, 1267–1275. https://doi.org/10.1080/02640414.2014.999699

Mountjoy, M., Miller, S., Vallini, M., Foster, J., & Carr, J. (2017). International sports federation's fight to protect the clean athlete: Are we doing enough in the fight against doping? *British Journal of Sports Medicine*, *51*(17), 1241–1242. https://doi.org/10.1136/bjsports-2017-097870

Nicholls, A. R., Cope, E., Bailey, R., Koenen, K., Dumon, D., Theodorou, N. C., Chanal, B., Saint Laurent, D., Müller, D., Andrés, M. P., Kristensen, A. H., Thompson, M. A., Baumann, W., & Laurent, J.-F. (2017). Children's first experience of taking anabolic-androgenic steroids can occur before their 10th birthday: A systematic review identifying 9 factors that predict doping among young people. *Frontiers in Psychology*, *8*, 1015. https://doi.org/10.3389/fpsyg.2017.01015

Ntoumanis, N., Gucciardi, D., Backhouse, S., Barkoukis, V., Quested, E., Patterson, L., Smith, B. J., Whitaker, L., Pavlidis, G., & Kaffe, S. (2018). An intervention to optimize coach motivational climates and reduce athlete willingness to dope (CoachMADE): Protocol for a cross-cultural cluster randomized control trial. *Frontiers in Psychology*, *8*. https://doi.org/10.3389/fpsyg.2017.02301

Ntoumanis, N., Ng, J. Y., Barkoukis, V., & Backhouse, S. (2014). Personal and psychosocial predictors of doping use in physical activity settings: A meta-analysis. *Sports Medicine*, *44*(11), 1603–1624. https://doi.org/10.1007/s40279-014-0240-4

Paternoster, R. (1987). The deterrent effect of the perceived certainty and severity of punishment: A review of the evidence and issues. *Justice Quarterly*, *4*(2), 173–217. https://doi.org/10.1080/07418828700089271

Patterson, L. B., & Backhouse, S. (2018). "An important cog in the wheel", but not the driver: Coaches' perceptions of their role in doping prevention. *Psychology of Sport and Exercise*, *37*, 117–127. https://doi.org/10.1016/j.psychsport.2018.05.004

Patterson, L. B., Backhouse, S., & Duffy, P. J. (2016). Anti-doping education for coaches: Qualitative insights from national and international sporting and anti-doping organisations. *Sport Management Review*, *19*(1), 35–47. https://doi.org/10.1016/j.smr.2015.12.002

Peters, S., Schulz, T., Oberhoffer, R., & Michna, H. (2009). Doping and doping prevention: Knowledge, attitudes and expectations of athletes and coaches. *Deutsche Zeitschrift für Sportmedizin*, *60*(3), 73–78.

Petróczi, A. (2021). Why clean sport is more than just drug-free. *Nature*, *592*(7852), 16. https://doi.org/10.1038/d41586-021-00820-7

Petróczi, A., & Aidman, E. (2008). Psychological drivers in doping: The life-cycle model of performance enhancement. *Substance Abuse Treatment, Prevention, and Policy*, *3*(7), 1–12.

Petróczi, A., Heyes, A., Thrower, S. D., Martinelli, L. A., Backhouse, S. H., Boardley, I. A., & The Respect Consortium. (2021). Understanding and building clean(er) sport together: Community-based participatory research with elite athletes and anti-doping organisations from five European countries. *Psychology of Sport and Exercise*, *55*. https://doi.org/10.1016/j.psychsport.2021.101932

Ryan, R. M., & Deci, E. L. (2000). Self-determination theory and the facilitation of intrinsic motivation, social development, and well-being. *American Psychologist*, *55*, 68–78.

Smrdu, M., Makuc, N., & Kajtna, T. (2018a). *Gamsek Miha in prvo tekmovanje*. Slovenian Anti-Doping Organisation.

Smrdu, M., Makuc, N., & Kajtna, T. (2018b). *Gams Miha in čudežne jagode*. Slovenian Anti-Doping Organisation.

Stewart, B., & Smith, A. C. (2008). Drug use in sport. Implications for public policy. *Journal of Sport & Social Issues*, *32*(3), 278–298.

Stojanović, E., & Radocanović, D. (2020). Educative aspects of doping prevention in school aged children and adolescents. *Physical Education and Sport*, *18*(2), 305–310. https://doi.org/10.22190/FUPES200520028S

Strelan, P., & Boeckmann, R. J. (2003). A new model for understanding performance-enhancing drug use by elite athletes. *Journal of Applied Sport Psychology*, *15*(2), 176–183. https://doi.org/10.1080/10413200390213795

U.S. Anti-Doping Agency. (2020). *Annual Report 2019*. U.S. Anti-Doping Agency.

Vitzthum, K., Mache, S., Quarcoo, D., Groneberg, D. A., & Schoffel, N. (2010). Interdisciplinary strategies versus doping. *Wiener Klinische Wochenschrift*, *122*(11–12), 325–333. https://doi.org/10.1007/s00508-010-1383-4

WADA. (2015). *World Anti-Doping Code 2015*. World Anti-Doping Agency.

WADA. (2021a). *International Standard for Education*. World Anti-Doping Agency.

WADA. (2021b). *2021 Code Implementation Support Program. Guidelines for the International Standard for Education (ISE)*. World Anti-Doping Agency.

WADA. (2021c). *WADA signs memorandum of understanding with the Central European Anti-Doping Organization to collaborate on anti-doping program development*. https://www.wada-ama.org/en/media/news/2021-06/wada-signs-memorandum-of-understanding-with-the-central european-anti-doping

Westmattelmann, D., Dreiskamper, D., Strauss, B., Schewe, G., & Plass, J. (2018). Perception of the current anti-doping regime – A quantitative study among German top-level cyclists and track and field athletes. *Frontiers in Psychology*, *9*, 1890. https://doi.org/10.3389/fpsyg.2018.01890

PART 2

HEALTH AND RISKS

Chapter 4

THE USE OF ANABOLIC ANDROGENIC STEROIDS AS A PUBLIC HEALTH ISSUE

Jim McVeigh, Geoff Bates and Gemma Anne Yarwood

ABSTRACT

In recent years there have been increasing calls for the use of anabolic androgenic steroids (AAS) and associated drugs to be recognized as a public health issue. In the domain of the competitive athlete and professional body-builder, recent decades have seen the diffusion of AAS from the hardcore gyms of the 1980s and 1990s to the mainstream exercise and fitness environments of the twenty-first century. Alongside the apparent increases in the use of these drugs, there is a growing evidence base in relation to harms – physical, psychological and (to some extent) social. But is this form of drug use a public health issue? What criteria should we use to make this judgement? What is the available evidence and has our understanding of the issue improved? By drawing on the authors' research in the United Kingdom and the wider international literature this chapter will explore these issues and attempt to answer the fundamental question – is the use of anabolic steroids a public health issue?

Keywords: Anabolic androgenic steroids; image and performance enhancing drugs; public health; harm reduction; evidence review; doping interventions

CRITERIA AND DEFINITIONS

This chapter will examine the growing recognition of doping within the general population as a public health issue. The focus will be on the use of AAS; however, this term will also be used to include a range of additional drugs that are used as

Doping in Sport and Fitness
Research in the Sociology of Sport, Volume 16, 71–91
Copyright © 2023 by Emerald Publishing Limited
ISSN: 1476-2854/doi:10.1108/S1476-285420220000016005

anabolic agents (e.g. human growth hormone, insulin, growth hormone-releasing peptides), prevent or mitigate the adverse effects of AAS (e.g. tamoxifen, human chorionic gonadotrophin [hCG]) or promote weight loss (e.g. dinitrophenol, clenbuterol). Over the years, many different substances have entered the repertoire of drugs used for muscular enhancement (McVeigh et al., 2020). For instance, human growth hormone has steadily increased in popularity, from use by competitive athletes and elite bodybuilders in the 1980s, to become easily available and commonly used within gyms around the world (Brennan et al., 2017; Evans-Brown & McVeigh, 2009; Holt & Ho, 2019). Some drugs have maintained a level of use despite scant evidence of effectiveness, for example, gamma hydroxybutyrate (GHB) (Takahara et al., 1977), taken to enhance the release of human growth hormone (Assael, 2007; McVeigh et al., 2020). While for other drugs, use has been transient, for instance, nalbuphine hydrochloride (Nubain©) gained popularity for a relatively short period in the 1990s based on an unfounded reputation for having anti-catabolic properties (Duchaine, 1988; Wines et al., 1999) and is now rarely reported as being used (Begley et al., 2017; McBride et al., 1996; McElrath & Connolly, 2006). However, while various drugs have gained popularity with those looking to enhance musculature, the AAS have remained a constant feature and the basis of drug regimens for muscular enhancement around the world (Bonnecaze et al., 2020; Cohen et al., 2007).

It is important to recognize that this chapter relates predominantly to the situation in the United Kingdom. While much of the international evidence relating to the use of AAS is generalizable, for example, the pharmacological actions and associated harms, the situation in the United Kingdom is unique in relation to its policy response to this form of substance use. When AAS and associated drugs were brought under control of the Misuse of Drugs Act (1971) during the 1990s, personal possession remained legal and only the manufacture, distribution and possession with intent to supply were categorized as class C offences (Druglink, 1993). The rationale for this decision, as stated by the Advisory Council on the Misuse of Drugs (ACMD), was to avoid driving AAS further underground and to avoid criminalizing large numbers of young men (ACMD, 2010b). This approach has continued following subsequent reviews by the ACMD, who advocate a public health approach to preventing or mitigating the harms associated with AAS use. Globally, no country other than the United Kingdom has significant criminal penalties for supply offences (up to 14 years and an unlimited fine) but no personal possession offence, and a comprehensive network of needle and syringe programmes (NSPs) available to AAS users (Henning & Andreasson, 2020; McVeigh & Begley, 2017).

This chapter will examine the evidence relating to the use of AAS and associated image and performance enhancing drug (IPED) use in the United Kingdom. Specifically, we will look at the epidemiology, motivations for use, range of potential harms and the public policy responses, in an attempt to answer the question: *is the use of anabolic steroids a public health issue?* This chapter builds upon and for the first time publishes the ongoing work of the lead author. Since commencing work on this topic in the early 1990s, McVeigh has collated the relevant published academic work on the use of AAS and associated IPED use in the UK on an annual basis. The 'state of the evidence base' has then been informally summarized at various times for inclusion in conference presentations and lectures. In collaboration with the co-authors and through discussion to find consensus, this process has been refined to identify 'state of the evidence base' at the end of each decade. The intention is to not only answer the question *is the use of anabolic steroids a public health issue?* but also to pose the question in relation to the categories of evidence 'are we there yet?' The chapter will discuss the required criteria for defining the use of AAS as a public health issue before grading our current understanding of each of the criterion. We will then summarize the evidence that informed our decision.

BACKGROUND

Since the identification and synthesis of testosterone in the 1930s, numerous variations of the hormone have been developed (although many have never been commercially developed, forming the 'family' of AAS) (for further details, see https://www.anabolicsteroids.org.uk/anabolic-steroids-and-associated-drugs/). All possess both anabolic (muscle-building) properties and androgenic (masculinizing) properties (Kanayama & Pope, 2018), with their potential for performance enhancement in sport being recognized by the 1950s, particularly those sports relying on power and strength (Dimeo, 2007; Kruskemper, 1968; Voy & Deeter, 1991). The use of AAS within the gym culture was well established in parts of the United States by the 1970s (Evans-Brown et al., 2012; Hoberman & Yesalis, 1995) and relatively common in parts of the United Kingdom by the late 1980s (Lenehan & McVeigh, 1997).

The last 30 years has seen unprecedented advances in pharmacology and technology, not least, the expansion of the internet resulting in increased availability and affordability of human enhancement drugs (Evans-Brown et al., 2012). Alongside our technological advances, our society has a dwindling requirement for physical size and strength in our everyday lives; however, this has not diminished the drive for muscularity amongst sections of the population. For some, the physical transformation through increased musculature has the potential to change their relationship and interaction with the world around them (Christiansen, 2019). This powerful motivation, among a complex environment of factors at an individual, social, institutional, community and societal level, has contributed to the widespread use of AAS (Bates et al., 2018). Those choosing to use AAS are by no means a homogenous group, not only in their drivers and motivations for use but in their behaviours and associated risks (Christiansen et al., 2016; Zahnow et al., 2018). These risk behaviours are diverse and may by associated with maximizing muscle growth through a broad pharmacopeia of substances (Sagoe et al., 2015) or extremely high dosages for prolonged periods (Chandler & McVeigh, 2014). However, other risks may be linked to broader lifestyle choices as psychoactive drug use, risky sexual behaviour (Hope et al., 2013).

What Constitutes a Public Health Issue?

There are no predetermined criteria to be met or formal grading by which we can define a public health issue in the United Kingdom. A public health issue is often characterized as a specific infectious agent causing an immediate impact on a substantial section of the population. Person-to-person transmission is not necessary to have a public health threat. Food safety, sanitation, water fluoridation, insect and vermin control, and pollution control are examples of public health issues for which measures have been taken to address health threats to the public (Rothstein, 2002). Alongside these examples are a range of behaviours which may be considered a public health issue, including substance use (Ashton & Seymour, 2010). It is within this context that we examine the use of AAS, consider the associated behaviours and judge if they cross a threshold to be classed as a public health issue. In general terms it is a basic assessment of the severity of harm at a population level. The recognition of AAS as a public health issue is the first stage of developing effective interventions. There are a range of public health intervention models, incorporating the identification of risk and protective factors, the testing of interventions and the implementation of effective programmes (Centers for Disease Control and Prevention, 2021; Wight et al., 2016). However, they all require the problem to be initially defined and the collation of available epidemiological data relating to prevalence, characteristics and behaviours.

To monitor our recognition of AAS as a growing public health issue, McVeigh has recorded his subjective opinion relating to our understanding of AAS across a number of specific areas of concern since commencing research in these fields in the early 1990s. The headings reflect the domains required to form a basic assessment of AAS as a public health issue. The four domains incorporating nine categories were derived to summarize our understanding of the phenomenon of AAS use, its potential for causing harms and the development of interventions (e.g. the prevention of initiation of use, the mitigation of adverse effects and support for the cessation of use).

While the following table and key for grading evidence is subjective and shaped by the author's personal view of the evolving evidence base, it does provide a consistent assessment over time of the size of the issue and the potential harms, sometimes referred to as the magnitude and severity of an issue (Rychetnik et al., 2004), the two primary criteria in the assessment of public health importance (World Health Organization, 1997) together with the progress in developing effective responses. Based on the published literature, the strength of evidence was assessed for each of the nine categories, providing a structure to examine this broad and complex topic. Where evidence was available, each category was assigned to one of four categories reflecting the strength of the evidence base.

Key to grading of evidence.

- No evidence (No evidence) = no evidence available.
- Very weak (very little, very limited etc.) = evidence from very small number of studies only or methodological quality of evidence is very poor.

- Weak (early stages, basics) = evidence is inconsistent, methodologically weak or considerable gaps remain.
- Moderate (Good, data to debate) = evidence from a range of studies but lacking in consistency or quality.
- Strong (Realization, confident) = consistent and comprehensive evidence base.

Table 1 provides the author's perception of the strength of evidence at the end of 1999, 2009 and 2019. While the level of evidence and understanding of these key elements relating AAS has undoubtedly increased over time, in several cases this has led to an appreciation that the issue is far more complex than previously recognized and the confidence of what we 'know' has diminished. However, this provides a basic framework to assess the use of AAS and conclude if we have the evidence to suggest that this is a public health issue by considering AAS use against the nine included criteria. One glaring omission from the outset of these reflections is the 'illicit market' and the public health consequences of the uncontrolled, illegal supply of AAS and associated drugs. This point will be reflected upon following the examination of the nine areas indicated in Table 1. These will be considered under the groupings of epidemiology, motivations and methods, harms and effective responses, respectively.

EPIDEMIOLOGY

For AAS to be considered a public health issue, it must either impact on a significant proportion of the population or be increasing at a rate that will impact significant numbers of the population. Estimating the number of people engaged in clandestine behaviours is notoriously difficult and at present we do not have robust estimates of AAS prevalence for the United Kingdom, although outputs from a current research programme will provide the foundation for these

Table 1. Review of the Anabolic Androgenic Steroid Evidence Base 1999–2019.

Category	Evidence Base	1999	2009	2019
Epidemiology	Prevalence	Very weak	Very weak	Moderate
Motivations and methods	Characteristics	Moderate	Strong	Moderate
	Reasons for use	Strong	Strong	Moderate
	Methods of use	Strong	Strong	Moderate
Associated harms	Harms	Moderate	Moderate	Strong
	Efficacy	Weak	Weak	Weak
Effective responses	Treatment	Very weak	Very weak	Very weak
	Prevention	No evidence	No evidence	Very weak
	Harm reduction	Very weak	Very weak	Weak

calculations (McVeigh, 2021). Even without robust prevalence estimations, there are clear indications at both national level in the United Kingdom and through global meta-analysis to justify public concerns regarding the levels of use. In the United Kingdom, the Crime Survey for England and Wales (CSES), and its forerunner, the British Crime Survey, produces estimates of drug use; however, these are recognized as a gross under representation of AAS use (ACMD, 2010b). That said, they estimated in excess of a quarter of a million people had used AAS in England and Wales during the lifetime (Office for National Statistics, 2021). Meanwhile, in the United States it has been estimated that between 2.9 and 4.0 million people had used AAS at some time in their lives (Pope, Kanayama et al., 2014). Drawing on studies from around the world, a global estimate has been calculated as lifetime prevalence of 3.3% (men: 6.4%, women: 1.6%), with higher rates in Western societies, the Middle East and South America (Sagoe & Pallesen, 2018).

Caution is required when interpreting these prevalence estimates, with some of the confounding factors well documented (e.g. gaining access to a clandestine AAS culture, the limitations of a household survey and practicalities of accessing a population who are predominantly working full time and spending a considerable amount of time in the gym) (ACMD, 2010b; Kanayama & Pope, 2018; Sagoe & Pallesen, 2018). However, even allowing for the limitations within these estimates, these studies demonstrate the magnitude of the use of AAS, clearly illustrating that the issue reaches the threshold of impacting on substantial numbers of general population and therefore potentially a public health issue. Current work being undertaken by academics in the United Kingdom aims to strengthen our understanding of the extent of AAS use. Funded by the National Institute for Health Research (NIHR), the work utilizes two approaches, secondary analyses of available UK data (including Crime Survey for England and Wales (CSEW), NSP data, United Kingdom Anti-Doping data and private injecting equipment sales), together with a Delphi survey technique, capturing the expertise and experience of a broad range of experts and stakeholders (McVeigh, 2021). This work will produce a plausible range of the extent of use and form the basis for the estimation of AAS and IPED use in the United Kingdom and have implications for prevalence estimates in other countries.

All evidence points towards a disproportionately high level of use amongst men compared to women in the United Kingdom (Begley et al., 2017; Hope et al., 2013; Korkia & Stimson, 1993) and internationally (Sagoe et al., 2014), and this is reflected in the focus of much of the published research. However, while prevalence is much lower in women, harms can be significantly greater (Havnes et al., 2020). Notably, media interest has focused on young men rather than their older male counterparts, often attributing perceived increases in the use of AAS to specific television programmes despite the lack of epidemiological evidence to support this (Hamilton & Sumnall, 2017). While much of the epidemiological work of the 1980s, particularly in the United States, focused on young males (teenaged and early 20s) and the use of AAS (Buckley & Yesalis, 1989; Buckley et al., 1988; Pope et al., 1988; Yesalis et al., 1989), recent evidence also indicates use in later life. A recent UK survey identified as many people using AAS in the

40 + age group as those under the age of 25 (Begley et al., 2017). Similarly, data from NSPs show an increasing average age of clients using AAS (McVeigh & Begley, 2017). Little research has been conducted regarding the use of AAS within Black, Asian and Minority Ethnic communities. While one small study identified significant differences relating to supply and use of AAS within British South Asian community (Van Hout & Kean, 2015), there is a clear need for further research to inform policy and practice.

Clearly, the number and sophistication of epidemiological studies on AAS have increased over time; however, we have unearthed a more diverse picture of use than previously recognized. Use is not restricted to gender age, race, sexuality or socioeconomic group. While we can say with confidence that AAS use is disproportionately higher amongst males, even this must be qualified with evidence of high use of weight loss and tanning agents by women (Germain et al., 2019). Rather than an easily identifiable group of young hyper-muscular men, (although this group of users still clearly exists (Goldman et al., 2018)), the use of AAS or associated IPEDs has been identified wherever and amongst whomever have been researched resulting in the recognition of a much more complex epidemiological landscape, which we are at only the early stages of exploration.

MOTIVATIONS AND METHODS OF USE

Closely associated to the diversity of populations of AAS users is the range of motivations for use. Building on the classifications of AAS users of the 1990s (Dawson, 2001; Lenehan & McVeigh, 1998), a typology of AAS in the twenty-first century has been developed (Christiansen et al., 2016). Utilizing previously collected qualitative interview data and supplemented by the observations of the authors, four ideal types of users were identified based on the effectiveness of AAS use and associated risks: the Expert type, the Well-being type, the 'YOLO' type and the Athlete. Using the data from the National IPED study (Bates & McVeigh, 2016) and working with colleagues in the United Kingdom and Australia, detailed cluster analyses and logistic regression were conducted and published (Zahnow et al., 2018). Findings closely reflected the four categories hypothesized by Christiansen et al. (2016).

While the aforementioned US prevalence studies of AAS use identified young males as the predominant group, this was closely aligned to sporting ambition at either high school (Buckley et al., 1988) or college level (Pope et al., 1988). Current research illustrates a more complex picture. With the identification of older men who use AAS, it appears that for some, this represents a prolonged career of 20 years use or more while for others, the decision to use AAS has been taken in later life, (Havnes et al., 2019), in one case at the age of 69 (Ip et al., 2015). The most recent UK national survey of IPED use provides some insight to the varied motivations of use, illustrating a complex picture of multiple rationales and ambitions for use. Of the total sample of 684 people using AAS, 6.5% were highly motivated by wanting to maintain a youthful appearance while 7.8% of the sample were using as a form of self-directed hormone replacement therapy (Begley et al., 2017).

While we propose that the use of AAS is a public health issue, it is also (at least for some) a sports issue. The latest UK national survey of IPED use demonstrates the diversity of motivations for use. While 27% of the sample felt that AAS was very important for their sporting performance (excluding bodybuilding), 33% felt it was unimportant. So, while the majority of users felt AAS use was very important for their cosmetic appearance/body image (56%), others felt it was very important for sex drive (8.4%), occupational performance (10%) and competitive bodybuilding (22%) (Begley et al., 2017).

Over time there has been a gradual recognition of the multiple subgroups of users and complex reasons for the use of AAS and associated drugs. In the 1990s there was a confidence within policy and legislation on both sides of the Atlantic that AAS use was driven by competitive sport (including bodybuilding) (Anabolic Steroid Control Act, 1990; Misuse of Drugs, 1996). Recently there has been a broadening of our understanding and an appreciation of the extent and variation of use of these substances. The complexity of AAS use highlighted by the broad range of motivating and influencing factors, substances used, and associated behaviours amongst diverse subgroups supports our understanding that AAS use is a public health issue. With the vast majority of IPED research focused on anabolic steroid use by males, we have even less data to guide a public health approach when we examine the use of drugs other than AAS (for example, human growth hormone and a range of other peptide hormones or clenbuterol etc. or the use of AAS by women).

HARMS

A key element in the recognition of AAS use as a public health issue is the identification of the extent and severity of actual or potential harms caused. These harms may be described as either direct or indirect harms.

AAS and Direct Harms

Direct harms are those adverse consequences directly linked to the pharmaco-logical effects of the drugs. As with much of our knowledge regarding AAS use, the majority of data relating to direct health harms are derived from 'weak evidence', that is, case reports/series and cross-sectional studies that are observational in nature, limiting their application to population-based health (Evans-Brown et al., 2009). However, since testosterone was first popularized in the twentieth century (de Kruif, 1945), we have gained an understanding of the drugs mechanisms of action and therefore the organs and systems of the body which are most likely to be damaged. These well-established deleterious effects may be described as cardiovascular effects, haematologic effects, psychiatric and neuropsychologic effects, and hormonal and metabolic effects (ACMD, 2010a;

Pope, Wood et al., 2014). Example of the harms that AAS may cause to specific organs and systems can be seen in Table 2.

As is often the case within AAS research and published literature, the data in Table 2 use the male as the template for harms, for example, the neuroendocrine condition of gynaecomastia, caused by increased levels of oestrogen in men, in this case du e to aromatization of excess testosterone (Niewoehner & Schorer, 2008). For women the neuroendocrine effect of virilization results in masculinization, gonadal and sexual effects (Havnes et al., 2020). While it remains an under-researched area of AAS use, there is compelling evidence that in addition to the adverse effects common to men women experience the additional masculinization of increased facial and body hair, deeper voice, reduced breast volume, enlarged clitoris, irregular/absent menstruation and reduced fertility (Andreasson & Henning, 2021; Borjesson et al., 2016; Korkia et al., 1996; Strauss et al., 1985).

In recent years, much of the research regarding the direct harms relating to AAS has been confirmatory in nature, for example, the growing evidence base related to mechanisms associated with untoward cardiovascular events and AAS (Bigi et al., 2020; McCullough et al., 2020; Sidelmann et al., 2021). A notable exception to this is the growing evidence base in relation to the effects of AAS and the brain. Descriptions of the psychological effects of AAS are rooted in the 1980s and 1990s, for example, personality disorder (Cooper et al., 1996), narcissism (Porcerelli & Sandler, 1995) and impulsivity (Pope & Katz, 1992), and it continues in current research (Aknouche et al., 2021; Chegeni et al., 2021; Hauger et al., 2021; Pope et al., 2021). However, it is the evidence of structural changes to the brain that provides a compelling explanation of the mechanism of action of AAS (Bjornebekk et al., 2017, 2021; Westlye et al., 2017), leading to changes in cognitive performance (Bjornebekk et al., 2019), dependence (Hauger et al., 2019) and the ultimate impact on public health. The relationship between these changes to the brain, dependence, cognitive function and anti-social behaviour (including aggression) is complex, requiring ongoing research.

Table 2. Conditions Commonly Attributed to the Use of AAS.

Organ/System Effect	Examples of Conditions Commonly Associated With Anabolic Androgenic Steroid Use
Cardiovascular	Atherosclerosis, hypertension and cardiomyopathy
Haematological	Coagulation and thrombosis
Neuroendocrine	Gynaecomastia, prostatic hypertrophy, hypogonadism, withdrawal
Neuropsychiatric	Depression, dependence irritability and mania
Hepatic	Inflammatory and cholestatic effects[a]
Musculoskeletal	Tendon/ligament damage
Renal	Rhabdomyolysis
Immunity	Immunosuppression
Dermatological	Acne, striae

[a]Usually associated with oral α-alkylated ASS.

However, these findings and their potential impact on communities have implications for society as a whole, adding considerable weight to the argument that
AAS is now a public health issue.

Indirect Harm

Indirect harms associated with AAS are those untoward effects other than the
pharmacological actions on the drugs. The presence of blood-borne viruses
(BBV) amongst AAS users is an issue that has been identified within the last
decade, although not uniformly recognized as a public health concern. Until
relatively recently, cases of HIV or viral hepatitis amongst AAS users were
extremely rare within the literature (Cook et al., 2000; Henrion et al., 1992; Scott
& Scott, 1989; Sklarek et al., 1984). While the potential for transmission was clear
(Dickinson & Rich, 1996; Midgley et al., 2000), the prevalence of BBV amongst
people who use AAS was generally considered relatively low (Crampin et al.,
1998; Day et al., 2008), although issues related to local infection have been a
consistent concern (Hope et al., 2015) However, this changed with the publication
of the largest study of BBV among people who use AAS, identifying a similar
prevalence of HIV amongst this cohort as that observed in people who inject
psychoactive drugs (Hope et al., 2013). Subsequent work supported this finding,
indicating the enduring presence of HIV amongst people who inject AAS and
associated IPEDs (Hope et al., 2016). Furthermore, research has also identified
elevated levels of hepatitis C within this population (Hope et al., 2013, 2016;
Hope & Iversen, 2019), often remaining undiagnosed (Hope et al., 2017, 2020).
However, the route of transmission remains unclear, with sharing of injecting
equipment during previous psychoactive drug injecting behaviour or sexual
transmission likely routes of at least some infections (Hope et al., 2013; Hope &
Iversen, 2019). This lack of clarity regarding the transmission of BBV has
contributed to the dismissal of BBV as a public health concern amongst some
users of AAS and the argument that this should not be a focus of harm reduction
(Underwood, 2019); however, the presence of BBV within at least some populations of people who use AAS is a genuine cause for concern (McVeigh, 2019).

Issues related to the illicit market were an omission from the initial assessment
of the AAS evidence base in 1999 and therefore not explicitly considered in
subsequent reviews (Table 1). However, the illicit market can result in negative
consequences for people who use AAS and therefore will be considered here,
under the domain *indirect harms*. As this chapter is focussed primarily on the
United Kingdom, the specific harms associated with the criminalization and
potential imprisonment of people who use AAS will not be considered due to the
specific UK legislation and the decision to exclude personal possession as a
criminal offence, a situation in stark contrast to countries such as Australia (Van
de Ven & Zahnow, 2017). However, the illicit market can still have a profound
negative impact on health. The uncontrolled illicit market and inevitable sale of
substandard products has long been an issue (Duchaine, 1989; Korkia & Stimson,
1993; McVeigh & Lenehan, 1994). However, over time as the availability of
legitimately manufactured products has decreased, the market has seen an influx

of products purportedly manufactured in countries such as China, often of questionable quality (Evans-Brown et al., 2009). In the absence of systematic purchasing and testing of products, a reliance on convenience samples provides an inexact picture of the extent of the issue (Fabresse et al., 2021; Graham et al., 2009; Shapira et al., 2018) and therefore the actual harms. However, with examples of gross misrepresentation of drugs, inexact dosages and high levels of contamination (Breindahl et al., 2015; Kimergard, Breindahl et al., 2014; Kimergard, McVeigh et al., 2014; Stensballe et al., 2015), it is clear that the illicit market presents significant challenges to public health.

EFFECTIVE RESPONSES

The final section on AAS and its recognition as a public health issue relates to the effective prevention, treatment and harm reduction associated with use. There remains a dearth of evidence in relation to effective interventions to prevent the onset of AAS use, mitigate the harms associated with use or support the successful cessation of use. There are few studies that have examined the effectiveness of strategies to prevent the use of AAS and associated drugs. Interventions that have been evaluated are predominantly delivered within school sport settings and limited to information provision (Bates & Backhouse, 2019). They are often hampered by the short-term nature of the follow ups and a lack of robust behavioural outcome measures (Bates, Begley et al., 2019). As we have outlined, there are diverse populations with a variety of motivations for using AAS, with this broadening further when the full range of IPEDs are concerned (McVeigh et al., 2012). It is clear that comprehensive interventions that address the complexity of the lived experience are required if prevention efforts are to be successful (Bates & Backhouse, 2019). At present, we remain some way off developing multi-layered responses with rigorous outcome measures, to reduce the initiation of this form of drug use.

Similarly, there is a lack of evidence on treating dependence, managing withdrawal, or initiating behaviour change in AAS users (Bates, Van Hout et al., 2019). While there are plentiful case reports of complications and adverse consequences of AAS use including psychiatric, neuroendocrine, hepatic, kidney, cardiovascular, musculoskeletal and infectious, together with their clinical management, there is little evidence on the successful management of the cessation of AAS use. Similarly, since the effects of testosterone on an individual's size and strength were proven scientifically (Bhasin et al., 1996), we have made little progress in understanding the potential benefits or the optimal dosages of specific AAS either in isolation or in combination. This lack of evidence regarding the efficacy of AAS limits the possibility of providing acceptable evidence-based advice on, for example, dosage, frequency of use and cycle length to reduce the risk of harm.

The clinician, health practitioner or even peer AAS user has little scientific evidence therefore on which to base harm reduction advice or guidance, with experiential or anecdotal information of varying reliability filling the void. This lack of evidence upon which health promotion guidance can be drawn can be seen clearly regarding the issue of post cycle therapy (PCT), the practice of using drugs such as tamoxifen and hCG to mitigate the effects of low levels of testosterone or stimulate the production of testosterone following a course of AAS. While the potential benefits of various substances have been identified in small scale studies (Anawalt, 2019; Tan & Scally, 2009) and supported by anecdotal evidence (Griffiths et al., 2016; Llewellyn, 2017), there has been little research conducted in relation to PCT. In fact, direct contradiction regarding the benefits of PCT and suggestions from a recent study of 80 users of PCT concluded that there was hardly any evidence to support its use, that tamoxifen had negligible effects on the actions of AAS and that hCG had no detectable effect on testicular size or spermatogenesis (Smit et al., 2021). Caution is required in the interpretation of research with relatively small sample sizes and the use of illicitly obtained medications with a lack of data on drug provenance; however, this illustrates the lack of progress in relation to answering a key question regarding AAS and a tenet of any harm reduction activity.

Recent publications have attempted to inform and develop the evidence base in relation to harm reduction in the United Kingdom. With a focus on health professionals and effective engagement, qualitative research has attempted to identify and contribute to the community of health practice (Atkinson et al., 2021; van de Ven et al., 2021) and to establish the need for a broader range of harm reduction interventions to be offered to address the determinants of the varied harms associated with AAS in addition to tackling the risk of BBVs (Bates et al., 2021; Harvey et al., 2020; Jacka et al., 2020).

CONCLUSION

Based on our assessment of the evidence we conclude that AAS use certainly meets the threshold to be considered a public health issue. The evidence highlights not only the extent of AAS use but also its complexity, diversity within the AAS using community, and the clear potential for harm to the AAS using community and wider population. Of concern is that despite the extent of AAS use and our understanding of associated direct and indirect harms, there remains a lack of evidence in relation to effective responses to this form of drug use. The complexity of AAS use through the diversity of the population, the nature of the illicit market and the range of additional IPEDs used present a significant challenge to developing effective responses that will address this multifaceted issue and ultimately reduce the associated harms.

While we may be still at the early stages of gaining a comprehensive picture of the complex epidemiology of AAS, we have enough data to be concerned by the extent of this phenomenon and to be clear that it will not simply go away. We now have compelling data on the long-term harms of AAS use. We can now add concerns regarding the effects of AAS on the brain (Bjornebekk et al., 2017, 2021; Westlye et al., 2017) to the established evidence related to cardiovascular risks.

While data related to BBV amongst this population are largely restricted to the United Kingdom (Hope & Iversen, 2019; Hope et al., 2013; Hope et al., 2016; Hope et al., 2017; Hope et al., 2020), this is also a cause for concern. The additional indirect harms caused by adulterated and contaminated products from the illicit market (Evans-Brown et al., 2009) merely compound the issue.

As the evidence base has developed in recent decades, it has highlighted our knowledge gaps and resulted in the recognition that this is a far more complex and multifaceted issue than many had previously imagined. We argue that the United Kingdom is ideally placed to develop our understanding of factors driving the use of the drugs and the regimes and behaviours employed, together with the potential harms and ultimately how society may implement a public health approach leading to the reduction of harm. The United Kingdom took the deliberate step of avoiding the criminalization of AAS use (ACMD, 2010b), combining this with a network of NSPs (NICE, 2014) and the recognition that AAS and associated IPED use is an issue, that for some, requires clinical management (Clinical Guidelines on Drug Misuse and Dependence Update 2017; Independent Expert Working Group, 2017). It is within this environment that we are hopeful of seeing significant developments across all the domains of evidence in relation to AAS use in the coming decade. Furthermore, we are hopeful that new approaches to complex issues such as systems mapping (ASUK, 2021) may support our understanding of the factors that contribute to problems and that working with stakeholders, in particular those who use of AAS and associated IPEDs, will support the development of interventions that will reduce harm.

KEY READINGS

(1) Pope, H. G., Jr., Wood, R. I., Rogol, A., Nyberg, F., Bowers, L., & Bhasin, S. (2014). Adverse health consequences of performance-enhancing drugs: An endocrine society scientific statement. *Endocrine Reviews*, *35*(3), 341–375.

This important scientific statement synthesizes the available evidence on the harms associated with AAS and other commonly used IPEDs. This provides a summary of what we knew at that point and is a useful starting point for those interested in the topic including policymakers, practitioners and those using or contemplating the use of AAS or other IPEDs.

(2) Hope, V. D., McVeigh, J., Marongiu, A., Evans-Brown, M., Smith, J., Kimergard, A., Croxford, S., Beynon, C. M., Parry, J. V., Bellis, M. A., & Ncube, F. (2013). Prevalence of, and risk factors for, HIV, hepatitis B and C infections among men who inject image and performance enhancing drugs: A cross-sectional study. *BMJ Open*, *3*(9), e003207.

Similarly, to work of Bjornebekk et al. (2017), this provided evidence of the presence of BBV amongst those who use IPEDs. Although not demonstrating how the viruses were contracted, it again illustrated the presence of a previously unrecognized public health issue.

(3) McVeigh, J., & Begley, E. (2017). Anabolic steroids in the UK: An increasing issue for public health. *Drugs-Education Prevention and Policy*, *24*(3), 278–285.

This paper identified the changes in the extent and patterns of anabolic steroid use in the United Kingdom between 1995 and 2015 providing an indication of the public health implications within the context of the health-related evidence base.

(4) Bjornebekk, A., Walhovd, K. B., Jorstad, M. L., Due-Tonnessen, P., Hullstein, I. R., & Fjell, A. M. (2017). Structural brain imaging of long-term anabolic-androgenic steroid users and nonusing weightlifters. *Biol Psychiatry*, *82*(4), 294–302.

This work provided compelling evidence of a significant health issue which up until then had not been recognized. This illustrates that we may not be aware of harms that we, as the scientific community, have not actively looked for.

(5) Bates, G., Tod, D., Leavey, C., & McVeigh, J. (2018). An evidence-based socioecological framework to understand men's use of ASS and inform interventions in this area. *Drugs: Education, Prevention and Policy*, *26*(6), 484–492.

This work provided a framework to view complex behaviours associated with AAS use together with the many influential environments and relationships that impact on a diverse population, in different ways and at different times. This was the basis of the subsequent systems mapping approach to considering the issues associated with the use of AAS.

REFERENCES

ACMD. (2010a). *Annex for the ACMD Anabolic Steroids Report; A-F*. https://assets.publishing.service. gov.uk/government/uploads/system/uploads/attachment_data/file/119133/ananbolic-steroids-annexes.pdf. Accessed on April 21, 2022.

ACMD. (2010b). *Consideration of the anabolic steroids*. https://assets.publishing.service.gov.uk/ government/uploads/system/uploads/attachment_data/file/119132/anabolic-steroids.pdf. Accessed on April 21, 2022.

Aknouche, F., Gheddar, L., Kernalleguen, A., Maruejouls, C., & Kintz, P. (2021). Anabolic steroids and extreme violence: A case of murder after chronic intake and under acute influence of metandienone and trenbolone. *International Journal of Legal Medicine*. https://doi.org/10.1007/s00414-021-02587-y

Anabolic Steroids Control Act. (1990). https://www.congress.gov/bill/101st-congress/house-bill/4658. Accessed on April 21, 2022.

Anawalt, B. D. (2019). Diagnosis and management of anabolic androgenic steroid use. *The Journal of Cinical Endocrinology and Metabolism*. https://doi.org/10.1210/jc.2018-01882

Andreasson, J., & Henning, A. (2021). Challenging hegemony through narrative: Centering women's experiences and establishing a sis-science culture through a women-only doping forum. *Communication & Sport*. https://doi.org/10.1177/21674795211000657

Ashton, J. R., & Seymour, H. (2010). Public health and the origins of the Mersey model of harm reduction. *International Journal of Drug Policy*, *21*(2), 94–96. https://doi.org/10.1016/j.drugpo. 2010.01.004

Assael, S. (2007). *Steroid nation*. ESPN Books.

ASUK. (2021). Systems map illustrating the influences on harmful image and performance enhancing drug use. https://www.anabolicsteroids.org.uk/influences-on-harmful-image-and-performance-enhancing-drug-use/. Accessed on April 21, 2022.

Atkinson, A. M., van de Ven, K., Cunningham, M., de Zeeuw, T., Hibbert, E., Forlini, C., Barkoukis, V., & Sumnall, H. R. (2021). Performance and image enhancing drug interventions aimed at increasing knowledge among healthcare professionals (HCP): Reflections on the implementation of the Dopinglinkki e-module in the HCP workforce in Europe and School of Pyschology, University of New South Wales, Australia. *International Journal of Drug Policy*, 103141. https://doi.org/10.1016/j.drugpo.2021.103141

Bates, G., & Backhouse, S. (2019). Preventing image and performance enhancing drug use: It's not all chalk and talk. In K. Van de Ven, K. Mulrooney, & J. McVeigh (Eds.), *Human enhancement drugs*. Routledge.

Bates, G., Begley, E., Tod, D., Jones, L., Leavey, C., & McVeigh, J. (2019). A systematic review investigating the behaviour change strategies in interventions to prevent misuse of anabolic steroids. *Journal of Health Psychology*, *24*(11), 1595–1612. https://doi.org/10.1177/1359105317737607

Bates, G., & McVeigh, J. (2016). *Image and Performance Enhancing Drugs 2015 Survey Results*. https://bit.ly/3xKyCO2. Accessed on April 21, 2022.

Bates, G., McVeigh, J., & Leavey, C. (2021). Looking beyond the provision of injecting equipment to people who use anabolic androgenic steroids: Harm reduction and behavior change goals for UK policy. *Contemporary Drug Problems*. https://doi.org/10.1177/0091450921998701

Bates, G., Tod, D., Leavey, C., & McVeigh, J. (2018). An evidence-based socioecological framework to understand men's use of anabolic androgenic steroids and inform interventions in this area. *Drugs: Education, Prevention & Policy*, *26*(6), 484–492. https://doi.org/10.1080/09687637.2018.1488947

Bates, G., Van Hout, M. C., Teck, J. T. W., & McVeigh, J. (2019). Treatments for people who use anabolic androgenic steroids: A scoping review. *Harm Reduction Journal*, *16*(1), 75. https://doi.org/10.1186/s12954-019-0343-1

Begley, E., McVeigh, J., Hope, V., Bates, G., Glass, R., Campbell, J., Tanner, C., Kean, J., Morgan, G., Acreman, D., & Smith, J. (2017). *Image and Performance Enhancing Drugs: 2016 National Survey Results*. https://bit.ly/3CD0dAp. Accessed on April 21, 2022.

Bhasin, S., Storer, T. W., Berman, N., Callegari, C., Clevenger, B., Phillips, J., Bunnell, T. J., Tricker, R., Shirazi, A. & Casaburi, R. (1996). The effects of supraphysiologic doses of testosterone on muscle size and strength in normal men. *New England Journal of Medicine*, *335*(1), 1–7. https://doi.org10.1056/Nejm199607043350101

Bigi, M. A. B., Abtahi, F., Namdar, Z. M., Amirhakimi, A., Hosseinpour, A., Shahrzad, S., & Aslani, A. (2020). Aortopathic effect of androgenic anabolic steroids. *Journal of Echocardiography*. https://doi.org/10.1007/s12574-020-00495-5

Bjornebekk, A., Kaufmann, T., Hauger, L. E., Klonteig, S., Hullstein, I. R., & Westlye, L. T. (2021). Long-term anabolic-androgenic steroid use is associated with deviant brain aging. *Biol Psychiatry Cogn Neurosci Neuroimaging*. https://doi.org/10.1016/j.bpsc.2021.01.001

Bjornebekk, A., Walhovd, K. B., Jorstad, M. L., Due-Tonnessen, P., Hullstein, I. R., & Fjell, A. M. (2017). Structural brain imaging of long-term anabolic-androgenic steroid users and nonusing weightlifters. *Biological Psychiatry*, *82*(4), 294–302. https://doi.org/10.1016/j.biopsych.2016.06.017

Bjornebekk, A., Westlye, L. T., Walhovd, K. B., Jorstad, M. L., Sundseth, O. O., & Fjell, A. M. (2019). Cognitive performance and structural brain correlates in long-term anabolic-androgenic steroid exposed and nonexposed weightlifters. *Neuropsychology*, *33*(4), 547–559. https://doi.org/10.1037/neu0000537

Bonnecaze, A. K., O'Connor, T., & Aloi, J. A. (2020). Characteristics and attitudes of men using anabolic androgenic steroids (AAS): A survey of 2385 men. *American Journal of Men's Health*, *14*(6). https://doi.org/10.1177/1557988320966536

Borjesson, A., Garevik, N., Dahl, M. L., Rane, A., & Ekstrom, L. (2016). Recruitment to doping and help-seeking behavior of eight female AAS users. *Substance Abuse Treatment, Prevention, and Policy*, *11*. https://doi.org/ARTN.1110.1186/s13011-016-0056-3

Breindahl, T., Evans-Brown, M., Hindersson, P., McVeigh, J., Bellis, M., Stensballe, A., & Kimergard, A. (2015). Identification and characterization by LC-UV-MS/MS of melanotan II skin-tanning products sold illegally on the Internet. *Drug Testing and Analysis*, *7*(2), 164–172. https://doi.org/10.1002/dta.1655

Brennan, R., Wells, J. S. G., & Van Hout, M. C. (2017). The injecting use of image and performance-enhancing drugs (IPED) in the general population: A systematic review. *Health and Social Care in the Community*, *25*(5), 1459–1531. https://doi.org/10.1111/hsc.12326

Buckley, W. E., & Yesalis, C. E. (1989). Anabolic steroid use among male high-school seniors-reply. *JAMA, the Journal of the American Medical Association*, *261*(18), 2640. https://doi.org10.1001/jama.1989.03420180063032

Buckley, W. E., Yesalis, C. E., Friedl, K. E., Anderson, W. A., Streit, A. L., & Wright, J. E. (1988). Estimated prevalence of anabolic-steroid use among male high-school seniors. *JAMA, the Journal of the American Medical Association*, *260*(23), 3441–3445.

Centers for Disease Control and Prevention. (2021). *Injury prevention and control*. https://www.cdc.gov/injury/about/approach.html. Accessed on April 21, 2022.

Chandler, M., & McVeigh, J. (2014). *Steroids and Image Enhancing Drugs: 2013 Survey Results*. https://bit.ly/390qWwF. Accessed on April 21, 2022.

Chegeni, R., Pallesen, S., McVeigh, J., & Sagoe, D. (2021). Anabolic-androgenic steroid administration increases self-reported aggression in healthy males: A systematic review and meta-analysis of experimental studies. *Psychopharmacology (Berl)*. https://doi.org/10.1007/s00213-021-05818-7

Christiansen, A. V. (2019). Civilized muscles: Building a powerful body as a vehicle for social status and identity formation. *Social Sciences*, *8*(10). https://doi.org/10.3390/socsci8100287

Christiansen, A. V., Vinther, A. S., & Liokaftos, D. (2016). Outline of a typology of men's use of anabolic androgenic steroids in fitness and strength training environments. *Drugs: Education, Prevention & Policy*, *24*(3), 295–305.

Clinical Guidelines on Drug Misuse and Dependence Update 2017 Independent Expert Working Group. (2017). Drug misuse and dependence: UK guidelines on clinical management. https://assets.publishing.service.gov.uk/government/uploads/system/uploads/attachment_data/file/673978/clinical_guidelines_2017.pdf. Accessed on April 21, 2022.

Cohen, J., Collins, R., Darkes, J., & Gwartney, D. (2007). A league of their own: Demographics, motivations and patterns of use of 1,955 male adult non-medical anabolic steroid users in the United States. *Journal of the International Society of Sports Nutrition*, *4*. https://doi.org/10.1186/1550-2783-4-12

Cook, P., McVeigh, J., Patel, A., Syed, Q., Mutton, K., & Bellis, M. (2000). *Hepatitis C in injecting drug users in the North West-Executive Summary*. http://www.cph.org.uk/wp-content/uploads/2012/08/hepatitis-c-in-injecting-drug-users-in-the-north-west—executive-summary.htm. Accessed on April 21, 2022.

Cooper, C. J., Noakes, T. D., Dunne, T., Lambert, M. I., & Rochford, K. (1996). A high prevalence of abnormal personality traits in chronic users of anabolic-androgenic steroids. *British Journal of Sports Medicine*, *30*(3), 246–250.

Crampin, A. C., Lamagni, T. L., Hope, V. D., Newham, J. A., Lewis, K. M., Parry, J. V., & Gill, O. N. (1998). The risk of infection with HIV and hepatitis B in individuals who inject steroids in England and Wales. *Epidemiology and Infection*, *121*(2), 381–386. https://doi.org10.1017/S0950268898001265

Dawson, R. T. (2001). Drugs in sport-the role of the physician. *Journal of Endocinology*, *170*, 55–61.

Day, C. A., Topp, L., Iversen, J., Maher, L., & Collaboration of Australian, N. (2008). Blood-borne virus prevalence and risk among steroid injectors: Results from the Australian needle and syringe program survey. *Drug and Alcohol Review*, *27*(5), 559–561. https://doi.org/10.1080/09595230801956132

Dickinson, B. P., & Rich, J. D. (1996). Infections secondary to anabolic steroid misuse and their prevention. *Journal of Perfomance Enhancing Drugs*, *1*(4), 146–150.

Dimeo, P. (2007). *A history of drug use in sport 1876–1976: Beyond good and evil*. Routledge.

Druglink. (1993). ACMD recommends new controls on steroids. Druglink, September/October 1993.

Duchaine, D. (1988). *Underground steroid handbook*. Duchaine.

Duchaine, D. (1989). *Underground steroid handbook II*. HLR Technical Books.

Evans-Brown, M., Kimergard, A., & McVeigh, J. (2009). Elephant in the room? The methodological implications for public health research of performance-enhancing drugs derived from the illicit market. *Drug Testing and Analysis*, *1*(7), 323–326. https://doi.org/10.1002/dta.74

Evans-Brown, M., & McVeigh, J. (2009). Injecting human growth hormone as a performance-enhancing drug-perspectives from the United Kingdom. *Journal of Substance Use, 14*(5), 267–288. https://doi.org/10.3109/14659890903224383

Evans-Brown, M., McVeigh, J., Perkins, C., & Bellis, M. (2012). *Human enhancement drugs: The emerging challenges to public health*. North West Public Health Observatory.

Fabresse, N., Gheddar, L., Kintz, P., Knapp, A., Larabi, I. A., & Alvarez, J. C. (2021). Analysis of pharmaceutical products and dietary supplements seized from the black market among bodybuilders. *Forensic Science International, 322*, 110771. https://doi.org/10.1016/j.forsciint.2021.110771

Germain, J., McLean, C., & Leavey, C. (2019). One size does not fit all: Tackling the issue of weight-loss drug use. In K. van de Ven, K. Mulrooney, & J. McVeigh (Eds.), *Human enhancement drugs*. Routledge.

Goldman, A. L., Pope, H. G., Jr., & Bhasin, S. (2018). The health threat posed by the hidden epidemic of anabolic steroid use and body image disorders among young men. *The Journal of Cinical Endocrinology and Metabolism*. https://doi.org/10.1210/jc.2018-01706

Graham, M. R., Ryan, P., Baker, J. S., Davies, B., Thomas, N.-E., Cooper, S.-M., Evans, P., Easmon, S., Walker, C. J., Cowan, D., & Kicman, A. T. (2009). Counterfeiting in performance-and image-enhancing drugs. *Drug Testing and Analysis, 1*(3), 135.

Griffiths, S., Henshaw, R., McKay, F. H., & Dunn, M. (2016). Post-cycle therapy for performance and image enhancing drug users: A qualitative investigation. *Performance Enhancement & Health*. http://doi.org/10.1016/j.peh.2016.11.002

Hamilton, A., & Sumnall, H. (2017, July 28). Number of young Britons using anabolic steroids is rising as latest drug use survey reveals changing habits. *The Independent*. https://www.independent.co.uk/news/uk/home-news/drug-use-latest-figures-uk-2017-anabolic-steroids-rise-young-britons-changing-habits-cocaine-heroin-cannabis-a7864706.html. Accessed on April 21, 2022.

Harvey, O., Parrish, M., van Teijlingen, E., & Trenoweth, S. (2020). Support for non-prescribed anabolic androgenic steroids users: A qualitative exploration of their needs. *Drugs: Education, Prevention & Policy, 27*(5), 377–386. https://doi.org/10.1080/09687637.2019.1705763

Hauger, L. E., Havnes, I. A., Jorstad, M. L., & Bjornebekk, A. (2021). Anabolic androgenic steroids, antisocial personality traits, aggression and violence. *Drug and Alcohol Dependence, 221*, 108604. https://doi.org/10.1016/j.drugalcdep.2021.108604

Hauger, L. E., Westlye, L. T., Fjell, A. M., Walhovd, K. B., & Bjornebekk, A. (2019). Structural brain characteristics of anabolic-androgenic steroid dependence in men. *Addiction*. https://doi.org/10.1111/add.14629

Havnes, I. A., Jorstad, M. L., Innerdal, I., & Bjornebekk, A. (2020). Anabolic-androgenic steroid use among women-a qualitative study on experiences of masculinizing, gonadal and sexual effects. *International Journal of Drug Policy, 102876*. https://doi.org/10.1016/j.drugpo.2020.102876

Havnes, I. A., Jorstad, M. L., & Wisloff, C. (2019). Anabolic-androgenic steroid users receiving health-related information; health problems, motivations to quit and treatment desires. *Substance Abuse Treatment, Prevention, and Policy, 14*(1), 20. https://doi.org/10.1186/s13011-019-0206-5

Henning, A., & Andreasson, J. (2020). Preventing, producing, or reducing harm? Fitness doping risk and enabling environments. *Drugs: Education, Prevention & Policy*, 1–10. https://doi.org/10.1080/09687637.2020.1865273

Henrion, R., Mandelbrot, L., & Delfieu, D. (1992). Contamination par le VIH a la suite d'injections d'anabolisants. *La Presse Médicale, 21*(5), 218.

Hoberman, J. M., & Yesalis, C. E. (1995). The history of synthetic testosterone. *Scientific American, 272*(2), 76–81.

Holt, R. I. G., & Ho, K. K. Y. (2019). The use and abuse of growth hormone in sports. *Endocrine Reviews, 40*(4), 1163–1185. https://doi.org/10.1210/er.2018-00265

Hope, V. D., Harris, R., McVeigh, J., Cullen, K. J., Smith, J., Parry, J. V., DeAngelis, D., & Ncube, F. (2016). Risk of HIV and hepatitis B and C over time among men who inject image and performance enhancing drugs in England and Wales: Results from cross-sectional prevalence surveys, 1992–2013. *Journal of Acquired Immune Deficiency Syndromes, 71*(3), 331–337. https://doi.org/10.1097/QAI.0000000000000835

Hope, V., & Iversen, J. (2019). Infections and risk among people who use image and performance enhancing drugs. In K. Van de Ven, K. Mulrooney, & J. McVeigh (Eds.), *Humam enhancement drugs*. Routledge.

Hope, V. D., McVeigh, J., Begley, E., Glass, R., Edmundson, C., Heinsbroek, E., Kean, J., Campbell, J., Whitfield, M., Morgan, G., Acreman, D., & Smith, J. (2020). Factors associated with hepatitis C and HIV testing uptake among men who inject image and performance enhancing drugs. *Drug and Alcohol Review, 40*(4), 586–596. https://doi.org/10.1111/dar.13198

Hope, V. D., McVeigh, J., Marongiu, A., Evans-Brown, M., Smith, J., Kimergard, A., Croxford, S., Beynon, C. M., Parry, J. V., Bellis, M. A., & Ncube, F. (2013). Prevalence of, and risk factors for, HIV, hepatitis B and C infections among men who inject image and performance enhancing drugs: A cross-sectional study. *BMJ Open, 3*(9), e003207. https://doi.org/10.1136/bmjopen-2013-003207

Hope, V. D., McVeigh, J., Marongiu, A., Evans-Brown, M., Smith, J., Kimergard, A., Parry, J. V., & Ncube, F. (2015). Injection site infections and injuries in men who inject image- and performance-enhancing drugs: Prevalence, risks factors, and healthcare seeking. *Epidemiology and Infection, 143*(1), 132–140. https://doi.org/10.1017/S0950268814000727

Hope, V. D., McVeigh, J., Smith, J., Glass, R., Njoroge, J., Tanner, C., Parry, J. V., Ncube, F., & Desai, M. (2017). Low levels of hepatitis C diagnosis and testing uptake among people who inject image and performance enhancing drugs in England and Wales, 2012–2015. *Drug and Alcohol Dependence, 179*, 83–86. https://doi.org/10.1016/j.drugalcdep.2017.06.018

Ip, E. J., Trinh, K., Tenerowicz, M. J., Pal, J., Lindfelt, T. A., & Perry, P. J. (2015). Characteristics and behaviors of older male anabolic steroid users. *Journal of Pharmacy Practice, 28*(5), 450–456. https://doi.org/10.1177/0897190014527319

Jacka, B., Larance, B., Copeland, J., Burns, L., Farrell, M., Jackson, E., & Degenhardt, L. (2020). Health care engagement behaviors of men who use performance-and image-enhancing drugs in Australia. *Substance Abuse, 41*(1), 139–145. https://doi.org/10.1080/08897077.2019.1635954

Kanayama, G., & Pope, H. G. (2018). History and epidemiology of anabolic androgens in athletes and non-athletes. *Molecular and Cellular Endocrinology, 464*(C), 4–13. https://doi.org/10.1016/j.mce.2017.02.039

Kimergard, A., Breindahl, T., Hindersson, P., & McVeigh, J. (2014). The composition of anabolic steroids from the illicit market is largely unknown: Implications for clinical case reports. *QJM, 107*(7), 597–598. https://doi.org/10.1093/qjmed/hcu101

Kimergard, A., McVeigh, J., Knutsson, S., Breindahl, T., & Stensballe, A. (2014). Online marketing of synthetic peptide hormones: Poor manufacturing, user safety, and challenges to public health. *Drug Testing and Analysis, 6*(4), 396–398. https://doi.org/10.1002/dta.1636

Korkia, P., Lenehan, P., & McVeigh, J. (1996). Non-medical use of androgens among women. *The Journal of Preformance Enhancing Drugs, 1*(2), 71.

Korkia, P., & Stimson, G. V. (1993). *Anabolic steroid use in Great Britain: An exploratory investigation: Final report to the departments of health for England, Scotland and Wales*. Centre for Research on Drugs Health Behaviour.

de Kruif, P. (1945). *The male hormone*. Brace and Company.

Kruskemper, H. (1968). *Anabolic steroids*. Academic Press.

Lenehan, P., & McVeigh, J. (1997). *Anabolic steroids: A guide for professionals*. Drugs & Sport Information Service.

Lenehan, P., & McVeigh, J. (1998). *Anabolic steroids: A guide for professionals*. University of Liverpool.

Llewellyn, W. (2017). *Anabolics* (11th ed.). Molecular Nutrition.

McBride, A. J., Williamson, K., & Petersen, T. (1996). Three cases of nalbuphine hydrochloride dependence associated with anabolic steroid use. *British Journal of Sports Medicine, 30*(1), 69–70.

McCullough, D., Webb, R., Enright, K. J., Lane, K. E., McVeigh, J., Stewart, C. E., & Davies, I. G. (2020). How the love of muscle can break a heart: Impact of anabolic androgenic steroids on skeletal muscle hypertrophy, metabolic and cardiovascular health. *Reviews in Endocrine & Metabolic Disorders, 22*(2), 389–405. https://doi.org/10.1007/s11154-020-09616-y

McElrath, K., & Connolly, D. (2006). Nalbuphine (nubain): Non-prescribed use, injecting, and risk behaviors for bloodborne viruses. *Contemporary Drug Problems*, *33*, 321–340.

McVeigh, J. (2019). Engaging with people who use image and performance enhancing drugs: One size does not fit all. *International Journal of Drug Policy*, *71*, 1–2.

McVeigh, J. (2021). Application development award image and performance enhancing drugs (IPEDs): Assessment of available intelligence and research gaps to inform intervention evaluation. *NIHR Journal Library*. https://www.journalslibrary.nihr.ac.uk/programmes/phr/NIHR132730/#/21/04/2022

McVeigh, J., & Begley, E. (2017). Anabolic steroids in the UK: An increasing issue for public health. *Drugs: Education, Prevention & Policy*, *24*(3), 278–285. https://doi.org/10.1080/09687637.2016.1245713

McVeigh, J., Evans-Brown, M., & Bellis, M. A. (2012). Human enhancement drugs and the pursuit of perfection. *Adicciones*, *24*(3), 185–190.

McVeigh, J., & Lenehan, P. (1994). Counterfeits and fakes: A growing problem. *Relay*, *1*(1), 8–9.

McVeigh, J., Salinas, M., & Ralphs, R. (2020). A sentinel population: The public health benefits of monitoring enhanced body builders. *International Journal of Drug Policy*, 102890. https://doi.org/10.1016/j.drugpo.2020.102890

Midgley, S. J., Heather, N., Best, D., Henderson, D., McCarthy, S., & Davies, J. B. (2000). Risk behaviours for HIV and hepatitis infection among anabolic-androgenic steroid users. *Aids Care-Psychological and Socio-Medical Aspects of AIDS/HIV*, *12*(2), 163–170. https://doi.org/10.1080/09540120050001832

Misuse of Drugs Act 1971 (Modification) Order 1996. (1996).

NICE. (2014). Needle and syringe programmes NICE public health guidance. www.nice.org.uk/guidance/ph52

Niewoehner, C. B., & Schorer, A. E. (2008). Gynaecomastia and breast cancer in men. *BMJ*, *336*(7646), 709–713. https://doi.org/10.1136/bmj.39511.493391.BE

Office for National Statistics. (2021). Crime survey for England and Wales - Drug misuse in England and Wales: Year ending March 2020. https://www.ons.gov.uk/peoplepopulationandcommunity/crimeandjustice/articles/drugmisuseinenglandandwales/yearendingmarch2020. Accessed on April 21, 2022.

Pope, H. G., Jr., Kanayama, G., Athey, A., Ryan, E., Hudson, J. I., & Baggish, A. (2014). The lifetime prevalence of anabolic-androgenic steroid use and dependence in Americans: Current best estimates. *American Journal on Addictions*, *23*(4), 371–377. https://doi.org/10.1111/j.1521-0391.2013.12118.x

Pope, H. G., Jr., Kanayama, G., Hudson, J. I., & Kaufman, M. J. (2021). Review article: Anabolic-androgenic steroids, violence, and crime: Two cases and literature review. *American Journal on Addictions*. https://doi.org/10.1111/ajad.13157

Pope, H. G., Jr., Wood, R. I., Rogol, A., Nyberg, F., Bowers, L., & Bhasin, S. (2014). Adverse health consequences of performance-enhancing drugs: An endocrine society scientific statement. *Endocrine Reviews*, *35*(3), 341–375. https://doi.org/10.1210/er.2013-1058

Pope, H. G., & Katz, D. L. (1992). Psychiatric effects of anabolic-steroids. *Psychiatric Annals*, *22*(1), 24–29.

Pope, H. G., Katz, D. L., & Champoux, R. (1988). Anabolic-androgenic steroid use among 1,010 college men. *The Physician and Sportsmedicine*, *16*(7), 75.

Porcerelli, J. H., & Sandler, B. A. (1995). Narcissism and empathy in steroid users. *American Journal of Psychiatry*, *152*(11), 1672–1674.

Rothstein, M. A. (2002). Rethinking the meaning of public health. *Journal of Law Medicine & Ethics*, *30*, 144–149.

Rychetnik, L., Hawe, P., Waters, E., Barratt, A., & Frommer, M. (2004). A glossary for evidence based public health. *Journal of Epidemiology & Community Health*, *58*(7), 538–545. https://doi.org/10.1136/jech.2003.011585

Sagoe, D., Andreassen, C. S., & Pallesen, S. (2014). The aetiology and trajectory of anabolic-androgenic steroid use initiation: A systematic review and synthesis of qualitative research. *Substance Abuse Treatment, Prevention, and Policy*, *9*. https://doi.org/10.1186/1747-597x-9-27

Sagoe, D., McVeigh, J., Bjornebekk, A., Essilfie, M. S., Andreassen, C. S., & Pallesen, S. (2015). Polypharmacy among anabolic-androgenic steroid users: A descriptive metasynthesis. *Substance Abuse Treatment, Prevention, and Policy*, *10*, 12. https://doi.org/10.1186/s13011-015-0006-5

Sagoe, D., & Pallesen, S. (2018). Androgen abuse epidemiology. *Current Opinion in Endocrinology Diabetes and Obesity*, *25*(3), 185–194. https://doi.org/10.1097/MED.0000000000000403

Scott, M. J., & Scott, M. J. (1989). HIV infection associated with injections of anabolic-steroids. *JAMA, the Journal of the American Medical Association*, *262*(2), 207–208.

Shapira, B., Poperno, A., Arieli, M., & Berkovitz, R. (2018). Label misrepresentation in seized anabolic steroids and performance-enhancing substances. *The European Journal of Public Health*, *28*, 128.

Sidelmann, J. J., Gram, J. B., Rasmussen, J. J., & Kistorp, C. (2021). Anabolic-androgenic steroid abuse impairs fibrin Clot Lysis. *Seminars in Thrombosis and Hemostasis*, *47*(1), 11–17. https://doi.org/10.1055/s-0040-1714398

Sklarek, H. M., Mantovani, R. P., Erens, E., Heisler, D., Niederman, M. S., & Fein, A. M. (1984). AIDS in a bodybuilder using anabolic-steroids. *New England Journal of Medicine*, *311*(26), 1701.

Smit, D. L., Buijs, M. M., de Hon, O., den Heijer, M., & de Ronde, W. (2021). Disruption and recovery of testicular function during and after androgen abuse: The Haarlem study. *Human Reproduction*. https://doi.org/10.1093/humrep/deaa366

Stensballe, A., McVeigh, J., Breindahl, T., & Kimergard, A. (2015). Synthetic growth hormone releasers detected in seized drugs: New trends in the use of drugs for performance enhancement. *Addiction*, *110*(2), 368–369. https://doi.org/10.1111/add.12785

Strauss, R. H., Liggett, M. T., & Lanese, R. R. (1985). Anabolic steroid use and perceived effects in ten weight-trained women athletes. *JAMA*, *253*. https://doi.org/10.1001/jama.1985.03350430083032

Takahara, J., Yunoki, S., Yakushiji, W., Yamauchi, J., Yamane, Y., & Ofuji, T. (1977). Stimulatory effects of gamma-hydroxybutyric acid on growth-hormone and prolactin-release in humans. *Journal of Clinical Endocrinology and Metabolism*, *44*(5), 1014-1017. https://doi.org10.1210/jcem-44-5-1014

Tan, R. S., & Scally, M. C. (2009). Anabolic steroid-induced hypogonadism – Towards a unified hypothesis of anabolic steroid action. *Medical Hypotheses*, *72*(6), 723–728. https://doi.org/10.1016/j.mehy.2008.12.042

Underwood, M. (2019). The unintended consequences of the current approach to blood borne virus prevention amongst people who inject image and performance enhancing drugs: A commentary based on enhanced bodybuilder perspectives. *International Journal of Drug Policy*, *67*, 19–23.

Van Hout, M. C., & Kean, J. (2015). An exploratory study of image and performance enhancement drug use in a male British South Asian community. *International Journal of Drug Policy*, *26*(9), 860–867. https://doi.org/10.1016/j.drugpo.2015.03.002

Van de Ven, K., & Zahnow, R. (2017, May 15). Australia should stop beefing up its steroid laws – That won't help users. *The Conversation*.

van de Ven, K., Boardley, I., & Chandler, M. (2021). Identifying best-practice amongst health professionals who work with people using image and performance enhancing drugs (IPEDs) through participatory action research. *Qualitative Research in Sport, Exercise and Health*, 1–18. https://doi.org/10.1080/2159676X.2021.1898457

Voy, R., & Deeter, K. D. (1991). *Drugs, sport, and politics*. Leisure Press.

Westlye, L. T., Kaufmann, T., Alnaes, D., Hullstein, I. R., & Bjornebekk, A. (2017). Brain connectivity aberrations in anabolic-androgenic steroid users. *Neuroimage Clin*, *13*, 62–69. https://doi.org/10.1016/j.nicl.2016.11.014

Wight, D., Wimbush, E., Jepson, R., & Doi, L. (2016). Six steps in quality intervention development (6SQuID). *Journal of Epidemiology & Community Health*, *70*(5), 520–525. https://doi.org/10.1136/jech-2015-205952

Wines, J. D., Gruber, A. J., Pope, H. G., & Lukas, S. E. (1999). Nalbuphine hydrochloride dependence in anabolic steroid users. *American Journal on Addictions*, *8*(2), 161–164.

World Health Organization (1997). Protocol for the evaluation of epidemiological surveillance systems. https://apps.who.int/iris/handle/10665/63639

Yesalis, C. E., Streit, A. L., Vicary, J. R., Friedl, K. E., Brannon, D., & Buckley, W. (1989). Anabolic-steroid use-indications of habituation among adolescents. *Journal of Drug Education*, *19*(2), 103–116. https://doi.org10.2190/Ng9c-0wea-8au8-Gua4

Zahnow, R., McVeigh, J., Bates, G., Hope, V., Kean, J., Campbell, J., & Smith, J. (2018). Identifying a typology of men who use anabolic androgenic steroids (AAS). *International Journal of Drug Policy*, *55*, 105–112. https://doi.org/10.1016/j.drugpo.2018.02.022

Chapter 5

THE EXPERIENCES OF HEALTHCARE PROFESSIONALS WITH PIED CONSUMERS AND THE EXPERIENCES OF PIED CONSUMERS WITH HEALTHCARE PROFESSIONALS: A SYSTEMATIC LITERATURE REVIEW

Matthew Dunn

ABSTRACT

The aim of this review was to amalgamate the extant literature that has investigated the experiences of healthcare professionals with PIED consumers and the experiences of PIED consumers with healthcare professionals, with a specific focus on medical practitioners. A systematic search was undertaken to identify studies that explored the experiences and perspectives of healthcare providers working with clients who use PIEDs, as well as to identify studies that explored the experiences and perspectives of PIED consumers with healthcare providers. Ten studies were included, of which four explored the experiences of healthcare providers with PIED consumers, and six explored the experiences of PIED consumers with healthcare providers. A sizeable proportion of healthcare providers come into contact with PIED consumers, with these interactions mostly related to consumers asking for information, though a small but significant proportion indicate they have been asked to prescribe doping agents. Of the six studies which focused on the consumer experience, five focused on PIED consumers; these studies found that while

Doping in Sport and Fitness
Research in the Sociology of Sport, Volume 16, 93–110
Copyright © 2023 by Emerald Publishing Limited
All rights of reproduction in any form reserved
ISSN: 1476-2854/doi:10.1108/S1476-285420220000016006

large proportions reporting accessing a medical practitioner, larger pro-
portions did not, with the doctor's lack of knowledge cited as one reason. More
research is needed to investigate how they come into contact with this group of
consumers, their level of knowledge and any training that they may need.
Given the harms associated with PIED use, and the lack of disclosure of use to
healthcare providers, more research is needed to understand the barriers and
facilitators for consumers to accessing health care.

Keywords: Performance and image enhancing drugs; anabolic–androgenic
steroids; medical practitioners; consumers; healthcare; systematic review

INTRODUCTION

Much sensationalism surrounds an athlete who admits to or is caught using performance and/or image enhancing drugs (PIEDs; also known as image and/or performance enhancing drugs [IPEDs] or appearance and/or performance enhancing drugs [APEDs]). Amidst the acrimony, accusations and emotion, an inevitable question is posed: who knew? Athletes and those competing at the highest level of competition exist in what Thomas et al. (2011) describe as an '...environment of complex networks or relationships (e.g. fellow athletes, coaches and team doctors) that may encourage the supply and demand of illicit and performance enhancing drugs' (p. 281). Rightly or wrongly, suspicion inevitably falls on the medical personnel, and high-profile cases such as Lance Armstrong only serve to demonstrate the role that a healthcare professional can have in preventing or – in his case, facilitating – PIED use. In testifying before a jury about doping in cycling, specifically in relation to Lance Armstrong, former professional cyclist Tyler Hamilton explains that he had to convey that there was a whole system in place that facilitated doping in the peloton – 'I made them [the jury] understand how the whole system worked, got developed over the years, and how you couldn't single one person out. It was everybody. Everybody' (Hamilton & Coyle, 2012). In USADA's Reasoned Decision regarding Lance Armstrong, the role of the team and in particular that of the team doctor, Michele Ferrari, is consistently highlighted (United States Anti-Doping Agency, 2012); the doctor prescribed a plan for doping for the team riders and also administered banned substances to them. Other recent examples from elite sport, such as the systematic doping of Russian Olympic athletes and the Nike Oregon Project (World Anti-Doping Agency, 2021b), have further highlighted the role that team members, including the healthcare professionals, can play in facilitating and supporting the doping behaviours of the athlete.

The term PIED encapsulates a wide variety of substances. These can include legal, widely available substances such as multivitamins and supplements such as protein powders and protein shakes, glucosamine, creatine, branch-chain amino acids (BCAAs) and energy drinks; illegal substances, such as cannabis, amphetamine and cocaine; and scheduled substances that have legitimate therapeutic uses which require a valid prescription but which are used for non-medical purposes, such as human growth hormones (HGH) and the most widely researched, anabolic–androgenic steroids (AAS). Most of these PIEDs are also on the World Anti-Doping Agency's (WADA's) Prohibited List (World Anti-Doping Agency, 2021a) and may be prohibited at all times (that is, in- and out-of-competition, such as AAS) or in-competition (e.g. stimulants). The wide variety of substances used for enhancement purposes makes understanding and responding to any associated harms challenging. Most legal PIEDs result in little or no harm when taken as directed; those which have resulted in harm have generally been reformulated or, as was the case with DMAA (an ephedrine-like vasoconstricting substance which had been included in many popular sports supplements), re-scheduled (Dunn, 2017). Most illegal substances, such as cannabis and amphetamine, may result in harm though perhaps not to the same extent as legal substances such as alcohol (Bonomo et al., 2019; Nutt et al., 2010; van Amsterdam et al., 2015). Furthermore, compared to the general population, their use among sporting populations is low; for example, Dunn et al. (2011) and Dunn and Thomas (2012) found that the prevalence of illicit 'recreational' drug use was lower among elite Australian athletes compared to the Australian general population.

PIEDs such as AAS are a unique group of substances. They are prescribed medications with legitimate therapeutic uses, and health professionals may be familiar with these substances' medical indications. However, their use for enhancement purposes may involve doses which are much higher than thera-peutic levels, which may pose challenges for medical professionals unfamiliar with the regimes that consumers may follow. The medical community and those who consume PIEDs have historically had a contentious relationship, commencing in the 1970s when the American College of Sports Medicine deemed steroids to be ineffective (Bahrke & Yesalis, 2002). That the bodybuilding com-munity had already been successfully using these substances for enhancement purposes conveyed a degree of naivety at best and condescension at worst and may have been the start of the schism that still exists. Despite this, medical professionals play a unique role within the PIED using community. Given the pharmaceutical status of these substances, the diversion from hospitals or other healthcare settings, or misprescribing from medical practitioners, has always been a cause for concern. While medical practitioners have not been nominated by consumers as the main source of PIEDs, they are one source; one study exam-ining court cases to ascertain what groups were involved in the production and supply of PIEDs in Australia found that the healthcare sector was involved in 17% of cases, second only to the fitness industry (22%) (van de Ven et al., 2018). In some countries where PIEDs such as AAS are scheduled substances, there is strict monitoring of the prescribing of these substances by general practitioners (GPs); in Australia, some doctors have been struck off for prescribing AAS to patients for body building and physical conditioning (e.g. Medical Board of Australia v Singh). The concern about medical practitioner involvement in the supply of PIEDs to athletes led WADA to include medical practitioners (along with other athlete support personnel) in their anti-doping Code; section 21.2 outlines the roles and responsibilities for athlete support personnel, of which the failure to comply may lead to disciplinary action (World Anti-Doping Agency,

2021c). Taken together, medical practitioners may face disciplinary action from medical boards, governments, anti-doping agencies or a combination of these if they prescribed these drugs for reasons other than what they have been approved or if they fail to act to prevent someone from taking them.

PIEDs are also unique in that while harm may result from use, there is no evidence of widespread individual or social harm comparable with other substances (Dunn et al., 2013). For example, intravenous injection of drugs such as heroin may result in a number of physical and psychological harms, with the most pressing being the risk of immediate overdose. Other harms may be related to the way the drug is used; injection drug use may lead to harms such as abscesses or place a consumer at risk for blood-borne virus through needle or syringe sharing. PIEDs such as AAS are either consumed orally or, if injected, are done so intramuscularly, which may place the consumer at a lower risk for blood-borne viruses. Harms such as the diminishment of the body's natural testosterone production, are known to reverse once exogenous testosterone is ceased. Most side effects experienced by PIED consumers, such as fluid retention, acne and even gynecomastia, are anticipated, with harm reduction strategies put in place to address them (Frude et al., 2020; Tighe et al., 2017). Due in part because the harms from these substances differ substantially to those of other substances, and in part because the motivations underlying the use of these substances differ from those of other substances, research has shown that healthcare professionals lack knowledge about these substances, even those who work in the alcohol and other drugs field (Dunn et al., 2014); additionally, research with PIED consumers has consistently shown that consumers believe that medical practitioners lack knowledge about PIED use and harm (Griffiths et al., 2016; Tighe et al., 2017; Underwood et al., 2020). While PIED consumers are concerned about their health and do seek medical advice when experiencing harm (Tighe et al., 2017), they are not the first group that consumers turn to; instead, social networks involving other PIED consumers appear to be more preferred and trusted options. This may not be a surprise, given that peers and social networks have consistently been important components of this community. As Tighe et al. (2017) discuss, the networks within the PIED consuming com munity have been important not only for the sharing of information regarding what compound to use, when to use it, and why, but also in facilitating access to actual compounds themselves as well as injecting equipment. While information sharing traditionally took them from of underground handbooks, magazines, as well as scientific literature, this information sharing has now moved online. So why is a consumer's work-out buddy, or a faceless person at the other end of an internet connection, trusted more than a medical doctor? There are a number of reasons why this may be the case, although the predominant reason appears to be related to trust. PIED consumers do not trust that most medical professionals possess the specific knowledge to help them if they encounter harm from their PIED use; they do trust others within their community of other PIED consumers, whatever this PIED community may be, however it is constructed and whomever fits within it. Monaghan (2012), in discussing bodybuilders in South Wales, writes that they '...usually only admitted to taking steroids when among people whom

Goffman (1968) would term "the own and the wise" – that is, people of like body and/or mind who understand the social situation of pro-steroid bodybuilders'. The shared experience, and understanding of that experience, may facilitate trust in a way that any doctor–patient relationship could hope to achieve.

The role medical practitioners may play in facilitating or preventing doping, or responding to the harms that come from doping, appears to vary depending on the lens which is adopted to investigate the behaviour. In elite sport, healthcare workers and those in the (human) organized sports world play a major part in the illegal supply of doping products. In their examination of the supply of doping products in Italy, Paoli and Donati (2013) identify five main categories of suppliers of doping products in Italy. Of those, one was 'health care' and the other '(human) organised sports world'. The former category includes pharmacists and physicians. The authors note that pharmacists sell doping products but may also produce their own. Their involvement in illegally selling doping products may be unwitting – they may sell products which have been obtained through stolen or false prescriptions, or prescriptions written by 'accommodating or corrupt physicians' (Paoli & Donati, 2013, p. 14). The inclusion of physicians also makes intuitive sense, and the authors note two high-profile Italian physicians who have been involved in doping: Francesco Conconi, and his student Michele Ferrari. In the latter category, the authors include staff members of sports teams and federations. However, elite sports is a small part of the doping 'world' and is often a closed system which is difficult to penetrate to understand how doping operates. Outside of this world, and more relevant for 'grassroots' and non-competitive athletes, there is a good volume of literature exploring the opinions and beliefs of medical practitioners towards doping (Backhouse & McKenna, 2011), and there is some literature exploring either attitudes of consumers towards medical practitioners (Pope et al., 2004). In their review of medical practitioners' knowledge, beliefs and attitudes towards doping in sport, Backhouse and McKenna found '…a negative attitude towards doping in sport prevails but this is combined with a lack of doping knowledge, a feeling of insufficient anti-doping training and a limited confidence in current prevention efforts' (p. 201). This aligns with the findings from the study by Pope et al. which explored AAS consumers' attitudes towards physicians, which found that AAS consumers have little trust in physician's knowledge about AAS. The authors suggest that this finding might be related to the decades that the medical community has spent suggesting that AAS are ineffectual or only mildly effective in producing strength or muscular gains; they further suggest that AAS consumers may see medical practitioners as 'outsiders' to the bodybuilding community and possibly unworthy of respect.

In summation, the research suggests that medical practitioners lack knowledge about PIED use, and consumers experience this, which leads to consumers not engaging with medical practitioners. While it is important to investigate attitudes, opinions and beliefs, these may be different from actual experiences. As such, the aim of this review is to amalgamate the extant literature that has investigated the experiences of healthcare professionals with PIED consumers and the experiences of PIED consumers with healthcare professionals, with a specific focus on medical practitioners.

METHODOLOGY

A systematic search was undertaken to identify studies that explored the experiences and perspectives of healthcare providers working with clients who use PIEDs, as well as to identify studies that explored the experiences and perspectives of PIED consumers with healthcare providers. The key search terms were (doping OR steroid* OR 'performance enhanc*') AND (prevent* OR 'harm reduction' OR knowledge OR 'help seek*' OR 'harm minimi?ation') AND 'service provider*' OR clinician* OR doctor* OR 'general practitioner*' OR trainer*). Searched databases included EBSCOhost (including Academic Search Complete, CINAHL Complete, Global Health, MEDLINE and SPORTDiscus). No limits were placed on publication dates. Only peer-reviewed articles published in English were considered; unpublished articles, books, theses, dissertations and non-peer-reviewed articles were excluded. Studies which explored only opinions, attitudes or beliefs from either healthcare providers or consumers, and did not include any measure of actual engagement, were excluded.

The author reviewed all articles to identify relevant studies. Articles underwent a three-step process (see Fig. 1). All articles were downloaded into Endnote X9, with duplicates identified and removed. Articles were first screened by title and abstract based on the inclusion and exclusion criteria, and any article that clearly did not meet the criteria was removed at this stage; any that did, or could possibly meet the criteria on further inspection, was retained. The full text of the remaining articles was obtained for further assessment. Any article which at this stage did not clearly meet the criteria was excluded. Where the author was unsure whether an article met the criteria, a colleague with expertise in conducting systematic reviews but not in the field of PIEDs was consulted. Articles were included if they contained data obtained from surveys or interviews with either healthcare professionals who come into contact with PIED consumers (including professional athletes) or data obtained from surveys or interviews with PIED consumers regarding their interactions with healthcare professionals. For the purposes of this review, a healthcare professional was defined as a GP/medical doctor, clinician or sports/athletic trainer.

Data were extracted from each article by the author. Data extracted at this stage included author/s and year; country; sample; design and method of data collection; and key findings relevant to this review.

FINDINGS

The search identified 2,592 articles, of which 789 were duplicates. The titles and abstracts of the 1,803 remaining articles were read, with 1,700 articles excluded as they did not meet the criteria, leaving 103 articles for further investigation. The full text of the 103 articles was reviewed; of these, 93 were excluded as they did not meet the inclusion criteria on closer inspection. The remaining 10 studies were included. Of these, four were focused on healthcare professionals (see Table 1)

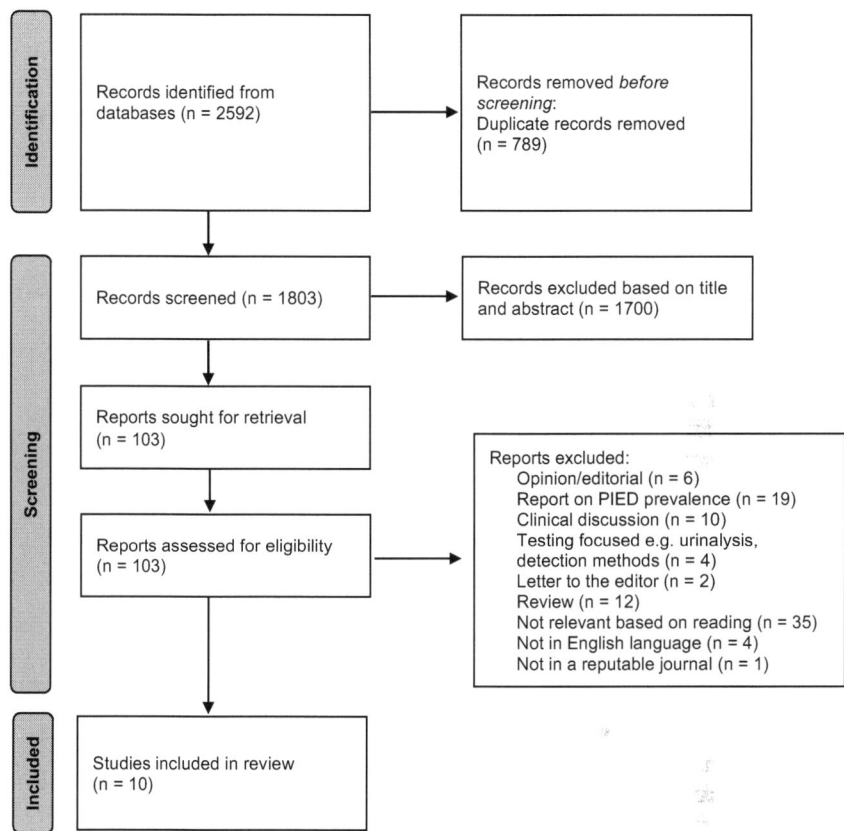

Fig. 1.   Search Strategy.

and six were focused on consumers (Table 2). The reference list of all the included articles was searched, though no new studies were identified.

Healthcare Professionals

Four studies focused on the experiences of healthcare professionals with PIED consumers. One study each came from Australia (Gupta & Towler, 1997), France (Laure et al., 2003), Ireland (Woods & Moynihan, 2009) and Slovenia (Auersperger et al., 2012). In terms of the samples, GPs were the sole focus of three studies (Gupta & Towler, 1997; Laure et al., 2003; Woods & Moynihan, 2009) while one study included GPs and pharmacists (Auersperger et al., 2012). Males represented an average of 59% of respondents. Two studies reported the mean age of participants (Laure et al., 2003; Woods & Moynihan, 2009); one study reported the median age (Gupta & Towler, 1997), while one study reported the percentage of participants within a specific age range (Auersperger et al., 2012),

Table 1. Health Professional Studies Included in This Review.

Authors (Year)	Country	Sample	Design and Method	Findings
Gupta and Towler (1997)	Australia	143 general practitioners (GPs) from the Central Business District of Sydney, Australia Response rate = 87% Median age = 46 years (range 26–80); 69% male; 70% practising full-time; 17% reporting an interest in sports medicine	• Cross-sectional • Survey	• 53% reported seeing at least one patient in the past year who told them they had used AAS for non-medical purposes • 34% suspected AAS usage by at least one patient in the past year • 2% ($n = 3$) stated explicitly that they had prescribed AAS for bodybuilding purposes • 21% knew of at least one GP in New South Wales (NSW) who prescribed AAS for non-medical purposes
Laure et al. (2003)	France	202 GPs Response rate 51% Mean age = 45.6 years; 75.5% male; 18% claimed a sports medicine qualification	• Cross-sectional • Telephone interview	• 37% reported being directly confronted by a request for information about doping agents in the past 12 months • 11% reported being directly confronted with a request for the prescription of doping agents in the past 12 months; these were mainly anabolic steroids, stimulants and corticosteroids • 14% believed that they had prescribed a medication to a patient for treatment that was really used by an athlete to improve sporting performance in the past 12 months
Woods and Moynihan (2009)	Ireland	771 GPs Response rate = 37% Mean age = 46 years (range 28–74); 62% male 12% had completed specific modules in doping or sport 24% currently connected with a specific sport as a team doctor or advisor	• Cross-sectional • Survey	• 28% had previously been consulted for advice on doping, with respondents listing advice on areas such as nutritional supplementation ($n = 162$), particular banned substances ($n = 130$), list of prohibited substances ($n = 95$), health risks of doping ($n = 84$), anti-doping regulations ($n = 59$), side effects of doping ($n = 57$) and other ($n = 16$) • 12% indicated they had received a request for anabolic steroids from a coach or an athlete without medical indications • 6% had received requests for other prohibited substances without medical indications

| Auersperger et al. (2012) | Slovenia | 204; 133 GPs and 71 Pharmacists
Overall response rate 21%; 65.2% response rate for GPs, 34.8% Pharmacists
About 70% in both groups were female
78.3% of GPs aged between 36 and 55 years
60% of pharmacists aged between 26 and 45 years | • Cross-sectional
• Survey | • 3% felt they had prescribed medication for what may have been deemed legitimate medical reasons but subsequently felt the substance was used by an athlete to improve sporting performance
• 8.4% reported personally knowing an athlete using doping agents (12.2% GPs, 1.4% Pharmacists)
• 36.6% of GPs and 46.2% of Pharmacists had been directly confronted with a request for information about doping in the past 12 months
• 12.2% had a direct request for prescription of doping agents during the previous 12 months (stimulants, 24%; anabolic agents, 18%; hormones, 22%; corticosteroids, 10%) |

Table 2. Consumer Studies Included in This Review.

Authors (Year)	Country	Sample	Design and Method	Findings
Pope et al. (2004)	United States	80 weightlifters, of which 43 were AAS users Mean age AAS users = 29.7 years 100% male 100% heterosexual	• Cross-sectional • Survey	• 44% ($n = 16$) of AAS users disclosed their AAS use to any physician they had ever seen (Pope et al., 2004)
Nieper (2005)	United Kingdom	32 track and field athletes selected for the Great Britain junior team and participating at the IAAF 2004 World Junior Championships Response rate = 94% Mean age = 18 years 63% male	• Cross-sectional • Survey	• 58% checked with the medical team before taking supplements
Hope et al. (2015)	United Kingdom	366 PIED injectors Median age = 28 years [of those who reported their age]; 28% < 25 years 100% male	• Cross-sectional • Survey	• 43% had seen a GP in the preceding year about their health, with 14% reporting a visit to a GP that was related to their PIED use • 15% had received advice from an emergency clinic in the preceding year, and 41% had done so more than once • 7% of the entire sample had sought treatment for having redness, tenderness and swelling at an injection site; this was most often done through a GP (59%) or emergency clinic (48%) or self-treatment (48%)
Rowe et al. (2017)	Australia	605 PIED injectors Mean age = 28.8 years 100% male 71.1% from culturally and linguistically diverse backgrounds; 86% born in Australia 976.6% heterosexual	• Cross-sectional • Survey	• 63.1% had disclosed their PIED use to a doctor • 51.6% had visited a doctor with one month • For PIEDs and injecting advice, 42.9% went to 'mates', 40.1% went to the internet, 33.9% went to doctors, 21.2% went to needle and syringe program staff, and 15.7% went to nurses • Men who had told a doctor about using PIEDs were more likely to have had PIEDs-related blood tests (N = 551, 82.2% vs. 29.1%, $p < 0.001$), and more likely to have ever been tested for hepatitis B (N = 502, 53.6% vs. 35.1%, $p < 0.001$), hepatitis C (N = 502, 52.1% vs. 35.1%, $p < 0.001$) or HIV (N = 502, 48.9% vs. 30.3%, $p < 0.001$)

Zahnow et al. (2017)	Global	195 AAS consumers who reported past 12 month AAS use + experienced concerns with adverse effects related to PIED use, from a sample of 1,000 lifetime AAS consumers representing 1.1% of the Global Drug Survey respondents Mean age 29.8 years (range 17–72) 79.56% male Region of residence: Europe 52.2%, North America 10.69%, South America 19.18%, Oceania 16.04% 82.70% Caucasian Only AAS in past year 54.72%	• Cross-sectional • Survey	• 35.23% reported visiting a doctor within the last year in relation to AAS use; 86.76% male; AAS users who engaged with health services were significantly older than those who did not • Of those who reported visiting a doctor in the past year, 79.41% reported receiving a physical examination and 80.88% reported receiving blood tests to assess liver function; 33.82% reported having a discussion about their mood and 38.42% reported receiving an ECG to assess cardiac health • 67.36% did not visit a doctor despite being worried about adverse effects from AAS use; most frequently cited reason was that the condition was not significant enough (53.85%), not confident the doctor had the knowledge to help (23.85%) or concerned about shame/stigma associated with use (22.31%); 13.85% did not think their doctor would be willing to help
Hill and Waring (2019)[a]	United Kingdom	216 AAS users 90% completion rate	• Cross-sectional • Survey	• 24 of 108 (22%) respondents relied on a National Health Service (NHS) doctor to interpret lab data, whereas 50% consulted a private specialist, 6% relied upon interpretation by a nonmedical friend and 22% relied on other general resources to interpret the lab data • 49% cited barriers to accessing health care, including fear of judgement by healthcare professionals (26%), perceived lack of knowledge of AAS by medical community (7.5%), healthcare professionals unwilling to arrange testing (13%), costs being prohibitive (13%), did not know where to get tests (8%), did not want AAS use on health records (7%) • 136 of 189 (72%) respondents reported a perceived judgemental attitude from their healthcare providers regarding AAS use, and 107 of 194 respondents held back seeking medical advice because of fear of judgement regarding AAS use

[a]Study surveyed consumers and professionals. The data presented here are from the consumer component only.
Source: Pope et al. (2004).

making it difficult to provide an average for the four studies. Small proportions of the samples reported either having completed a sports medicine course (Laure et al., 2003), having an interest in sports medicine (Gupta & Towler, 1997), or completing modules related to doping or sports (Woods & Moynihan, 2009). All the studies were quantitative, employing a cross-sectional design with surveys (Auersperger et al., 2012; Gupta & Towler, 1997; Woods & Moynihan, 2009) or interviews (Laure et al., 2003) utilized.

Despite the differences in focus, and thus reporting, the studies generally showed that GPs and pharmacists reported coming into contact with PIED consumers. Sizeable proportions from the studies reported being approached directly for information regarding PIEDs, ranging from 28% (Woods & Moynihan, 2009) to 36.6% (Auersperger et al., 2012) and 37% of GPs (Laure et al., 2003), and 46.2% of pharmacists (Auersperger et al., 2012). Three studies reported on whether participants had been asked for doping agents without a prescription. Eleven and 12% of GPs in the studies by Laure et al. (2003) and Auersperger et al. (2012) respectively reported having had a direct request for the prescription of doping agents during the previous 12 months; in the study by Woods and Moynihan (2009), 12% indicated they had received a request for anabolic steroids from a coach or an athlete without medical indication and 6% for other doping agents without medical indication. Fourteen percent of participants in the study conducted by Laure et al. (2003) and 34% of participants in the study conducted by Gupta and Towler (1997) suspected that they had prescribed substances which were subsequently used for enhancement purposes.

Consumers

Six studies focused on the experiences of PIED consumers with healthcare professionals. Three studies came from the United Kingdom (Hill & Waring, 2019; Hope et al., 2015; Nieper, 2005), while one study came from Australia (Rowe et al., 2017) and one from the United States (Pope et al., 2004); one study was based on data collected from participants located worldwide, with just over half of the respondents included in the analysis from Europe (Zahnow et al., 2017). Five studies focused upon AAS consumers in general (Hill & Waring, 2019; Hope et al., 2015; Pope et al., 2004; Rowe et al., 2017; Zahnow et al., 2017), whereas one study focused on junior athletes and focused on supplement use rather than doping (Nieper, 2005). Three studies had samples comprised solely of males (Hope et al., 2015; Pope et al., 2004; Rowe et al., 2017); two studies included both males and females, though both with a higher proportion of males than females (Nieper, 2005; Zahnow et al., 2017); and one study did not provide detailed demographics of the participants (Hill & Waring, 2019). All the studies were quantitative, employing a cross-sectional design with surveys.

While all five studies explored health professional engagement, their aims were sufficiently different to make comparisons difficult. For instance, the only study which explicitly included professional athletes (Nieper, 2005) focused on nutritional supplement practices rather than doping, and was focused on use, reasons for use, knowledge and sources of information. This study found that 58% of participants checked with the medical team before taking supplements. One study investigated perceptions between consumers and healthcare professionals (Hill & Waring, 2019); the consumer data relevant to this review indicated that while consumers use a variety of sources to interpret lab data from blood tests to monitor health, a quarter (22%) report using a National Health Seervice (NHS) doctor. This is lower than the proportion who reported using a private specialist (50%) (Hill & Waring, 2019).

Three studies investigated health service utilization among respondents, though again the aims of each study differed. Between 35% and 43% of respondents in two studies (Hope et al., 2015; Zahnow et al., 2017) reported seeing a GP in the preceding year about their health (Hope et al., 2015) or their AAS use (Zahnow et al., 2017). Half (51.6%) of participants in the study by Rowe et al. (2017) had visited a doctor within the past month. When seeking advice or treatment, a similar proportion of participants in the studies by Rowe, Berger and Copeland and Hope et al. went to some form of emergency or health service; however, the study by Rowe and colleagues demonstrated that participants seek advice from friends or the internet in higher proportions than from an actual health professional. Two studies explored lack of access or barriers to access to health services (Hill & Waring, 2019; Zahnow et al., 2017). Half of the participants in the study by Hill cited barriers to service access, with fear of judgement by healthcare professionals (26%) and perceived lack of knowledge of AAS by medical community (7.5%) cited as reasons. Almost 70% of participants in the study by Zahnow et al. reported not visiting a doctor despite being worried about adverse effects from AAS use, and while the largest proportion nominated that the condition was not serious enough to warrant seeking treatment, one quarter were not confident that the doctor had the knowledge to help, and a similar proportion were concerned about stigma/shame. One study, which investigated AAS consumers' attitudes towards physicians, found that 44% had never disclosed their AAS to any physician ever (Pope et al., 2004).

IMPLICATIONS

The aim of this systematic review was to amalgamate the extant literature that has investigated the experiences of healthcare professionals with PIED consumers and the experiences of PIED consumers with healthcare professionals, with a specific focus on medical practitioners. Only 10 articles were located, with four studies exploring the professionals' experiences and six exploring the consumers' experiences. The findings indicate that a sizeable proportion of healthcare providers come into contact with PIED consumers, with these interactions mostly related to consumers asking for information, though a small but significant proportion indicate they have been asked to prescribed doping agents, and a number indicating that they believe they have prescribed substances which have been used for non-medical purposes. Of the six studies which focused on the consumer experience, five focused on PIED consumers; these studies found that while large proportions reporting accessing a medical practitioner, larger proportions did not, with the doctor's lack of knowledge cited as one reason.

Healthcare professionals, in particular medical practitioners, operate in a unique space with regard to PIEDs. They often have the knowledge of the medical indications for those substances with therapeutic uses but lack the knowledge regarding how these substances are used non-medically for enhancement purposes. Furthermore, they may hold negative attitudes and beliefs towards PIED use for non-medical reasons. PIED consumers hold these beliefs about healthcare professionals, who are seen as lacking knowledge and being judgemental about PIED use. These attitudes and beliefs may impair a professional's ability to treat PIED consumers, who in turn may be reluctant to seek treatment for fear of judgement. This misalignment may create a tension, in that PIED consumers may want or need to seek medical attention, but medical practitioners may not be able to provide it.

A further tension exists within the healthcare community – and more specifically, the medical community – regarding the prescribing of and responding to harms associated with these substances. Some medical practitioners may be willing to work with those who take PIEDs, but work in a tight regulatory framework where medicines are approved for specific reasons to treat specific conditions which render them unable to work in this space. This thus hinders them to provide the type of care that PIED consumers may want, which in turn may present a negative perception to consumers. As Dunn et al. (2014) surmised, '…the stigma that [consumers] report experiencing may actually be an attempt by medical practitioners to engage in prevention, based on their belief that this is the best for the individual's health (p. 382)'.

Limitations

There are limitations to the current review. Firstly, the review had a broad remit, in that it sought to identify studies which focused on two groups (healthcare professionals and consumers), which are themselves both broad groups. As such, the search strategy was deliberately designed to reflect this. As with any review, it may be the case that studies were not identified; however, the number of databases and search terms utilized does lend credence to the idea that a large proportion of the relevant studies were identified. Secondly, grey literature was not included in the search, and while it could be presumed that any grey literature would have been cited in the included articles and picked up in a reference list search, the included studies are not recent, and thus grey literature published since 2012 would not have been cited. Thirdly, the review excluded certain healthcare professionals, such as needle and syringe programme (NSP) workers, and thus studies which focused on this group, or access to these services, were not included. The focus on professionals such as GPs was deliberate, in that they can prescribe substances considered PIEDs, but also fall under a country's laws regarding prescribing practices or be sanctioned under the WADA Code if they work with athletes. Finally, while the included studies had similar designs and broadly similar approaches to collecting data, the differences in questionnaires (and thus the questions asked) does make it difficult to make firm comparisons. That all the studies included in this review were quantitative is not a limitation of the review per se, but a limitation of the field of literature on this topic. Qualitative research provides us with the understanding of behaviours, experiences, intentions and attitudes; without these data, it is difficult to contextualize the quantitative data that has been collected. Why does a GP react to a patient asking them to prescribe steroids in a certain way? Why does stigma stop a PIED consumer from seeking medical assistance when they experience negative side effects? There are many gaps in our knowledge on this topic that need to be filled, and so this is a call to action for researchers in this field: we need qualitative research to unpack the quantitative data that have already been collected.

CONCLUSIONS

There is a small volume of literature exploring the experiences and perspectives of healthcare providers working with clients who use PIEDs, as well as studies exploring the experiences and perspectives of PIED consumers with healthcare providers. Given that medical practitioners may have a unique role when it comes to these substances and addressing associated harms, more research is needed to investigate how they come into contact with this group of consumers, their level of knowledge and any training that they may need. Given the harms associated with PIED use, and the lack of disclosure of use to healthcare providers, more research is needed to understand the barriers and facilitators for consumers to accessing health care.

KEY READINGS

(1) Backhouse, S. H., & McKenna, J. (2011). Doping in sport: A review of medical practitioners' knowledge, attitudes and beliefs. *International Journal of Drug Policy*, *22*(3), 198–202. https://doi.org/10.1016/j.drugpo.2011.03.002

This review, while slightly dated now, provides the reader with a good starting point for developing resources aimed at educating medical practitioners on their role and responsibilities when it comes to elite athletes and the WADA Code.

(2) Dunn, M., McKay, F. H., & Iversen, J. (2014). Steroid users and the unique challenge they pose to needle and syringe program (NSP) workers. *Drug and Alcohol Review*, *33*(1), 71–77. https://doi.org/10.1111/dar.12085

This study highlighted how many frontline health workers who come into contact with PIED consumer – in this case, needle and syringe programme workers – lack the knowledge to work effectively with this client group, and provides some suggestions for developing resources to support this workforce group.

(3) Pope, H. G., Kanayama, G., Ionescu-Pioggia, M., & Hudson J. I. (2004a). Anabolic steroid users' attitudes towards physicians. *Addiction*, *99*(9), 1189–94. https://doi.org/10.1111/j.1360-0443.2004.00781.x

This study provides the reader a good insight into why PIED consumers do not engage with the medical workforce.

(4) Tighe, B., Dunn, M., McKay, F. H., & Piatkowski, T. (2017). Information sought, information shared: Exploring performance and image enhancing drug user-facilitated harm reduction information in online forums. *Harm Reduction Journal, 14*(1), 48. https://doi.org/10.1186/s12954-017-0176-8

PIED consumers are quite knowledgeable about what compounds they intend to use, why they intend to use them and the effects (both positive and negative) that may arise, and the community is an important source of knowledge. This study gives the reader insight into how these online communities operate and how this knowledge can be incorporated into practice.

(5) Underwood, M., van de Ven, K., & Dunn, M. (2020, September). Testing the boundaries: Self-medicated testosterone replacement and why it is practised. *International Journal of Drug Policy, 95*, 103087. https://doi.org/10.1016/j.drugpo.2020.103087

This study gives the reader insight to an emerging issue – the use of these compounds not specifically for body or performance issues, but to help achieve optimal 'health'.

REFERENCES

Auersperger, I., Topič, M. D., Maver, P., Pušnik, V. K., Osredkar, J., & Lainščak, M. (2012). Doping awareness, views, and experience: A comparison between general practitioners and pharmacists. *Wiener Klinische Wochenschrift, 124*(1–2), 32–38. https://doi.org/10.1007/s00508-011-0077-x

Backhouse, S. H., & McKenna, J. (2011). Doping in sport: A review of medical practitioners' knowledge, attitudes and beliefs. *International Journal of Drug Policy, 22*(3), 198–202. https://doi.org/10.1016/j.drugpo.2011.03.002

Bahrke, M. S., & Yesalis, C. E. (2002). *Performance-enhancing substances in sport and exercise.* Human Kinetics.

Bonomo, Y., Norman, A., Biondo, S., Bruno, R., Daglish, M., Dawe, S., Egerton-Warburton, D., Karro, J., Kim, C., Lenton, S., Lubman, D. I., Pastor, A., Rundle, J., Ryan, J., Gordon, P., Sharry, P., Nutt, D., & Castle, D. (2019). The Australian drug harms ranking study. *Journal of Psychopharmacology, 33*(7), 759–768. https://doi.org/10.1177/0269881119841569

Dunn, M. (2017). Have prohibition policies made the wrong decision? A critical review of studies investigating the effects of DMAA. *International Journal of Drug Policy, 40*, 26–34. https://doi.org/10.1016/j.drugpo.2016.10.005

Dunn, M., Cooper, A., & Farrell, M. (2013). Performance and image enhancing drug users: The forgotten injectors? *Drug and Alcohol Review, 32*(S1), 34.

Dunn, M., McKay, F. H., & Iversen, J. (2014). Steroid users and the unique challenge they pose to needle and syringe program (NSP) workers. *Drug and Alcohol Review, 33*(1), 71–77.

Dunn, M., & Thomas, J. O. (2012). A risk profile of elite Australian athletes who use illicit drugs. *Addictive Behaviors, 37*, 144–147.

Dunn, M., Thomas, J. O., Swift, W., & Burns, L. (2011). Recreational substance use among elite Australian athletes. *Drug and Alcohol Review, 30*, 63–68. http://doi.org/10.1111/j.1465-3362.2010.00200.x

Frude, E., McKay, F. H., & Dunn, M. (2020). A focused netnographic study exploring experiences associated with counterfeit and contaminated anabolic-androgenic steroids. *Harm Reduction Journal, 17*(1), 42. https://doi.org/10.1186/s12954-020-00387-y

Griffiths, S., Henshaw, R., McKay, F. H., & Dunn, M. (2016). Post-cycle therapy for performance and image enhancing drug users: A qualitative investigation. *Performance Enhancement & Health, 5*(3), 103.

Gupta, L., & Towler, B. (1997). General practitioners' views and knowledge about anabolic steroid use-survey of GPs in a high prevalence area. *Drug and Alcohol Review, 16*(4), 373–379. https://ezproxy.deakin.edu.au/login?url=https://search.ebscohost.com/login.aspx?direct=true&db=edb&AN=63544664&site=eds-live&scope=site

Hamilton, T., & Coyle, D. (2012). *The secret race.* Transworld Publishers.

Hill, S., & Waring, W. (2019). Pharmacological effects and safety monitoring of anabolic androgenic steroid use: Differing perceptions between users and healthcare professionals. *Therapeutic Advances in Drug Safety, 10.* https://doi.org/10.1177/2042098619855291

Hope, V. D., McVeigh, J., Marongiu, A., Evans-Brown, M., Smith, J., Kimergard, A., Parry, J. V. & Ncube, F. (2015). Injection site infections and injuries in men who inject image-and performance-enhancing drugs: Prevalence, risks factors, and healthcare seeking. *Epidemiology and Infection, 143*(1), 132–140. https://ezproxy.deakin.edu.au/login?url=https://search.ebscohost.com/login.aspx?direct=true&db=edb&AN=99893647&site=eds-live&scope=site

Laure, P., Binsinger, C., Lecerf, T., Laure, P., Binsinger, C., & Lecerf, T. (2003). General practitioners and doping in sport: Attitudes and experience...including commentary by Ayotte C. *British Journal of Sports Medicine, 37*(4), 335–338. https://doi.org/10.1136/bjsm.37.4.335

Monaghan, L. F. (2012). Accounting for illicit steroid use: Bodybuilder's justifications. In A. Locks & N. Richardson (Eds.), *Critical readings in bodybuilding.* Routledge.

Nieper, A. (2005). Nutritional supplement practices in UK junior national track and field athletes. *British Journal of Sports Medicine, 39*(9), 645–649. https://doi.org/10.1136/bjsm.2004.015842

Nutt, D. J., King, L. A., & Phillips, L. D. (2010). Drug harms in the UK: A multicriteria decision analysis. *Lancet, 376*(9752), 1558–1565. https://doi.org/10.1016/s0140-6736(10)61462-6

Paoli, L., & Donati, A. (2013). The supply of doping products and the potential of criminal law enforcement in anti-doping: AN examination of Italy's experience. Retrieved from Montreal.

Pope, H. G., Jr., Kanayama, G., Ionescu-Pioggia, M., & Hudson, J. I. (2004). Anabolic steroid users' attitudes towards physicians. *Addiction, 99,* 1189–1194.

Rowe, R., Berger, I., & Copeland, J. (2017). "No pain, no gainz"? Performance and image-enhancing drugs, health effects and information seeking. *Drugs: Education, Prevention & Policy, 24*(5), 400–408. https://doi.org/0.1080/09687637.2016.1207752

Thomas, J. O., Dunn, M., Swift, W., & Burns, L. (2011). Illicit drug knowledge and information-seeking behaviours among elite athletes. *Journal of Science and Medicine in Sport, 14,* 278–282. https://doi.org/10.1016/j.jsams.2011.02.001

Tighe, B., Dunn, M., McKay, F. H., & Piatkowski, T. (2017). Information sought, information shared: Exploring performance and image enhancing drug user-facilitated harm reduction information in online forums. *Harm Reduction Journal, 14,* 48.

Underwood, M., van de Ven, K., & Dunn, M. (2020). Testing the boundaries: Self-medicated testosterone replacement and why it is practised. *International Journal of Drug Policy,* 103087. https://doi.org/10.1016/j.drugpo.2020.103087

United States Anti-Doping Agency. (2012). *Reasoned decision of the United States Anti-Doping Agency on disqualification and ineligibility.* Retrieved from Colorado.

van Amsterdam, J., Nutt, D., Phillips, L., & van den Brink, W. (2015). European rating of drug harms. *Journal of Psychopharmacology, 29*(6), 655–660. https://doi.org/10.1177/0269881115581980

van de Ven, K., Dunn, M., & Mulrooney, K. (2018). Performance and image enhancing drug (PIED) producers and suppliers: A retrospective content analysis of PIED-provider cases in Australia from 2010–2016. *Trends in Organized Crime.* https://doi.org/10.1007/s12117-018-9348-5

Woods, C. B., & Moynihan, A. (2009). General practitioners knowledge, practice and training requirements in relation to doping in sport. *Irish Medical Journal, 102*(1). https://ezproxy. deakin.edu.au/login?url=https://search.ebscohost.com/login.aspx? direct=true&db=edselc&AN=edselc.2-52.0-65349187523&site=eds-live&scope=site

World Anti-Doping Agency. (2021a). Prohibited list 2021. https://www.wada-ama.org/en/resources/ science-medicine/prohibited-list-documents

World Anti-Doping Agency. (2021b). Summary of the review of the USADA 'Nike Oregon Project' investigation. Retrieved from Montreal.

World Anti-Doping Agency. (2021c). *World Anti-Doping Code*. Retrieved from Montreal, Quebec.

Zahnow, R., McVeigh, J., Ferris, J., & Winstock, A. (2017). Adverse effects, health service engagement, and service satisfaction among anabolic androgenic steroid users. *Contemporary Drug Problems, 44*(1), 69–83. https://doi.org/10.1177/0091450917694268

Chapter 6

TAKING 'THE GOD OF ALL STEROIDS' AND 'MAKING A PACT WITH THE DEVIL': ONLINE BODYBUILDING COMMUNITIES AND THE NEGOTIATION OF TRENBOLONE RISK

Mair Underwood

ABSTRACT

Previous research has found that people who use anabolic androgenic steroids (hereafter 'steroids') typically describe these drugs as safe. However, research exploring the inside perspective on steroid risk has focussed on steroids in general, and failed to examine how particular steroids are viewed and experienced. During my online ethnographic research in bodybuilding communities, I found discussion of one particular steroid said to cause significant physical, psychological, social and sexual harm: trenbolone. Trenbolone is a veterinary drug used to increase muscle in beef cattle that has been found to have neurodegenerative and genotoxic effects on animals. It has been used by bodybuilders since the 1980s, and recent research has found it to be one of the most popular steroids used by bodybuilders. If trenbolone is described by bodybuilders as causing significant harm, why do so many bodybuilders use it? This chapter attempts to answer this question through a description of bodybuilder folk models of trenbolone risk. Using a social life of drugs approach it describes: (1) the effects of trenbolone; (2) how these effects are given meaning as either harms or benefits, and then weighed against each other; (3) how the risks of trenbolone are reduced through harm reduction strategies and

Doping in Sport and Fitness
Research in the Sociology of Sport, Volume 16, 111–136
Copyright © 2023 by Emerald Publishing Limited
All rights of reproduction in any form reserved
ISSN: 1476-2854/doi:10.1108/S1476-285420220000016007

(4) the role of online communities in negotiations of trenbolone risk. Trenbolone was found to occupy a mythical status in bodybuilding communities, in part because of the conflicted relationship bodybuilders have with the drug. This conflicted relationship illustrates the inherent ambivalence of drugs, which are always both remedy and poison.

Keywords: Anabolic androgenic steroids; trenbolone; bodybuilding; online/digital research; ethnography; harm reduction

INTRODUCTION

All drug use entails risk. Drug risks are typically discussed from an outside perspective, that is, by those with limited experience of the drug such as scientists, policy makers and the media. This 'official' or 'professional' perspective takes a realist approach, seeing risks as pre-existing in nature, objective and scientifically measurable (Hunt et al., 2007). The official discourse on risk tends to focus on the individual who is 'at risk' in a way that isolates them from their cultural context.

Throughout history, science has remained largely ignorant of the inside perspective on risk, or the lived experience of risk in social and cultural contexts (Lupton, 2013). Lay perceptions of risk have been considered unscientific, inferior and unsophisticated (Hunt et al., 2007). But an understanding of drug risk based solely on professional models is incomplete (Kelly, 2005). Furthermore, the perspective of those at risk is the most important because it is what informs risk behaviours. It is only through ascertaining fuller understandings of 'folk models' of risk that we can understand why the folk act as they do (Kelly, 2005). Understanding folk models of risk allows us to eliminate the assumptions inherent in professional models of risk, and is the only way to provide an adequate foundation for policy and health promotion efforts (Kelly, 2005).

Anabolic Androgenic Steroid Risk

The outside, or official, discourse on risk has dominated our understanding of steroid risk. That is, steroid risks have been primarily defined and discussed by those with no lived experience of these drugs. Efforts to understand steroid risk focus on the objective measurement of risks that are approached as individual, natural and independent of their sociocultural context. This field of study has been, and continues to be, dominated by epidemiological and structural functionalist perspectives, typically employing quantitative measures (Andreasson & Johansson, 2019).

The steroid risk literature consists primarily of medical discussions of steroid risk, and surveys of harm and benefit (e.g. Cohen et al., 2007; Hope et al., 2013; Parkinson & Evans, 2006; Pope et al., 2014; Rowe et al., 2017; Smit & de Ronde, 2018; Van de Ven et al., 2018; Zahnow et al., 2018), and thus focusses on those risks (and benefits) deemed significant from an outside perspective. While this literature has contributed greatly to our understanding of steroid risk, those who actually face the risks of steroids sometimes disagree on the appropriateness of the focus of these outside discourses (Underwood, 2019).

In order to address the limitations of quantitative approaches, and to further understanding of the inside perspective on steroid risk, a significant amount of qualitative research has been conducted with those who use steroids (including Andreasson & Johansson, 2019; Dennington et al., 2008; Greenway & Price, 2018; Harris et al., 2016; Monaghan, 2011; Van Hout & Kean, 2015). This qualitative literature has added dimension to our understanding of steroid risk decisions by examining the diversity of steroid risk practices (e.g. Christiansen et al., 2017), by increasing the emphasis on the benefits of steroid use, and by examining steroid use in context.

One limitation of all literature on steroid risk, both quantitative and qualitative, is that it focusses on steroids in general. This places this literature at odds with the perspective of those who use steroids, who tend to discuss the risks of particular steroids. While there have been a few studies of specific image and performance enhancing drugs such as 2,4-Dinitrophenol (McVeigh et al., 2017), insulin (Ip et al., 2012), Ephedrine and Nubain (Monaghan et al., 2000), until now there has been no compound-specific study of a steroid.

Trenbolone

The dominant narrative in enhancement drug communities is that steroids are relatively safe and that most harms can be managed (Hanley Santos & Coomber, 2017; Kimergard, 2015; Kimergård & McVeigh, 2014; Monaghan, 2002). However, during my fieldwork I found many reports of harm from one particular steroid: trenbolone, or 'tren' as it is commonly termed in the community, so I set out to explore how trenbolone differed from other steroids.

Trenbolone, a non-17α-alkylated derivative of 19-nortestosterone, has three times the binding affinity of testosterone (Yarrow et al., 2010), making it one of the strongest injectable steroids ever commercially manufactured (Llewellyn, 2017). It is one of few steroids commonly used by bodybuilders that has been primarily manufactured for animals rather than humans (Equipoise and Winstrol are similar in this regard), and is primarily used to promote growth in beef cattle. Since the early 1970s trenbolone acetate has been used to increase weight gain and improve feed efficiency before slaughter in several countries such as Australia, New Zealand, The United States, Japan and various South American countries (Llewellyn, 2017). However, in many other parts of the world its use has been banned for decades. Trenbolone even caused an international trade dispute in 2014 when Russians claimed to have found traces of it in Australian beef.

Although trenbolone has primarily been manufactured for veterinary purposes, there was a period when a longer ester trenbolone, trenbolone hexahydrobenzylcarbonate, was manufactured for human consumption. From 1980 to 1997 the French pharmaceutical company Negma began manufacturing trenbolone hexahydrobenzylcarbonate (under the brand name 'Parabolan') to treat muscle wasting, malnutrition and osteoporosis.

Animal studies have demonstrated significant harms caused by trenbolone. For example, trenbolone has been found to have a neurodegenerative effect in rats (Ma & Liu, 2015). Trenbolone results in forced copulatory behaviours

(Bertram et al., 2015), complete sex reversal and increased mortality among fish exposed to it through agricultural run-off (Laggeson et al., 2019). Furthermore, trenbolone has been suggested to be genotoxic even at low concentrations (Boettcher et al., 2011).

Bodybuilders have been using trenbolone since the 1980s (Llewellyn, 2017). Veterinary pellets have been swallowed, inserted, snorted, or converted and injected (Llewellyn, 2011). Parabolan was also used during the period it was available. However, bodybuilders state that it was not until the increase in use of Chinese raw powders in underground steroid laboratories (c. 2005) that trenbolone became readily available and popular. Studies have found that trenbolone is one of the most frequently used anabolic compounds, with approximately 20% of enhanced bodybuilders reporting that they have used it within the last 12 months (Ip et al., 2011; Perry et al., 2005).

THE STUDY

This study is the first to pose the question: *why do bodybuilders use trenbolone?* It utilizes online sites as these are popular places for the discussion of steroid use decisions, the harms and benefits of use, and harm reduction strategies (Andreasson & Johansson, 2016; Harvey et al., 2019; Tighe et al., 2017; Underwood, 2017). Through an online ethnography of enhanced bodybuilding communities, this study explores trenbolone use decisions through three sub-questions:

(1) What are the benefits and risks/harms of trenbolone as understood/ experienced by bodybuilders?
(2) How are the risks/harms of trenbolone reduced through harm reduction practice?
(3) What role do online bodybuilding communities play in negotiations of trenbolone risk?

To understand the inside perspective on trenbolone risk, and to examine negotiations of this risk in context, I employ theory from two main areas: (1) sociocultural approaches to risk and (2) the social life of drugs.

Dichotomies such as person/thing, animate/inanimate and subject/object can impede the production of empirically nuanced accounts of drug use (Duff, 2013). The 'social life of things' (Appadurai, 1986) is an approach, developed within material culture studies, that is designed to challenge these dichotomies (Miller, 2010). When we approach drugs as having social lives it allows us to see not only the ways that people create drugs and give meaning to drugs through their interactions but also how drugs shape interactions between people (Whyte et al., 2002). That is, a social life of drugs approach allows us to examine both how people shape drugs, and how drugs shape people.

In order to examine the social life of trenbolone I approach risk from a sociocultural perspective. Although science has tended to focus on risks as objective, measurable and natural (as described above), social scientists have pointed out that judgements of relative safety or appropriate risk are almost entirely sociocultural (Oaks & Harthorn, 2003). That is, risk decisions are not made in a vacuum but are always social processes influenced by cultural frameworks (Kelly, 2005). Broader social, political, economic and cultural forces play themselves out at the local level, thus forming a context that shapes not only which dangers are faced but also perceptions of risk (Kelly, 2005). Following Douglas (1985, 1992) I argue that risks cannot be seen as uncontested facts isolated from their contexts, but rather certain dangers and hazards become defined as 'risks' within certain contexts. In what follows I therefore consider how the context shapes the dangers that are faced from trenbolone, how the risks of trenbolone are perceived, and how risks are defined.

APPROACH

In order to examine the social life of trenbolone, an ethnographic approach was taken. Ethnography allows for the examination of practices (like drug use) in context. It consists of both observation of a community and participation in that community. To explore trenbolone use decisions I created online profiles on social media and in online forums, and used them to participate in and observe (mostly closed) groups of enhanced bodybuilders for a period of four years. These groups are frequented by competitive and recreational bodybuilders and consist almost entirely of enhanced bodybuilders, although some bodybuilders use these sites to explore the possibility of enhancement. I also collected data from blogs, websites and YouTube videos.

While I have discussed steroid use with hundreds of bodybuilders (recreational and competitive), and observed thousands online, a core group of key cultural consultants informed this research. That is, in-depth interviews (face-to-face, phone and video conference) were conducted with 38 enhanced bodybuilders, all men, and all of whom were recreational bodybuilders, who acted as key cultural consultants and who I will refer to as 'participants'. These individuals were recruited primarily through online interactions in online enhanced bodybuilder communities, but some were recruited by other research participants, and some volunteered after the first author participated in a televised panel discussion. These participants were aged between 21 and 56 years (average 34 years) and were based in Australia ($n = 18$), the United States ($n = 12$), the United Kingdom ($n = 3$), Canada ($n = 2$), Germany ($n = 1$) and India ($n = 1$). These individuals had varying levels of experience with image and performance enhancing drugs, from a few months to decades, and three served as community experts advising other bodybuilders how to use steroids. In what follows I use pseudonyms for these participants so that individuals can be followed through the chapter and to distinguish them from the enhanced bodybuilders who I have had less in-depth contact with, or merely observed.

All of the data collected – interview transcripts, notes from observations and videos, and online interactions – concerned use of trenbolone by men (in enhanced bodybuilding communities trenbolone use by women is not advised because of its virilizing effects). These data were entered into NVivo 11, a qualitative analysis software program that aids coding and retrieval. Data were coded thematically with an emphasis on the enhanced bodybuilders' perspective. For example, I privileged bodybuilder definitions of things like risk and harm reduction over my own.

In what follows I attempt to prioritize the inside perspective on trenbolone in numerous ways. For example, I quote bodybuilders verbatim, with no correction of spelling or grammar (in the case of internet posts and online messages), so as to retain their authentic voices. In order to ensure that I represented the views of these communities as accurately as possible, drafts of the findings were circulated within enhanced bodybuilding communities for feedback. In this chapter I make no attempt to use scientific literature to critique bodybuilder understandings of the benefits and harms of trenbolone. Indeed, such efforts would be futile as the literature on trenbolone benefit and harm consists almost exclusively of animal studies. As a social scientist I am not trained to judge the transferability of animal studies to the human context, nor to judge bodybuilder efforts to theorize from this literature to their practice.[1]

Using the Association of Internet Researchers ethical guidelines for online research (Franzke et al., 2020), I made the following ethical decisions (which were approved by the University of Queensland Human Ethics Research Committee). I clearly identified myself as a researcher in all interactions through the use of the profile name 'Mair Underwood Researcher', and described the nature of the research in my profile, and to anyone I had ongoing interactions with. All participants gave their written consent to participate in the research. To protect the privacy and confidentiality of the enhanced bodybuilders I observed and interacted with, all identifying information was removed from the data prior to publication. Whilst there is a danger of re-identification posed by quoting individuals verbatim (as research participants could potentially be re-identified as a result of internet searches for their words), I have decided to use verbatim quotes because I deem re-identification unlikely. This is because: (1) social media comments are virtually impossible to find through internet searches; (2) most of the quotes were collected from groups that are closed to outsiders and (3) most individuals in online enhancement communities do not use their real names (because of the stigma, and, in some countries, illegality, of steroid use), so even if the original post was located it would not typically lead to identification of the individual.

FINDINGS

In this section I initially intended to describe the benefits and the harms of the drug, and how they are weighed and balanced through harm reduction efforts. However, this task was made difficult by the fact that sometimes the benefits of trenbolone could not easily be distinguished from the harms. Therefore, instead I describe the primary effects (the main reasons trenbolone is used) and the secondary effects (which may be unwelcomed or welcomed) of trenbolone. I then describe how these effects are assigned meaning through their categorization as benefits or harms, how the harms are reduced through harm reduction efforts, and how harms and benefits are weighed against each other in order to decide if trenbolone use is worth the risk. I then consider the place of trenbolone in bodybuilding culture and the role of online communities in the negotiation of trenbolone risk.

Primary Effects: 'The God of all Steroids'

Bodybuilders describe trenbolone as 'the most powerful anabolic', and sometimes as 'the perfect anabolic'. As trenbolone is more powerful than other steroids it can allow individuals more leeway in their bodybuilding practice:

> It [trenbolone] is so powerful it allows for so many holes in your approach to training and nutrition. It makes it an incredibly popular drug [Sean].

Trenbolone is also popular because of its versatility. Bodybuilding is done in two phases: a 'bulking' phase, when the bodybuilder gains muscle (typically with some unavoidable fat), and a 'cutting' phase, when the fat is stripped away to reveal the definition of the muscle (typically with some unavoidable muscle loss). Trenbolone is reported as being beneficial in terms of both preventing fat gain during bulking (i.e. bodybuilders can achieve a 'lean bulk') and preventing muscle loss during cutting. Indeed, trenbolone can allow bodybuilders to maintain, or even *gain*, muscle whilst cutting.

Another benefit of trenbolone is that it is a 'dry' compound in that there is no risk of water retention (whereas there is with other steroids). Trenbolone is described as producing a particularly valued look, which whilst achievable using other compounds, is particularly facilitated by trenbolone. Trenbolone is reported as making veins and muscles 'pop' [Edward, Carl, Robert], and as producing a '3D effect' [Robert, Brax, Oliver] or a 'comic book effect' [Leo] that is 'hard', 'dense' [Edward] and like 'granite' [Mark]. The incredibly defined aesthetic of trenbolone is valued in bodybuilding competitions, increasing the drugs appeal to competitive bodybuilders who use it as a hardening agent (Llewellyn, 2011). Indeed, some bodybuilders suggest that competitors who do not use trenbolone will fail to be competitive at the higher levels of bodybuilding competition [social media comments]. Furthermore, trenbolone may be particularly suited to changing bodybuilding ideals.

> Recently it's gone from big, massive, jacked dudes to sort of the model look. ... It's good for the compounds like tren, people are going to buy it more. Guys don't want to be massive bulky anymore. They want the dry compounds [Jock].

The power, versatility and particular aesthetic of this compound make trenbolone a very valuable tool for bodybuilding. These physical effects are the primary reason that trenbolone is used.

Secondary Effects

Whilst trenbolone is described as having powerful physical effects which are the primary reasons it is used, it also has secondary effects which may or may not be welcome. Welcome secondary effects may be described as secondary reasons for use. Secondary effects may be physical, psychological/social, sleep/energy-related, or related to sex and sexual relationships. There is incredible variation in the experience of these secondary effects, to the extent that sometimes descriptions of trenbolone appear to be contradictory.

Secondary Physical Effects: 'It's an Extremely Toxic Drug'
Trenbolone has significant physical effects in addition to those for which it is primarily used. Trenbolone is described by bodybuilders as having the same side effects as other steroids such as organ damage, an impact on cholesterol and blood pressure, acne, sweating and the exacerbation of male pattern hair loss. However, trenbolone is described as producing these side effects to a much greater degree, and at much lower doses, than other steroids.

> You have blood pressure spikes, blood noses ... It is a whole other level above everything else [Jack].

> It [trenbolone] causes damage to the liver, it blocks a bile duct, you can get acid reflux, upsets your blood pressure. I had to come off because my blood pressure got dangerously high and I had some side effects that weren't very conducive to staying alive, shall we say [Rocco].

Trenbolone is a steroid that is sometimes described in ways that run counter to the dominant narrative of steroids as 'safe'.

> It's an extremely toxic drug with a very wide range of far-reaching issues from direct kidney damage through to brain damage. It cannot be taken safely [Sean].

The increased sweating caused by steroids can become extreme with trenbolone use, with individuals describing it as embarrassing [Scott], and as looking 'suspicious' at work [social media post].

Trenbolone also has other side effects which it shares with 19-nortestosterone and its derivatives. One of those is neurotoxicity. Several bodybuilders complained about the impact of trenbolone on their cognitive functioning, for example:

> I swear tren made me dumber while on it. Like my IQ dropped to half [social media post].

There are some physical effects which were described as largely compound-specific. Firstly, trenbolone can cause a dry, persistent cough upon injection. This is known as 'tren cough'. Secondly, trenbolone can result in body fluids (sweat and urine) having a distinct smell: 'like a fucking corpse', like 'vinegar' or like a 'barnyard' [social media comments]. A third effect that I have seen attributed to trenbolone more than any other steroid is a significant decrease in cardiovascular fitness.

Effects on Sleep and Energy: 'Trensomnia', 'Trenergy' and 'Tren Lethargy'
Trenbolone has a complex relationship with energy levels as it can both increase ('trenergy') and reduce ('tren lethargy') energy.

> It was a mix of being completely tired and completely wired [i.e. elevated, excited or energised, especially from coffee or drugs] [forum comment].

The energizing effect of trenbolone is not always experienced as positive as some report an inability to relax or 'switch off'. Trenbolone is described as impacting on the quality and the quantity of sleep. Some individuals report only 2–3 hours' sleep per night on trenbolone (what has been termed 'trensomnia'), and many report disturbed sleep:

> It [trenbolone] always gave me horrible nightmares and really vivid dreams ... I'd literally wake up jumping just because it was that realistic, or I'd wake up screaming, or something [Brax].

> I had nightmares [on trenbolone] about being attacked one time I woke up to my gf [girlfriend] at the time clawing my face off because I was strangling her in my sleep! [forum comment].

While a reduction in the quality and quantity of sleep undoubtedly contribute to 'tren lethargy', other contributing factors could include the decreased cardiovascular fitness that accompanies trenbolone use, and the liver damaging effects of trenbolone.

Psychological/Social Effects: 'Tren: Like Being God, but Also With a Mental Illness'
This section describes both the psychological and social effects of trenbolone as bodybuilders typically describe the psychological effects in terms of their social impact. The psychological/social effects of trenbolone can vary widely from person to person, or even in the same individual across time (especially according to duration of use). There are some bodybuilders who describe trenbolone as 'euphoric'. The term 'alpha euphoria' will sometimes be used to describe the strong sense of self and the conviction that can come with trenbolone use. Some describe trenbolone as increasing their calmness and confidence, or making them more assertive and focussed. However, accounts of trenbolone having a positive impact on mental state are comparatively rare, and such individuals typically acknowledge that their positive experience is not the norm. The dominant discourse of trenbolone is one of increased anxiety, paranoia and aggression.

> A lot of people report really severe anxiety attacks when using tren, and it's what stops a lot of people from using tren [Sean].

> Tren is brutal. The anxiety and always being on edge, overthinking everything. You're fighting with yourself all the time [video comment].

> I'm fine on tren until someone starts giving me BS [bullshit] then the tren just takes over the conversation [social media post].

> Prone to fight, fuck, argue, maybe not seek conflict but almost perceive everything as a potential conflict [social media post].

For most bodybuilders, aggression was controllable and did not result in any incidents:

> I wasn't beating people up, or anything, but I started feeling like I wanted to [Alan].

Others were unable to control their increased aggressiveness, and accounts of losing control, especially with regards to other drivers, were not uncommon.

> I find tren is okay up until eight weeks and then your fucking brain falls out the back and road rage is really bad for me. I've chased people and fucking screamed at them, thrown shit at their car [Colin].

Finally, trenbolone impacts emotional independence/detachment. While some describe feeling more independent on trenbolone, others felt this to a greater, and more disturbing, extent.

> . . .it just made me kind of emotionally distant from everything and everyone, and even my Mrs and my kids, and that was horrible for her [Dave].

> It's not just like a rage, there's a cold calculation about it . . . it's unnerving . . . I have had anger issues with check drops [an oral steroid] and stuff like that where it's just been anger, it's just been a frustrating sort of rage, it's not been this cool, cold undertone of calculating what I'm going to do to get my revenge [Sean].

Trenbolone has pronounced effects on psychology that could exacerbate existing issues such as anxiety, obsessive compulsive tendencies and body image issues. However, in contrast, for a minority trenbolone resulted in a *decrease* in their pre-existing mental health problems. For example:

> Tren makes me god. Suffer with anxiety for 15 years don't give a shit about anything on tren [social media post].

Trenbolone has significant psychological and social effects, some of which are welcome, and may even be described as secondary reasons for use, but others are described as unwelcomed. Trenbolone is described as having a significantly greater impact on psychology, and therefore sociality, than any other steroid.

Effects on Sexuality: 'Tren Dick', Kinkiness and 'Rape-Like' Sex
The psychological effects of trenbolone also have an influence on sexuality. The aggression caused by trenbolone can manifest as sexual aggressiveness.

> . . .when you're on tren your brain is literally on kill/fuck mode. Every social interaction has only those 2 outcomes [social media post].

> I feel like fucking on tren is like one of the only good outlets for that fury. Great to let it out and not feel like you'll go to jail for it haha [social media post].

Trenbolone can result in a significant increase in sex drive, and sexual thoughts can become all-consuming and uncontrollable for some:

> . . .i can not run tren because i can have sex 8–10 times a day and it still will be hard to semi all day long i have had some boners last well over 6–8 hours straight which is bad.my wife gets so

sore we can not have sex and it gets to the point i can not sleep or work or anything because i am thinking the dirtiest nasty sex stuff you can think of. i can see how someone could rape someone while in this state it is out of my control and i would never ever rape anybody so i have to stop the tren [forum post].

The emotional distance that is characteristic of trenbolone use manifests as 'rape-like', 'animalistic' or 'primal' sex.

When I was on tren I turned into a rapist ... No emotional contact at all, it was just get it in there and do as much damage as I can and then job's done and that was it. ... It's totally emotional disassociation from the female and it turns you into a rapist, as simple as that [Rocco].

Not only is sex drive increased, but sexual adventurousness or 'kinkiness' is increased, and sexual interests may broaden to include people that would not have been considered potential sexual partners before trenbolone. One participant, Jock, even briefly considered sexual play with an elderly woman he was bathing whilst working in a nursing home.

Multiple guys have said they're definitely straight but on tren they've done things with men and then once they're off the tren they feel disgusted [Tony].

The term 'tren dick' is used to describe both (1) a trenbolone-induced erection (or 'tren boner') as described earlier and (2) the erectile dysfunction that can result from trenbolone use.

I had the nickname 'roll-up' because the girl I was sleeping with - she told everyone that she had to roll it up to get it inside of her [Scott].

Trenbolone can have a variety of significant effects on sexuality. Whilst other steroids impact on sexuality, no other steroid is described as having such an impact on sexuality.

Effects on Sexual Relationships: 'Tren: The Relationship Killer'

Given the psychological/social and sexual effects of trenbolone, it is probably unsurprising that it can place considerable strain on relationships. While the increased amount of sex, and the increased aggressiveness of sex, may be enjoyed by some partners, it may not be appreciated by others. The increased anxiety and paranoia (described above) could also manifest as sexual possessiveness and jealousy:

If you think your girlfriend is being loyal to you while you're on tren then it's fake gear [video comment].

Trenbolone is also described as leading to sexual infidelity. As a result trenbolone use can, and frequently does, result in the end of relationships, and tren is known in the enhancement community as 'the relationship killer':

That stupid fucking drug is what caused me to leave my wife. I was saying to myself that she doesn't make me happy because I felt nothing while around her and when I told her that I was done with the marriage she was in tears and devastated and I didn't feel an ounce of guilt, and I told myself that that means that I had made the right decision. Because if it was the wrong decision then I would have felt awful seeing her cry. But the whole time it was the tren keeping the feelings away :(... Once I had stopped the tren and it had all worn off what I had said had caused permanent damage to the marriage... I'd give anything in the world to go back and not break her heart. I'd live a thousand lives in hell ... I hate tren!!!! [Tony].

Trenbolone can ruin lives:

6 weeks in [to a trenbolone cycle], 10 Year relationship/marriage was thrown away, I was constantly horny, after a night of drinking I came onto my wife's cousin, I punched every wall in the house, to which I received a DVO [Domestic Violence Order] and AVO [Apprehended Violence Order], then lost custody of my two children, and lost my job as an armed guard [video comment].

The secondary effects of trenbolone are many and varied. Trenbolone may have the same physical effects as other steroids (e.g. organ damage), or the same effects as 19-nortestosterone and its derivatives (e.g. neurodegeneration). But it also has compound-specific effects such as 'tren cough', altered body odour and decreased cardiovascular fitness. Trenbolone can affect energy levels in a positive way, but can also interrupt or prevent sleep, and cause lethargy. It is reported to have pronounced effects on the psychology of some people who use it. These effects can be positive (euphoria, calmness, confidence, assertiveness, independence) but are more often described as negative (paranoia, anxiety, aggression and coldness). Trenbolone may be described as improving mental health, but is more likely to be described as exacerbating existing mental health conditions. Use of trenbolone can result in an increase in both sex drive and sexual aggressiveness, and a broadening of sexual interest to include individuals who are not normally sexually desired. Finally, because of the increased paranoia and emotional detachment associated with use, trenbolone is described as frequently destroying sexual relationships.

Distinguishing Benefit From Harm

The effects of trenbolone were sometimes not easily categorized as either 'benefits' or 'harms'. There were some that were described as clear benefits (such as the anabolic effect), and others that were described as clear harms (e.g. organ damage, gynecomastia, erectile dysfunction), but there were many that did not fall clearly on one side of the boundary or the other. For example, with regards to the psychological and sexual effects, whether or not they were considered a benefit or harm often depended on the degree or severity of the effect. An increase in assertiveness could be experienced as positive, but the same tendency towards assertiveness could become aggression at a different time, or under different circumstances, and become problematic. Emotional independence could be experienced as positive, but if this independence became detachment it could become problematic. Whether or not some effects were positive or negative could depend on context. For example, a level of aggression could be valued in some professions, or in some sexual encounters, but not others. Thus, the boundary between benefit and harm could be subjective.

Furthermore, some of the effects of trenbolone that from an outside perspective would be considered to be harms, can, from an inside perspective, be considered to be benefits. Because trenbolone is purchased on the black market, the quality of the trenbolone is variable. As a result, some 'harms' of trenbolone, such as 'tren cough' and the mental effects of trenbolone, may be defined as 'benefits' because they assure the person that they have consumed actual trenbolone.

> The good thing about trenbolone is that you can really tell you're on it right away because of all the side effects [video].

> The sides [side effects] are how i'm recognising if its [i.e. the trenbolone is] legit. When my wife's doing every day make up and it starts looking suspicious while never was im like 'yep, top notch gear i got here' [video comment].

Trenbolone is a drug that individuals can feel, unlike most enhancement drugs. Thus, the feelings of trenbolone, even those that from an outside perspective would be considered negative, can be defined as benefits as they assure the individual that the drug they have used is what it is purported to be.

Trenbolone Harm Reduction

Drug decisions are informed by the balance of benefit to harm, and people who use drugs actively negotiate this balance through self-directed harm reduction practice. There are many ways that online enhancement communities serve to alter the level of harm experienced from trenbolone use. Before we consider the ways that these communities may act to reduce harm, we must first acknowledge that they may also act to encourage drug use, and therefore increase harm. Communities may encourage drug use through the meanings they give to drug use.

> We [bodybuilders] gave it [trenbolone] this reputation as the god of steroids and expected inexperienced, not-ready-for-it bros to not flock to it like the second coming [forum comment].

Descriptions of the benefits of drug use obviously act to encourage use, and online communities are sites where descriptions of the benefits of trenbolone are shared. They are also sites for the encouragement of caution, the discouragement of use, and the discussion and dissemination of harm reduction practice.

Bodybuilders sometimes make videos discussing the mental health harms they have experienced as a result of trenbolone use (I have quoted some of these earlier). For example, one video described the potential harms of trenbolone, and when trenbolone use should be avoided:

> If you're going to use it [trenbolone] make sure you've got all your ducks in a row, financially, relationship wise, everything is like spot on, like nothing is like in the middle of being fucked up, because if you throw tren in when you are like in the middle of financial hardship or your relationship is iffy, the tren is going to make it much worse, and you'll get super paranoid and in your fuckin head about it. .... it's definitely not going to help. It's very unlikely that if you are facing any emotional turmoil that throwing tren into the mix will have zero impact on it [video].

These videos start a dialogue about trenbolone harm that others are inspired to contribute to:

> I can definitely attest to the psychological sides on Tren. I did 10 wk tren e [trenbolone enanthate] cycle (around 500mg/wk) with 12 wk test e [testosterone enanthate] as base. I WAS BATSHIT CRAZY. I thought my wife was cheating on me and could not stop other strange compulsions. I will say that I returned to normal a week after the cycle, but my wife said she will divorce me if I ever take it again. Just a PSA [public service announcement] [video comment].

These, descriptions of harm, or 'public service announcements', work to reduce harm. They are peer accounts that other bodybuilders can relate to and which can act to discourage use. One such video led other members of the community, who were considering using trenbolone for the first time, to comment:

> So glad you put this out. My life isnt in a great place and I was gonna throw tren into the last 4–6 weeks of my 20 week cycle and this has legit talked me out of it [video comment].

> Thanks for talking about this. Based on what you've stated I'm not compatible with Tren [video comment].

There are also other ways that online communities may act to discourage use, such as establishing circumstances under which trenbolone use is considered inappropriate, such as in a first cycle of steroids. Standard advice is to use only one type of testosterone in the first cycle, and then in subsequent cycles to either increase dose or add a compound, but never both. By doing so an individual can establish a baseline, and then more easily identify the cause of problems (i.e. increased dose or new compound) should they occur. As trenbolone is notorious for causing problems it is vital to be able to ascertain its impact, and monitor harms.

Trenbolone use is most acceptable if the individual is preparing for a bodybuilding competition. Indeed, there are some who consider trenbolone use a necessity in competitive bodybuilding (as mentioned previously). In response to a social media post which described first time use of trenbolone at 400 mg per week, another enhanced bodybuilder responded:

> Way too much tren for your first time with the drug. I got tremendous results from 120mg of tren E. ... Tren isn't a drug to just fuck around with. Unless you have a contest in the next 8 weeks I'd drop it completely or cut dose in half [social media comment].

Online sites can be sites for the discouragement of use or the encouragement of caution. They are also sites where strategies for reducing or preventing harm are shared. Bodybuilders will sometimes suggest individuals use the shorter ester (trenbolone acetate), rather than the longer ester (trenbolone enanthate), at least initially. Harm from trenbolone is unpredictable. Therefore, using the shorter ester ensures that if harms do occur the individual can cease use and rid their body of trenbolone in a shorter amount of time. However, some bodybuilders also state that the longer ester may produce less harm as it does not produce such sudden changes in hormone levels.

Bodybuilders frequently emphasize the fact that trenbolone is different from other steroids, and thus should be used differently. They advise lower doses and shorter cycles of trenbolone than other steroids, as trenbolone harm is described as increasing with dose and duration of use.

200g mg is plenty, beyond that it is diminishing returns [forum comment].

Eight weeks is probably the ideal amount for that drug before it starts affecting the mental state [Robert].

Some bodybuilders will suggest additional cardiovascular exercise and water consumption to counter the effects of trenbolone. Monitoring health before, during and after trenbolone use is also recommended. While much of the health monitoring advised for trenbolone applies to all steroids, some of it is compound-specific. For example, bodybuilders often suggest that trenbolone use increases prolactin which should be reduced through the use of dopamine agonists. Trenbolone can also confuse the results of testing if individuals are unaware of the compound-specific monitoring necessary.

When you take Trenbolone if you use ECLIA, electrochemiluminescence immunoassay, that's the normal testing methodology for blood tests, if you use that for estrogen when you're on tren, it'll give you a really, really high response, which normally you would say right, I've got to take a heap of aromatase inhibitor. ... But if you get it tested with LCMS, liquid chromatography mass spectrometry, you'll find that the results will be accurate [Bjorn].

Because trenbolone can have pronounced psychological and sexual effects that impact individuals socially, sometimes forms of social harm reduction may become necessary. For instance, one competitive bodybuilder I spoke to who felt that trenbolone use was necessary for the 6–8 weeks prior to a competition, socially isolated himself for this period so that other people would not suffer as a result of his trenbolone-induced mood change. I have seen numerous individuals suggest that trenbolone should only be used when single. For example:

Oh my god. Hyper sexuality on Trenbolone. Believe me it is very real and it's very dangerous. Anyone in a relationship should not take Trenbolone [Tony].

Online enhancement communities provide vital sites for sharing experiences of both benefit (thus encouraging use) and harm (thus deterring use). They are also sites where caution is encouraged and where harm reduction strategies are disseminated.

Weighing Benefit Against Harm

Decisions to use drugs involve a (conscious or subconscious) weighing of benefit against harm. This is a complex task which includes many factors (such as observable harms, understandings of risk, understandings and experiences of benefit) across numerous domains (such as physical, psychological, social, sexual etc.). People who use trenbolone may weigh the benefits and harms of trenbolone in online communities.

Well! I'm 18 weeks deep in my cycle with Tren and here's what has happened:

(1) Lost my girlfriend
(2) Got my gains appreciated by two of her friends
(3) Stood up against a senior bullying me in office
(4) For my courageous act I'm being considered for a promotion
(5) Got my first sponsorship deal
(6) Boner train is bang on!
(7) Sleep isn't as good as it used to be, but I manage [video comment].

The weighing of harm against benefit is a dynamic process. For example, context can, and does, change. Relationships may change, as may occupations. Individuals may also experience changes in the level of reward that bodybuilding provides them. For example, if an individual begins to compete in the sport of bodybuilding the reward they experience from bodybuilding may increase, thus altering the ratio of benefit to harm, and therefore allowing a tolerance of greater harm. The weighing of harm to benefit is also a dynamic process because awareness of harm may increase over time.

Trenbolone decisions are made even more complex by the huge variety of responses individuals have to the drug. Some people report that they cannot take trenbolone at any dose because the harms they experience are so great (and thus trenbolone use becomes a risk boundary). At the other end of the spectrum are individuals who report little or no harm as a result of trenbolone use (even at higher doses). It is often said that it is impossible to predict how one will react to trenbolone prior to use, and that protocols and harm reduction strategies must be individualized as everyone responds differently. The wide variety of responses to trenbolone result in much disagreement about the extent and nature of trenbolone harm.

While I have provided many descriptions of harm earlier, we have no idea how common these experiences of harm are. It may be that those who experience the most harm are the most vocal in online communities. It is possible, as some bodybuilders suggest, that some bodybuilders use trenbolone as an 'excuse for bad behaviour' and therefore overstate the harms. In contrast, some people who use trenbolone may be in denial about its harms. One community expert, Sean, was the most vocal about this, describing trenbolone as inherently unsafe. He felt that many people who use trenbolone deny the harms it causes in order to justify their use. As a provider of harm reduction services to people who use trenbolone he witnesses the extent of harm that this drug causes, and may be in less denial than others as he no longer uses drugs for enhancement. It is also possible that self-reported harms are underestimated due to lack of awareness. While some who use trenbolone do monitor their health and alter their use according to their health markers (e.g. shortening the cycle if lipid markers 'look bad' [forum comment]), others do not. Also, a lack of awareness of psychological/social effects has been noted by people who use trenbolone:

I used to work sales when I was into body building. Didn't notice tren changing my behavior when I was on it. Did notice I went from doing pretty good consistently to not selling anything at all whatsoever [video comment].

Often you don't realise how much it was screwing with you until after you're off it. And you're like 'wow I was a fuckin idiot when I was on that shit' [video].

Thus, it is very difficult to gauge the true extent of trenbolone harm.

The Place of Trenbolone in Bodybuilding Culture

Another factor influencing use decisions and the weighing of benefit against harm are the meanings attributed to trenbolone. Trenbolone use may foster a sense of belonging to the community as trenbolone has an 'almost mythical reputation within bodybuilding circles' [website]. This reputation was built in part by the older generation of bodybuilders who experienced a time when Parabolan was discontinued and thus became the 'holy grail' [Mark] because it was so difficult to obtain. I believe this mythical reputation is also due to the love/hate relationship bodybuilders have with trenbolone.

Trenbolone is like the bat shit crazy girlfriend you consider breaking up with daily, but you never do because the sex is so fucking good lol [laugh out loud] [forum comment].

Trenbolone is described as 'the god of all steroids' [website], and 'the nectar of the gods', but also as 'the devil in a bottle' and as 'making a pact with the devil' [video comments]. The conflicted relationship bodybuilders have with trenbolone is also evident in bodybuilding humour.

Tren is very hard on the heart. I've ended up in cardiac arrest, but I was lookin' shredded [i.e. muscular and lean] in that hospital bed [video comment].

In the humour of enhanced bodybuilder communities, trenbolone, in particular an increased dose of trenbolone, is presented as the solution to any and all problems. This most commonly manifests as the phrase 'up the tren' (i.e. increase the dose of trenbolone). For example, if a bodybuilder complains of experiencing side effects from enhancement drug use, others will suggest they 'up the tren'. Problems completely unrelated to bodybuilding will also provoke this response, for example, 'Car won't start? Up the tren'. One participant explained the humour of 'up the tren' by explaining the two possible uses of the phrase:

(1) Up the tren - this is an absurd option and I am making fun of people who take risks when it's not necessary, I am making fun of that.
(2) Up the tren - if your life is going badly then you may as well look like a freak, I am laughing at how that silver lining is something bodybuilders can relate to but other people can't.

Both are delivered with an implied understanding that it's an absurd suggestion.
Neither is seriously suggesting to up the tren [Bjorn via messenger].

Trenbolone is one of the most talked about and joked about steroids in online bodybuilding communities. It causes divides in the community with people frequently accusing one another of overstating or understating the harms and benefits (to the extent that it was difficult to ascertain the 'truth' about trenbolone). It is highly likely that the special and controversial place trenbolone has in bodybuilding culture influences trenbolone use decisions.

DISCUSSION

In this, the first study of a specific steroid, I have described a folk model of risk that runs counter to the dominant narrative of steroid use as safe (Hanley Santos & Coomber, 2017; Kimergard, 2015; Kimergård & McVeigh, 2014; Monaghan, 2002). In so doing I have eliminated some of the assumptions inherent in professional models of steroid risk, such as: (1) the assumption that steroid risk can be discussed in general ways that ignore the differences between specific steroid compounds, and (2) that risks are objective facts that can be isolated from their cultural context.

Previous steroid research has lumped all steroids together and failed to consider the differences between specific steroids. In so doing it has put itself at odds with the perspectives of those who use steroids who tend to discuss specific compounds. It has also failed to capture the nuance of folk models of risk and the specific meanings of these drugs to those who use them.

Previous steroid research has also tended to treat the boundary between harm and benefits as objective and clear-cut. Researchers have categorized steroid effects into harms and benefits and then surveyed people on this basis (e.g. Cohen et al., 2007; Hope et al., 2013; Parkinson & Evans, 2006; Pope et al., 2014; Rowe et al., 2017; Smit & de Ronde, 2018; Van de Ven et al., 2018; Zahnow et al., 2018). In many cases drug effects can be easily categorized as either harms or benefits. But with regards to other drug effects the boundary may be less easily defined. The increased sex drive and the animalistic nature of sex on trenbolone may be a harm in one context, but a benefit in another. The increased assertiveness that comes with trenbolone use may be a harm in one context and a benefit in another. Thus, the boundary between harm and benefit may be subjective and context-dependent.

Why Do Bodybuilders Use Trenbolone?

The obvious answer to the question of why bodybuilders use trenbolone is because it assists them to gain muscle. Previous research has found that steroids are used to achieve a 'better looking body' (Kimergard, 2015, p. 289), a bigger or 'ripped' body (Petrocelli et al., 2008), increased muscle mass and strength (Jennings et al., 2014, p. vi), and 'enhanced definition and density of muscle, and improved recovery from training and injuries' (Van Hout & Kean, 2015, p. 860). In this chapter I have described additional instrumental benefits that inform trenbolone use. Trenbolone is an extremely versatile compound which may be beneficial in both the bulking and cutting phases of the bodybuilding process. Trenbolone is more powerful than other steroids used by bodybuilders. Therefore, bodybuilders can typically achieve more muscular gains from trenbolone as compared to other steroids. Trenbolone is so effective that it may facilitate muscular gains despite flaws in training or diet. It may also allow for deliberate laxity in diet and training, which in such a demanding sport may be a welcome relief. Furthermore, the aesthetic trenbolone facilitates is particularly well-suited to current bodybuilding ideals. Trenbolone is used as a hardening agent, and some suggest that the 'tren look' has become so ingrained in bodybuilding ideals that failure to use trenbolone will lead to failure to produce a competitive physique.

The Benefits and Risks/Harms of Trenbolone

Drugs are used when the perceived benefits outweigh the perceived harms. The complexity of this process of distinguishing benefit from harm, and weighing and negotiating the ratio of benefit to harm, is the focus of this chapter. In this section I summarize the benefits and harms of trenbolone as described by bodybuilders. What makes this description difficult is that the experience of trenbolone is extremely varied. People who use trenbolone may even describe it in ways that appear contradictory. Some experience calmness, others anxiety. Some experience an energizing effect, others lethargy. Some experience confidence, others paranoia. As a result of the varied experiences of trenbolone people have very different perspectives on trenbolone harm. Thus, when the findings presented in this chapter were circulated in bodybuilding communities for comment they caused a great deal of debate. Some suggested that I was overstating the harms of trenbolone and contributing to the demonization of people who use steroids. Others suggested that the descriptions of harm I had collected were accurate, and yet others suggested that the harms of trenbolone were even greater than described. Never before have I presented findings to the community that have resulted in such oppositional views. Trenbolone is truly a drug that divides the bodybuilding community.

Whether individuals describe few or many harms from trenbolone, all bodybuilders acknowledge at least the greater potential for harm from trenbolone than other commonly injected steroids. Trenbolone causes significantly more harm than an equivalent dose of another steroid. There are more discussions of trenbolone harm in online bodybuilding communities, than there are discussions of harms from other steroids. This suggests that the compound specific harms of steroids, particularly trenbolone, should receive greater academic attention. Whilst we do not know how commonly harm is experienced as a result of trenbolone use, this chapter has demonstrated that some people who use it experience it as extremely harmful. Trenbolone is described as ruining lives, something that I have not seen reported in relation to other steroids. It is urgent that we understand trenbolone's harms and develop harm reduction strategies specific to this compound.

Trenbolone is described as causing significant organ damage, and negatively impacting on cognitive function and energy levels. It is also described as resulting in more 'rape-like' sexual behaviours by some people who use it, in a manner reminiscent of the forced copulatory behaviours found among fish exposed to trenbolone (Bertram et al., 2015). But the harms of trenbolone that are most frequently discussed are the psychological and social harms. Some of the most frequently mentioned harms were decreased connection with other people, and increased aggression. These factors result in trenbolone having the potential for significant social harm. Increased aggressiveness has been frequently noted among people who use steroids (Chegeni et al., 2021). This chapter has demonstrated that not all steroids are alike in this regard, and trenbolone may be more likely to cause an increase in aggression than other steroids. An understanding of the compound specific nature of steroid-induced aggression could be useful, as the societal harms of steroids may be reduced by directing individuals away from particularly problematic compounds (such as trenbolone) and towards others.

The perceived benefits of trenbolone are great, and thus efforts to discourage use of this particular compound may face a difficult task. Not only does trenbolone have tremendous instrumental effects (described above), but some experience psychological benefits from its use such as increased confidence. In addition to the physical and mental benefits, it is possible that bodybuilders may experience social benefits within the bodybuilding community as a result of use. Given the special place of trenbolone in bodybuilding communities, individuals may feel a greater sense of belonging to these communities if they use trenbolone. Indeed, in a world where it is not infrequent to hear the sport of bodybuilding described as a sport of 'out suffering' the competition, even descriptions of harm from trenbolone may increase social standing.

Trenbolone Harm Reduction

Bodybuilders primarily reduce the harms of trenbolone by acknowledging the fact that trenbolone is more powerful than other steroids and then treating it as such. Thus, most community-driven trenbolone harm reduction messages focus on reducing the dosage and duration of trenbolone use, relative to other steroids. I have seen more encouragement of caution with regards to trenbolone than any other steroid. Discussions of trenbolone harm in online bodybuilding communities act to discourage use. Thus, official harm reduction strategies, which tend to be designed by those outside of the community, could include bodybuilders' own words of caution and descriptions of harm. It is also vital that the harm reduction strategies practised by bodybuilders (such as the use of specific blood tests and ancillary drugs described earlier) are evaluated to determine their effectiveness. It is possible that over-zealous harm reduction efforts could actually be increasing harm. In short, trenbolone harm reduction strategies should ideally work to bridge the divide between enhanced bodybuilders and those who study and serve them, and work to transform two discourses of steroid harm reduction, the bodybuilder and professional discourses, into one (Underwood, 2019).

The Role of Online Bodybuilding Communities in the Negotiation of Trenbolone Risk

Online communities are important sites for drug harm reduction. Firstly, they operate as sites for the circulation of harm reduction strategies. This has been noted with regards to psychoactive drugs (Móró & Rácz, 2013; Soussan & Kjellgren, 2014) as well as with regards to steroids (Tighe et al., 2017).

Online drug communities are also places where drugs have social lives, and where boundaries, such as that between person and thing, animate or inanimate, and subject and object, are blurred. This study has highlighted that whilst people shape drugs, drugs also shape people (literally and not just metaphorically in the case of image and performance enhancing drugs). Trenbolone is used to create bodies that meet the ideals that trenbolone helped to create in the first place. Online sites are where drugs are given a personality and agency, or a 'life' (similarly advertising and marketing give life to pharmaceuticals; Martin, 2006). They are where trenbolone becomes a 'crazy girlfriend', a 'god' or a 'devil', or where trenbolone is given agency and possesses the individual (e.g. taking over conversations, switching the brain to 'kill/fuck mode', turning people into rapists or bisexuals). They are sites where drugs may even be personified. Indeed, some memes circulated in online enhancement communities depict trenbolone as a person, typically one that is monstrous and overwhelms the individual.

Online drug communities are sites where drugs and their effects are given meaning. These meanings shape folk models of risk, as risks and their perception are context-dependent (Rhodes, 2002). This study has demonstrated that online drug communities are sites where drug effects are defined as harms or benefits. For example, in online enhancement communities some of the effects of trenbolone that from an outside perspective would be deemed harms (such as 'tren cough' and paranoia) are redefined as benefits because they serve to prove that genuine trenbolone has been consumed. This is an example of how the boundary between harm and benefit is socially constructed. To say that risks or harms are socially constructed is not to say that they do not exist and have real consequences, but rather that notions of risk are situated value judgements (Duff, 2003). In order to make a risk decision an individual must first distinguish benefit from harm. Therefore, before a drug decision can be made the individual must first distinguish, in collaboration with others, the beneficial effects of the drug from its harmful effects, and then weigh these against each other. As Becker (1953) in his classic paper *Becoming a Marihuana User* explains, people who use drugs must first learn to experience their effects as enjoyable or pleasurable. To use trenbolone one first has to learn to value its effects. While there is an evolutionary dimension to the appeal of muscularity, the meaning of muscle is also always cultural (Gray & Ginsberg, 2007). Individuals who use trenbolone have first learnt to value the aesthetic it produces. They have learnt to value its hardening capacity and the '3D' or 'comic book' effect it produces. They have learnt to value vascularity, which would appear to be of no evolutionary benefit and indeed indicates fat levels so low that they may be detrimental to survival.

The Ambivalence of Drugs

Drug effects require meaning to be assigned to them because drugs are inherently ambivalent. They are what the ancient Greeks referred to as 'pharmakons' (Whyte et al., 2002). The term 'pharmakon', from which the term 'pharmaceutical' derives, translates as both 'remedy' and 'poison' (Rinella, 2010). All drugs are both therapeutic and poisonous:

> ... even in the case of drugs used exclusively for therapeutic ends, even when they are wielded with good intentions, and even when they are as such effective. There is no such thing as a harmless remedy. The pharmakon can never be simply beneficial. (Derrida, 1981, pp. 101–102)

There are two reasons for this: (1) the beneficial essence does not prevent it hurting, and (2) it is essentially harmful because it is artificial (Derrida, 1981). The pharmakon is both a solution for one particular problem and the cause of other problems. It is a remedy that is always already a poison.

The ambivalence of drugs is beautifully illustrated by trenbolone. People who use trenbolone have a love/hate relationship with it. They are conflicted about its use. Trenbolone is a god, but also the devil. It makes one energized but lethargic; erect but also flaccid. The ambivalence of trenbolone is highlighted in bodybuilder humour. Instructing others to 'up the tren' (as described earlier) as the solution to any and all problems is an instance of irony which therefore keeps both the explicit and implicit messages in play (Korobov, 2009). It presents trenbolone use as both beneficial and harmful, as reasonable yet absurd.

Given the ambivalent nature of drugs, when it comes to understanding drug decisions we must ask, as Martin (2006, p. 274) asks, 'how do people keep ambivalence about drugs at bay enough to take them?'. Decisions to take drugs, or the practice of keeping drug ambivalence at bay long enough to allow drug consumption, are social processes influenced by cultural frameworks. When it comes to the ambivalence of trenbolone, there are many factors at work that allow this drug to be consumed.

Some people who use trenbolone appear to suffer little harm and thus their relationship with trenbolone is less conflicted than others. We, as a society, need to increase the likelihood of this experience of trenbolone through the design and dissemination of compound-specific harm reduction strategies. However, some people who use trenbolone ignore or deny the harms they are experiencing, so accounts of little harm may not be accurate. We can increase understanding of the harms of trenbolone by disseminating the stories of those who have experienced harm. It is hoped that this chapter is a first step in this direction.

People who use trenbolone can lessen the ambivalence they feel about this drug by surrounding themselves with others who share the same folk model of risk and who place the same value on the drug's effects. More research into bodybuilder folk models of risk is needed so we can understand the role of bodybuilding communities in the negotiation of steroid risk. But we must also remember that bodybuilders have not created the muscular ideals they conform to in isolation. We, as a society, are complicit as we demand increasingly muscular actors, action toys and comic book heroes. It's likely that 'the comic book effect' is not just a result of trenbolone use, but also a cause.

KEY READINGS

(1) Becker, H. S. (1953). Becoming a Marihuana User. *The American Journal of Sociology*, *59*(3), 235–242.

In this classic paper that still has relevance today, Becker presents the benefits of drugs not as unmediated pharmacologically induced events, but rather as the result of users' interpretations of those effects.

(2) Franzke, A. S., Bechmann, A., Zimmer, M., Ess, C., & the Association of Internet Researchers. (2020). Internet Research: Ethical Guidelines 3.0. https://aoir.org/reports/ethics3.pdf

As there are no universally accepted formulae for ethical online research, this source is invaluable to those who wish to conduct an online study of enhancement drug use/doping, or any other topic.

(3) Llewellyn, W. (2017). *Anabolics* (11th ed.). Molecular Nutrition, LLC.

For an introduction to enhancement drugs, and how they are used, from a user perspective, you cannot go past Llewellyn's work. It is probably the reference guide that people who use enhancement drugs consult most.

(4) Martin, E. (2006). The pharmaceutical person. *BioSocieties*, *1*(3), 273–287. https://doi.org/10.1017/S1745855206003012

Martin explores how pharmaceutical drugs are given life, and personalities, and how effects are given meaning, with side effects being displaced. This is a great example of how material culture perspectives can enhance our understanding of the roles drugs play in our lives.

(5) Rhodes, T. (2002). The 'risk environment': A framework for understanding and reducing drug-related harm. *The International Journal of Drug Policy*, *13*(2), 85–94. https://doi.org/10.1016/S0955-3959(02)00007-5

For those who want to understand risk as not only an issue of individual behaviour change but as part of the environment, this classic work is the perfect introduction.

NOTE

1. Bodybuilders often engage with the scientific literature. During this research I found a bodybuilder analysis of trenbolone that cited literally hundreds of scientific studies and appeared (from my non-medical perspective) to engage with this literature in a very sophisticated manner. Judging how well they theorized from the results of animal studies to their own situation would require the analysis of someone with medical training, or indeed a multidisciplinary team.

REFERENCES

Andreasson, J., & Johansson, T. (2016). Online doping. The new self-help culture of ethnopharmacology. *Sport in Society*, *19*(7), 957–972. https://doi.org/10.1080/17430437.2015.1096246

Andreasson, J., & Johansson, T. (2019). (Un)Becoming a fitness doper: Negotiating the meaning of illicit drug use in a gym and fitness context. *Journal of Sport & Social Issues, 44*(1), 93–109. https://doi.org/10.1177/0193723519867589

Appadurai, A. (1986). *The social life of things.* Cambridge University Press.

Becker, H. S. (1953). Becoming a Marihuana User. *American Journal of Sociology, 59*(3), 235–242.

Bertram, M. G., Saaristo, M., Baumgartner, J. B., Johnstone, C. P., Allinson, M., Allinson, G., & Wong, B. B. M. (2015). Sex in troubled waters: Widespread agricultural contaminant disrupts reproductive behaviour in fish. *Hormones and Behavior, 70*, 85–91. https://doi.org/10.1016/j.yhbeh.2015.03.002

Boettcher, M., Kosmehl, T., & Braunbeck, T. (2011). Low-dose effects and biphasic effect profiles: Is trenbolone a genotoxicant? *Mutation Research/Genetic Toxicology and Environmental Mutagenesis, 723*(2), 152–157. https://doi.org/10.1016/j.mrgentox.2011.04.012

Chegeni, R., Pallesen, S., McVeigh, J., & Sagoe, D. (2021). Anabolic-androgenic steroid administration increases self-reported aggression in healthy males: A systematic review and meta-analysis of experimental studies. *Psychopharmacology, 238*(7), 1911–1922. https://doi.org/10.1007/s00213-021-05818-7

Christiansen, A. V., Vinther, A. S., & Liokaftos, D. (2017). Outline of a typology of men's use of anabolic androgenic steroids in fitness and strength training environments. *Drugs: Education, Prevention & Policy, 24*(3), 295–305. https://doi.org/10.1080/09687637.2016.1231173

Cohen, J., Collins, R., Darkes, J., & Gwartney, D. (2007). A league of their own: Demographics, motivations and patterns of use of 1,955 male adult non-medical anabolic steroid users in the United States. *Journal of the International Society of Sports Nutrition, 4*, 12. https://doi.org/10.1186/1550-2783-4-12

Dennington, V., Finney-Lamb, C., Dillon, P., Larance, B., Vial, R., Copeland, J., & Newcombe, D. (2008). Qualitative field study for users of performance and image enhancing drugs. *Drug and Alcohol Services South Australia.*

Derrida, J. (1981). *Dissemination* (B. Johnson, Trans.). Continuum.

Douglas, M. (1985). *Risk acceptability according to the social sciences.* Russell Sage Foundation.

Douglas, M. (1992). *Risk and blame: Essays in cultural theory.* Routledge.

Duff, C. (2003). The importance of culture and context: Rethinking risk and risk management in young drug using populations. *Health, Risk & Society, 5*(3), 285–299. https://doi.org/10.1080/13698570310001606987

Duff, C. (2013). The social life of drugs. *International Journal of Drug Policy, 24*(3), 167–172.

Franzke, A. S., Bechmann, A., Zimmer, M., Ess, C., & the Association of Internet Researchers (2020). *Internet Research: Ethical Guidelines 3.0.* https://aoir.org/reports/ethics3.pdf

Gray, J., & Ginsberg, R. (2007). Muscle dissatisfaction: An overview of psychological and cultural research and theory. In K. Thompson & G. Cafri (Eds.), *The muscular ideal: Psychological, social, and medical perspectives* (pp. 15–39). American Psychological Association.

Greenway, C. W., & Price, C. (2018). A qualitative study of the motivations for anabolic-androgenic steroid use: The role of muscle dysmorphia and self-esteem in long-term users. *Performance Enhancement & Health, 6*(1), 12–20. https://doi.org/10.1016/j.peh.2018.02.002

Hanley Santos, G., & Coomber, R. (2017). The risk environment of anabolic–androgenic steroid users in the UK: Examining motivations, practices and accounts of use. *International Journal of Drug Policy, 40*, 35–43. https://doi.org/10.1016/j.drugpo.2016.11.005

Harris, M. A., Dunn, M., & Alwyn, T. (2016). A qualitative exploration of the motivations underlying anabolic-androgenic steroid use from adolescence into adulthood. *Health Psychology Report, 4*, 315–320. https://doi.org/10.5114/hpr.2016.61669

Harvey, O., Keen, S., Parrish, M., & van Teijlingen, E. (2019). Support for people who use anabolic androgenic steroids: A systematic scoping review into what they want and what they access. *BMC Public Health, 19*(1), 1024. https://doi.org/10.1186/s12889-019-7288-x

Hope, V. D., McVeigh, J., Marongiu, A., Evans-Brown, M., Smith, J., Kimergård, A., Croxford, S., Beynon, C. M., Parry, J. V., Bellis, M. A., & Ncube, F. (2013). Prevalence of, and risk factors for, HIV, hepatitis B and C infections among men who inject image and performance enhancing drugs: A cross-sectional study. *BMJ Open, 3*(9). https://doi.org/10.1136/bmjopen-2013-003207

Hunt, G. P., Evans, K., & Kares, F. (2007). Drug use and meanings of risk and pleasure. *Journal of Youth Studies, 10*(1), 73–96. https://doi.org/10.1080/13676260600983668

Ip, E. J., Barnett, M. J., Tenerowicz, M. J., & Perry, P. J. (2011). The anabolic 500 survey: Characteristics of male users versus nonusers of anabolic-androgenic steroids for strength training. *Pharmacotherapy: The Journal of Human Pharmacology and Drug Therapy, 31*(8), 757–766. https://doi.org/10.1592/phco.31.8.757

Ip, E. J., Barnett, M. J., Tenerowicz, M. J., & Perry, P. J. (2012). Weightlifting's risky new trend: A case series of 41 insulin users. *Current Sports Medicine Reports, 11*(4), 176–179. https://doi.org/10.1249/JSR.0b013e31825da97f

Jennings, C., Patten, E., Kennedy, M., & Kelly, C. (2014). *Examining the profile and perspectives of individuals attending harm reduction services who are users of performance and image enhancing drugs.* Merchants Quay Ireland.

Kelly, B. C. (2005). Conceptions of risk in the lives of club drug-using youth. *Substance Use & Misuse, 40*(9–10), 1443–1459. https://doi.org/10.1081/JA-200066812

Kimergard, A. (2015). A qualitative study of anabolic steroid use amongst gym users in the United Kingdom: Motives, beliefs and experiences. *Journal of Substance Use, 20*(4), 288–294. https://doi.org/10.3109/14659891.2014.911977

Kimergård, A., & McVeigh, J. (2014). Environments, risk and health harms: A qualitative investigation into the illicit use of anabolic steroids among people using harm reduction services in the UK. *BMJ Open, 4*(6). e005275. https://doi.org/10.1136/bmjopen-2014-005275

Korobov, N. (2009). Expanding hegemonic masculinity: The use of irony in young men's stories about romantic experiences. *American Journal of Men's Health, 3*, 286–299. https://doi.org/10.1177/1557988308319952

Lagesson, A., Saaristo, M., Brodin, T., Fick, J., Klaminder, J., Martin, J. M., & Wong, B. B. M. (2019). Fish on steroids: Temperature-dependent effects of 17β-trenbolone on predator escape, boldness, and exploratory behaviors. *Environmental Pollution, 245*, 243–252. https://doi.org/10.1016/j.envpol.2018.10.116

Llewellyn, W. (2011). *Anabolics* (E-book ed.). Molecular Nutrition, LLC.

Llewellyn, W. (2017). *Anabolics* (11th ed.). Molecular Nutrition, LLC.

Lupton, D. (2013). *Risk: Key ideas* (2nd ed.). Routledge.

Ma, F., & Liu, D. (2015). 17β-trenbolone, an anabolic–androgenic steroid as well as an environmental hormone, contributes to neurodegeneration. *Toxicology and Applied Pharmacology, 282*(1), 68–76. https://doi.org/10.1016/j.taap.2014.11.007

Martin, E. (2006). The pharmaceutical person. *BioSocieties, 1*(3), 273–287. https://doi.org/10.1017/S1745855206003012

McVeigh, J., Germain, J., & Van Hout, M. C. (2017). 2,4-Dinitrophenol, the inferno drug: A netnographic study of user experiences in the quest for leanness. *Journal of Substance Use, 22*(2), 131–138. https://doi.org/10.3109/14659891.2016.1149238

Miller, D. (2010). *Stuff.* Polity Press.

Monaghan, L. F. (2002). Vocabularies of motive for illicit steroid use among bodybuilders. *Social Science & Medicine, 55*(5), 695–708.

Monaghan, L. F. (2011). Accounting for illicit steroid use: Bodybuilders justifications. In A. Locks & N. Richardson (Eds.), *Critical readings in bodybuilding.* Taylor & Francis.

Monaghan, L., Bloor, M., Dobash, R. P., & Dobash, R. E. (2000). Drug-taking, 'risk boundaries' and social identity: Bodybuilders' talk about Ephedrine and Nubain. *Sociological Research Online, 5*(2), 1–12. https://doi.org/10.5153/sro.489

Móró, L., & Rácz, J. (2013). Online drug user-led harm reduction in Hungary: A review of "Daath". *Harm Reduction Journal, 10*(1), 18. https://doi.org/10.1186/1477-7517-10-18

Oaks, L., & Harthorn, B. H. (2003). Health and the social and cultural construction of risk. In B. H. Harthorn & L. Oaks (Eds.), *Risk, culture, and health inequality: Shifting perceptions of danger and blame* (pp. 3–12). Praeger.

Parkinson, A. B., & Evans, N. A. (2006). Anabolic androgenic steroids: A survey of 500 users. *Medicine & Science in Sports & Exercise, 38*(4), 644–651. https://doi.org/10.1249/01.mss.0000210194.56834.5d

Perry, P. J., Lund, B. C., Deninger, M. J., Kutscher, E. C., & Schneider, J. (2005). Anabolic steroid use in weightlifters and bodybuilders: An internet survey of drug utilization. *Clinical Journal of Sport Medicine*, *15*(5), 326–330. https://doi.org/10.1097/01.jsm.0000180872.22426.bb

Petrocelli, M., Oberweis, T., & Petrocelli, J. (2008). Getting huge, getting ripped: A qualitative exploration of recreational steroid use. *Journal of Drug Issues*, *38*(4), 1187–1205. https://doi.org/10.1177/002204260803800412

Pope, H. G., Jr., Wood, R. I., Rogol, A., Nyberg, F., Bowers, L., & Bhasin, S. (2014). Adverse health consequences of performance-enhancing drugs: An endocrine society scientific statement. *Endocrine Reviews*, *35*(3), 341–375. https://doi.org/10.1210/er.2013-1058

Rhodes, T. (2002). The 'risk environment': A framework for understanding and reducing drug-related harm. *International Journal of Drug Policy*, *13*(2), 85–94. https://doi.org/10.1016/S0955-3959(02)00007-5

Rinella, M. A. (2010). *Pharmakon: Plato, drug culture, and identity in ancient Athens*. Lexington Books.

Rowe, R., Berger, I., Yaseen, B., & Copeland, J. (2017). Risk and blood-borne virus testing among men who inject image and performance enhancing drugs, Sydney, Australia. *Drug and Alcohol Review*, *36*(5), 658–666. https://doi.org/10.1111/dar.12467

Smit, D. L., & de Ronde, W. (2018). Outpatient clinic for users of anabolic androgenic steroids: An overview. *The Netherlands Journal of Medicine*, *76*(4), 167–175.

Soussan, C., & Kjellgren, A. (2014). Harm reduction and knowledge exchange—A qualitative analysis of drug-related Internet discussion forums. *Harm Reduction Journal*, *11*(1), 25. https://doi.org/10.1186/1477-7517-11-25

Tighe, B., Dunn, M., McKay, F. H., & Piatkowski, T. (2017). Information sought, information shared: Exploring performance and image enhancing drug user-facilitated harm reduction information in online forums. *Harm Reduction Journal*, *14*(1), 48. https://doi.org/10.1186/s12954-017-0176-8

Underwood, M. (2017). Exploring the social lives of image and performance enhancing drugs: An online ethnography of the Zyzz fandom of recreational bodybuilders. *International Journal of Drug Policy*, *39*(C), 78–85. https://doi.org/10.1016/j.drugpo.2016.08.012

Underwood, M. (2019). The unintended consequences of emphasising blood-borne virus in research on, and services for, people who inject image and performance enhancing drugs: A commentary based on enhanced bodybuilder perspectives. *International Journal of Drug Policy*, *67*, 19–23. https://doi.org/10.1016/j.drugpo.2018.11.005

Van Hout, M. C., & Kean, J. (2015). An exploratory study of image and performance enhancement drug use in a male British South Asian community. *International Journal of Drug Policy*, *26*(9), 860. https://doi.org/10.1016/j.drugpo.2015.03.002

Van de Ven, K., Maher, L., Wand, H., Memedovic, S., Jackson, E., & Iversen, J. (2018). Health risk and health seeking behaviours among people who inject performance and image enhancing drugs who access needle syringe programs in Australia. *Drug and Alcohol Review*, *0*(0). https://doi.org/10.1111/dar.12831

Whyte, S., van der Geest, S., & Hardon, A. (2002). *Social lives of medicines*. Cambridge University Press.

Yarrow, J. F., McCoy, S. C., & Borst, S. E. (2010). Tissue selectivity and potential clinical applications of trenbolone (17β-hydroxyestra-4,9,11-trien-3-one): A potent anabolic steroid with reduced androgenic and estrogenic activity. *Steroids*, *75*(6), 377–389. https://doi.org/10.1016/j.steroids.2010.01.019

Zahnow, R., McVeigh, J., Bates, G., Hope, V., Kean, J., Campbell, J., & Smith, J. (2018). Identifying a typology of men who use anabolic androgenic steroids (AAS). *International Journal of Drug Policy*, *55*, 105–112. https://doi.org/10.1016/j.drugpo.2018.02.022

PART 3

DOPING ARENAS AND COMMUNITIES

Chapter 7

STEROID USE AMONG INMATES IN BELGIAN PRISONS

Bertrand Fincoeur and Jessica Rullo

ABSTRACT

While steroid use in the sports context has already been extensively studied by academic researchers, its patterns and implications in the prison context have received scant attention. Why do inmates use androgenic–anabolic steroids (AAS)? How does this use relate to sports activities, in particular fitness training, and what does it mean vis-à-vis the body image that is promoted in this environment? Does it even relate to fitness or sport? How do prison authorities regulate or prevent prisoners' AAS use? This empirical study is based on 28 interviews with 19 inmates and nine staff members (guards, managers) of four Belgian prisons. We showed that steroid use is largely connected with fitness activities and that it has an instrumental, goal-oriented dimension. AAS are used for athletic/performance purposes, e.g. increasing muscular strength. They also help gain or maintain a satisfactory body (self-) image, which has implications on the own identity, prestige and power relations within the prison community. In jail, the body is a major type of symbolic capital that is intended to reinforce status and cope with the difficulties and actual conditions of incarceration. We also observed differences in the perceived legitimacy of the various drugs that are used in prison. While guards are more tolerant towards AAS than other drugs, prisoners are less prone to openly confess to using AAS. Admitting to using AAS would damage the inmate's reputation, the legitimacy of his muscled body, and the subsequent goals of individual power and prestige.

Keywords: Image and performance-enhancing drugs; steroid use; prison; sports; fitness; body

Doping in Sport and Fitness
Research in the Sociology of Sport, Volume 16, 139–153
Copyright © 2023 by Emerald Publishing Limited
All rights of reproduction in any form reserved
ISSN: 1476-2854/doi:10.1108/S1476-285420220000016008

INTRODUCTION

While steroid use in the sports context (e.g. fitness doping: see Andreasson & Johansson, 2020; Christiansen et al., 2017) has already been extensively studied by academic researchers, its patterns and implications in the prison context have received scant attention. Although prison is known to be a hub for drug use and trafficking (Fazel et al., 2017; O'Hagan & Hardwick, 2017), it is unclear how important illegal image and performance-enhancing drug (IPED) use, in particular androgenic–anabolic steroid (AAS) use, is among inmates. Why do inmates use IPEDs or AAS? How does this use relate to sports activities, in particular fitness activities (e.g. bodybuilding, powerlifting), and what does it mean vis-à-vis the body image that is promoted in this environment? Finally, how do prison authorities regulate or prevent prisoners' IPED/AAS use? These issues were the focus of an empirical research study we conducted between June and November 2019 within four Belgian prisons, and this chapter reports on several main results of this project (Fincoeur & Rullo, 2021).

Imprisonment is commonly considered stressful and disruptive, both for physical and mental health, and sports activities may help reduce its global negative impact, which is subsumed under the concept of 'prisonization' (Thomas, 1977). Most prisons offer inmates the opportunity to do some physical activity in often precarious facilities whose opening hours basically vary from one prison to another, depending on their internal policies and constraints. A European Commission-funded project (Devis-Devis et al., 2012) has analyzed and compared physical and sports activities in 153 prisons in five countries (Belgium, Denmark, the Netherlands, Romania and Spain). It identified no fewer than 61 various sports activities, the most frequent ones being football and fitness/bodybuilding. The prison staff massively associated these activities with positive occupational, health and educational expected outcomes. In fact, this simply mirrors what has been evidenced in the scholarly literature regarding the impact of physical activities on inmates' physical (Nelson et al., 2006) and mental health (Buckaloo et al., 2009; Cashin et al., 2008), and reduction of aggressiveness (Martos-Garcia et al., 2009). Importantly, although there is some evidence about the positive effects of sports on drug use and addiction in general (Collingwood et al., 2000), there is a lack of empirical research on such possible effects among drug users within prison.

However, sports activities do not only endorse positive effects. In particular, they may involve several risks related to IPED/AAS use, including among inmates. Although several sources report an unquantified AAS use in prison (Meek, 2014, p. 158), the analyses on drug use in prison have so far focused on, and were limited to, cannabis, cocaine and heroin (Fazel et al., 2017; Mjåland, 2016). For example, the 2018 European Monitoring Centre for Drugs and Drug Addiction report on drug use in prison did not include IPED or ASS use at all (EMCDDA, 2019), which may suggest that the authorities did not see IPED use as a serious issue to investigate. Moreover, the illegal use of IPEDs, in particular AAS, is no longer a problem for only elite athletes. It has become an increasing concern for public health in general (McVeigh & Begley, 2017) since these products are used in various settings, such as student life, the sex industry and security businesses/occupations (e.g. bouncers, policemen) (Kiepek & Baron, 2019; Lucke et al., 2011; Wiegel et al., 2015).

A better understanding and analysis of AAS use among inmates is of high relevance because several scholars have shown that AAS use increases aggressiveness and the risk of violent behaviour (Beaver et al., 2008; Lundholm et al., 2010; Schulte et al., 1993). AAS use thus raises concerns not only vis-à-vis the reasons that may send an individual to prison but also about the consequences of potential violent conflict among inmates who use AAS and/or between inmates and prison guards. Inmates may also use IPEDs/AAS for muscular strength and bodily appearance purposes (Klötz et al., 2010) because the body is a major symbolic resource in the prison environment, which is often ruled by masculinity norms (Ricciardelli et al., 2015). The body is thus a tool of power and recognition in the interactions among peers (Jewkes, 2005). The specific role of sports activities and IPED/AAS use in the construction process of these masculinity norms therefore needs to be addressed and further explored (Sabo, 2001).

METHODS

This chapter relies on the results of a qualitative research study carried out in four French-speaking Belgian prisons between June and November 2019. The research design involved peripheral observations and semi-directed interviews among inmates and prison staff. The selection of the four prisons was made because they all had various sports facilities and because they hosted a substantial number of inmates. Among the 35 Belgian prisons, the four selected hosted about 20% of the whole prison population in Belgium (i.e. about 10,000 prisoners). The sports facilities available in the prisons were very heterogeneous. For example, while one prison had a dedicated room with more than 20 fitness machines in relatively good condition, another prison had no real fitness room and half of fitness machines (stored in former cells) were defective. The access to those facilities for inmates was also unequal from one prison to another: number of days and/or hours per week, number of inmates who could use the sports facilities etc.

Since we aimed at better understanding and analyzing inmates' attitudes towards and experience with IPED use, we took the seminal decision to focus on inmates participating in fitness and bodybuilding activities in prison. We were fully aware there was a risk of selection bias, and thus did not deeply investigate other forms of sports activities in prison such as football, table tennis or yoga. We then obtained the authorization from the prison authorities to access the fitness rooms. A prison guard briefly introduced us to the fitness participants, we presented them with objectives of the project, and asked if we could do some fitness training with them. Because prison is known to be a low-trust environment (Liebling & Arnold, 2004), our aim was to establish some confidence with inmates before conducting individual interviews. While inmates often experience the loss of any other identity outside of their 'criminal' one (Jewkes, 2005), we were only interested in 'inmates as athletes.' As a result, we did not ask questions about the reasons for which they were incarcerated. This may have contributed to a better acceptance of our presence as a mixed duo of researchers (Gurney, 1985) in sports sciences (and not, for example, in criminology) from a foreign university (i.e. Switzerland).

Each fitness participant was free to decide whether he agreed to take part in an individual interview. Several inmates refused to be interviewed for various reasons: insufficient knowledge of French language, lack of motivation etc. Surprisingly, although possessing substances in prison is itself an offence, the inmates were very open to discussing drugs in general. The widespread use and culture of acceptance of drugs in prison (Carpentier et al., 2018) may serve as an explanation for this. Despite the guarantee of confidentiality and anonymity, we are also aware that several inmates might have agreed to take part in the project because they supposedly (but mistakenly) expected some positive impact on the conditions of their incarceration (Hanson et al., 2015). The selection of interviewees followed the rules of purposive sampling; hence the size of our sample was determined by data saturation (Fusch & Ness, 2015). The interviews with the prison staff (guards, directors) were conducted either face-to-face or by phone. In total, we conducted 19 interviews with inmates, and nine interviews with prison staff members. Of the inmates we interviewed, all were male. We focused on male inmates for two reasons. First, because according to the statistics from the Belgian Ministry of Justice men represent 96% of the prison population in Belgium. Second, because the academic literature indicates a higher prevalence of IPED users among males (Henne & Livingstone, 2020).

The interview guide covered five main topics: inmates' sports backgrounds, sports activities in prison, IPED and drug use, body image and experience of detention (including the relationships with guards and other inmates). Each interview was recorded then transcribed. In addition, we took field notes which helped further contextualize and validate our results. Finally, we employed a thematic analysis with the data (Braun & Clarke, 2006), that is, we identified themes and patterns, and compared them with each other.

RESULTS

Our data analysis shows three main findings. First, while IPEDs and AAS in particular are factually used in prison, it is difficult to assess their prevalence, but they are largely associated with fitness and bodybuilding activities. Second, there are several significant differences in the use of, and attitudes towards, AAS and other drugs. Third, the reflection on the AAS issue needs to be considered together with the analysis of the challenges associated with sports activities and body image culture in prison.

The Extent of AAS Use and Its Link With Fitness Training Activities

In each of the four prisons studied, our interviewees reported on the existence of IPED users within the prison. First, several inmates reported self-use of some legal IPEDs, such as diet supplements, which are sold over the counter in the shop of the prison. All IPEDs are not legal, though, and AAS use was also reported, either by users or by inmates suspecting other users. However, we could not always interview these suspected users. As a result, the prevalence of AAS use was difficult to assess, and our qualitative research design did not aim or allow us to draw conclusions on this point. In addition, AAS use, just like any illegal drug use, often remains underestimated due to its illegal status. We nevertheless interviewed seven inmates who had ever used AAS in prison. One then needs to contextualize such use.

Although empirical research is scant, there is no real consensus regarding the link between sports activities in prison and AAS use (Meek, 2014). However, the inmates who self-reported AAS use did it systematically with reference to athletic purposes. Athletic purposes include either athletic performance or body achievements through fitness training. We will elaborate on this later. Since our methodological approach focused on users of sports facilities, it is obviously possible that we missed non-athlete AAS users, but this is very unlikely according to the prison staff members and inmates we interviewed. When considering AAS use among the various drugs that circulate in prison, it also seems that AAS use is very 'marginal' compared to other drugs, such as cannabis and heroin. Nevertheless, interviewees emphasized and reported less on the low prevalence of AAS use than the very high prevalence of other drugs, which is consistent with official figures and the academic literature (EMCDDA, 2019; Kolind & Duke, 2016). In addition, unlike products such as cannabis or heroin, AAS were described as less available – presumably because their use is less widespread – and more expensive when they are purchased in prison. Depending on the substances, retail prices would be at least twice higher inside than outside prison, but they decrease as more retailers enter the market (De Maere et al., 2000). Yet, the prevalence of AAS use and supply are not as high as for several other illicit drugs. This could thus explain why AAS do not appear as the main drug issue in prison.

Several inmates also considered that the very high prevalence of drugs in prison could explain the low participation in sports activities in general, and consequently the lower prevalence of AAS use, since such use was associated with fitness activities. Roughly said, the instrumental use of AAS (e.g. gaining muscle mass or reaching athletic performance) was considered not attractive enough for most inmates because they got caught up in health and/or addiction problems. Many prisoners could therefore not really participate in sports activities due to the various other problems they faced. One could, however, wonder whether, or to what extent, AAS use is part of a polydrug use phenomenon, which has already been evidenced among IPED users (Salinas et al., 2019). We unfortunately did not collect enough (or not unequivocal) data to seriously confirm or reject this hypothesis. We also need to contextualize AAS issue within the overall drug and sports issue that takes place in prison, which is the focus of the two following sections.

Are AAS Not Quite Like Any Other Drugs?

Although AAS and other drugs, such as cannabis, can all have harmful effects, they differ with regard to their perceived legitimacy and seriousness. First, in a context of prison overcrowding and lack of prison personnel, and unlike most illegal drugs, AAS were not presented as a policy priority by the prison staff members. They did not appear as a main health issue compared to other drugs, nor are they perceived as a major threat for prison security. In particular, the allegedly lower prevalence of AAS compared to that of other drugs did not justify an urgent need for regulation of AAS use and trafficking problems that take place in prison. According to our interviewees, the allegedly less widespread outbreak of AAS would provide fewer opportunities of uncontrollable trafficking activities among inmates. Tompkins (2016) distinguished two categories of black-market operators in prison: established enterprises and separate suppliers, that is, inmates who sell drugs in order to finance their own consumption. This echoes the distinction made by Coomber and Moyle (2014) between social supply and minimally commercial supply as an analysis of the transaction modes and supplying networks outside of the prison context. Unlike several other drugs, the AAS supply was not described as being supported by established enterprises. Instead, the ways to be provided with AAS seemed rather 'simple' and 'unorganized,' and they were basically made possible through the inventiveness of smugglers (e.g. complicity of prison guards, package delivery by friends and relatives, purchase in fitness centres etc.), but our interviewees did not report any real organization within the prison. For example, while several inmates reported they earn money by selling drugs to other inmates, we collected no such information regarding AAS.

We also observed different attitudes from the prison staff members vis-à-vis AAS compared with other types of drugs. Actually, the tolerance for AAS, which are perceived as less health damaging than, for example, heroin, seemed greater than that towards other drugs. As already stated earlier, the AAS issue is considered less problematic than other drug issues by the prison authorities, who must face the usual risks of overdose and settling of scores by inmates. This more tolerant attitude towards AAS then simply results in poor attention from the prison authorities to the treatment of this issue (EMCDDA, 2019). Surprisingly, our interviews with the inmates also indicated a different perceived legitimacy between IPEDs/AAS and other drugs. However, this perceived legitimacy among inmates was the opposite of that of the prison staff members. The latter were more permissive in their views about AAS, whereas inmates were much less prone to considering AAS as 'normal,' as developed in the following discussion. While our interviewees spoke very openly about, for example, cannabis use in prison, including the supplying networks, AAS use remained more hidden and was judged more severely. In fact, the instrumental use of AAS and other types of drugs seemed to significantly differ from each other: while cannabis or heroin use illustrates the extent of addiction among inmates and/or the negative effects of prisonization, AAS use challenges the importance of the bodily culture in prison, as outlined in the next section.

The Instrumental Use of AAS: Gaining a Status in Prison

Mike, one of our interviewees, reported that 'in prison, there are two behavioral options: doing sports or using drugs.' In this context, sports activities are not only intended to reduce boredom and sedentary lifestyles, they are also aimed to serve as a protective factor against drug use (Collingwood et al., 2000). The hybrid status of AAS is not uncontroversial, though, since AAS may be used for sports purposes and they can also have harmful effects (Horwitz & Christoffersen, 2019). While drugs other than AAS, such as cannabis, heroin etc., may be considered as an output of addiction, a reaction to anxiety or the integration of subcultural norms and values promoted in the prison environment (Connor & Tewksbury, 2016; Mjåland, 2016), AAS use seemed to be a goal-oriented behaviour. That is, as a strategy to better perform, gain muscular strength or personal pride, just like the motivation factors for AAS use outside of prison (Kimergard, 2015). Perhaps even more than in any other environment, the body in prison is symbolic capital that reinforces identity and masculinity, and consequently helps gain prestige and respect among inmates (Ricciardelli et al., 2015). AAS use, thus, has an instrumental function: obtaining a better (informal) status inside the prison.

Other individual, social and/or cultural factors also explain why there is a risk of AAS use among inmates. In particular, the prisoners' sports background (i.e. sports activities they did prior to their incarceration) likely have an impact on AAS use during incarceration. Among our interviewees, a substantial number were involved in fitness/bodybuilding and/or combat sports, that is, environments in which doping prevalence is allegedly higher compared to other sports (Christiansen et al., 2017; Coquet et al., 2018). Maintaining or improving athletic performance, including one's body image, is then a driver for using products intended to increase muscular strength, lose weight, burn fat etc.

Beyond their occupational purposes for inmates, sports activities can thus be considered as a means to reach or reinforce a status and a role that have an impact on the power relations inside the prison. These power relations are not limited to relationships between prisoners; they are also expressed in the relationships between prisoners and guards. In fact, this is why numerous guards are so sceptical about, and sometimes even averse to, fitness activities in prison, because this would increase inmates' strength, and consequently the perceived threat to their own integrity and safety. This then echoes the Foucauldian perspective of disciplined bodies (Foucault, 1975).

The AAS issue in prison is therefore at the crossroads of health, ethical and security challenges. Given their hybrid function in prison life, AAS raise a series of concerns related to the regulation of trafficking activities, the perceived legitimacy of the various drugs in jail, the power and leadership games between the actors and the global impact of sports activities in the prison ecology. We then discuss our main findings in the following section.

DISCUSSION

We present three levels of analysis in the next section. The micro-level refers to individual challenges related to inmates. The meso-level addresses issues related to the prison ecosystem. The macro-level focuses on challenges at the global policy level.

Micro-Level: Ambiguous Effects of Sports Activities in Prison

Our findings showed that although AAS are used in prison, though in unknown proportions, their consumption seems marginal compared to that of other drugs. Based on aggregated data from 59 studies from 31 countries, the lifetime prevalence of illicit drug use in prison ranges between 2% and 76% worldwide with, in most cases, cannabis being the most frequently reported substance. Up to 39% reported injecting illicit drugs during their stay in prison (Carpentier et al., 2018). The prevalence and patterns of drug use in prison seem to be the opposite of those outside of prison, as the academic literature has evidenced that the estimated prevalence of AAS use among the general population is higher than that of products such as cocaine and heroin (Pope et al., 2014). But what is the impact of incarceration on AAS use? Several scholars argued that the drug prevalence in prison would decrease as a result of the increased surveillance and the lower availability of the products (Shewan et al., 1994). Other studies indicated that incarceration may have an impact on the type of products that are used, depending on the duration of detention, the psychological profile of inmates or the availability of several products (Boys et al., 2002). In our study, AAS use was described as limited because of the availability and price of these products, but also because AAS use was basically understood as a goal-oriented behaviour and prison offers weak opportunities to reach the goals of such use. Several inmates serve long-term prison sentences and may struggle to develop coping strategies. In particular, the lack of motivation of most prisoners for physical or sports activities and the insufficient time slots allocated for sports activities in prison decrease the perceived utility of AAS use. This then echoes several conclusions made in the academic literature on athletic performance-driven IPED use by athletes (Christiansen et al., 2017).

The issue of AAS in prison then raises the question of access to sports activities and facilities. One could formulate the hypothesis that the more opportunities a prisoner has to do sports and pursue athletic objectives, the greater his propensity to use AAS in order to attain his objectives. Conversely, in theory, the more complicated the access to sports facilities, the lower the perceived utility of AAS use. However, one cannot seriously support the idea that a prison providing inmates with many opportunities to do fitness training would unduly encourage AAS use. Indeed, this would lead to a dilemma according to which either sports activities should be promoted with a risk of development of AAS use or preventing AAS use should be prioritized at the cost of sports activities in prison. Yet, involvement in regular sports activities in prison has positive health effects (Ross, 2013), especially as detention itself increases vulnerability to adverse physical and mental health outcomes (Fischer et al., 2012). Our interviewees then emphasized the positive outcomes of sports in prison, which help reduce harm from prisonization (Meek, 2014, pp. 30–31; Thomas, 1977). Since the prison environment is characterized by several forms of de-humanization and loss of identity, the fitness rooms and activities serve as a means to re-take control of the 'territories of the self' (Goffman, 1961). Doing bodybuilding or fitness training may thus be analyzed as a strategy that is intended to overcome the difficult conditions inmates do experience. Sports helps inmates get used to reduced bodily activity: tiny cells, limited movement etc. (Gras, 2003). In fact, the development of sports activities in jail contributes to transforming and modernizing the sentence's execution because it aims at rehabilitating prisoners' identity and dignity.

However, it would be both naïve and dangerous not to acknowledge that sports activities may also be a source of various risks. For example, several sports facilities and materials can be used as weapons or tools to facilitate evasion in case of lack of supervision (Meek, 2014, pp. 158–159). In addition, sports activities may cause injuries or, in some cases, be detrimental to health, especially when they are not properly realized or if they are driven by utopian expectations regarding athletic performance or body image (Nelson et al., 2006).

AAS are therefore ambiguous because they are often used for legitimate sports purposes, but they can result in safety risks and/or side effects such as sleep disorders and aggressiveness (Horwitz & Christoffersen, 2019). Given that sports activities likely convey promises of prevention or reduction of the use of various kinds of drugs, IPEDs/AAS excepted, it might nevertheless be acceptable to assume the risk of seeing the development of AAS use in prison if the global balance is judged positively. Policymaking in this respect calls for a global and integrated reflection addressing the various issues raised by the prison ecosystem.

Meso-Level: Impact on the Prison Ecosystem

The meso-level refers to the organizational functioning of, and interactions in, the prison. In this part, we address three points: the perceived legitimacy of AAS, the impact of fitness activities on inequalities between prisoners and the role of these activities on the various interactions between prisoners and guards.

The lower subcultural acceptance of AAS among inmates compared to other drugs can be interpreted at two levels. First, the differential perceived legitimacy could be explained because AAS use is not (yet) widespread enough to be fully culturally tolerated or even promoted within the inmates' community. From a Beckerian perspective (Becker, 1963), one could make the hypothesis that the more widespread a behaviour among a group of peers, no matter if it is illegal, the more likely this group of peers will see it as legitimate. Roughly said, openly discussing or widely using AAS should contribute to their banalization. Coakley (2015) elaborated the concept of positive deviance in sports to define the subcultural positive attitudes towards norms and values that go against social rules or laws, but that are tolerated or promoted by the insiders. Following our results, unlike cannabis, AAS use does not seem to have reached this stage of positive deviance within the inmates' community, hence its lower acceptance. Second, this relative omerta might convey the spread, including in prison, of the anti-doping propaganda, according to which doping is cheating. In fact, since the body is a symbolical resource of power and prestige, inmates cannot accept the value, merit or perceived image of their body being questioned. In particular, it is difficult to acknowledge that illegitimate means, such as AAS use, were adopted to shape this body. AAS issue in prison cannot be dissociated from the analysis of the construction of body cultures in general and its link with IPED use (Andreasson & Henning, 2021).

Although sports activities in prison have merits in terms of integration and socialization (Gallant et al., 2015; Meek & Lewis, 2014), they might also entail a series of side effects. For example, they likely increase the risk of inequalities and conflicts between inmates, which can result in abuse and (real or symbolic) violent behaviours (Ireland, 1999). Our results show that it is basically always the same prisoners who do fitness training. Those who were already the sportiest ones prior to incarceration and who have allegedly the most mental resilience to cope with incarceration 'monopolize' access to fitness rooms. The self-management of these rooms allows prisoners to take over several 'spaces of freedom,' as are prison yards too. However, these spaces are also areas where masculinities are often overemphasized, hence the need for further reflection on the opportunity for incentivizing the most vulnerable inmates to do sports activities. In addition, it is necessary to engage in open reflection and discussion about the presence and the role of professional coaches in prison. To date, such support is missing to a large extent while it could significantly contribute to regulate the power relations between prisoners, but also prevent possible misuse of IPEDs.

Finally, sports activities in jail often modify the nature of the relationships between inmates and guards. They help reduce, even fade, the distance, or sometimes the conflicts, between these actors (Crewe, 2011) because fitness activities are characterized by a more relaxed atmosphere, and informal exchanges are made easier there. However, they also provide guards with an additional control and regulation tool. For example, since fitness training activities appear as very valuable in the eyes of inmates, they may be suspended as a means of coercion for internal discipline purposes. This illustrates how complex and double-binding interactions in prison can be. Indeed, it is expected from guards that they establish a climate of confidence, which can then result in situations of manly camaraderie (Wacquant, 2002), while keeping their role of authority. This then raises a couple of final considerations about the nature of sports and drug policies in prison.

Macro-Level: Towards a Global Drugs and Sports Policy in Jail

We identify two discussion topics at the macro-level: the relevance and implementation of prevention measures against the (mis)use of AAS in prison, and the development of a global and integrated policy on sports activities in prison.

Our findings indicated poor knowledge among inmates regarding the risks and side effects of AAS. It appeared that IPED and AAS use primarily rely on self-administration, at most peer experience, but without any supervision from health professionals. In this respect, prison seems to be no real exception to what happens outside the prison (Kimergard, 2015). This, however, calls for a large educational program about drug use in prison, which needs to go far beyond the sole AAS issue, but which would include AAS as part of the problem. Yet, the AAS issue is still largely neglected in current drug policies in prison, as illustrated earlier by the lack of attention and data regarding IPEDs in the recent EMCDDA reports. It seems equally important to seriously consider the establishment of structures and experts in charge of detecting and treating the use and misuse of AAS in the prison environment (Havnes et al., 2019). Importantly, this raises the question about the opportunity of implementing or promoting harm reduction policies in prison (Hughes, 2003; Sander et al., 2016; Zurhold & Stöver, 2016) and including AAS in these policies. There could also be better monitoring of the use of the various substances in prison, and AAS should be systematically surveyed as are other types of drugs.

Our analysis has shown that there is to date no real consistent policy regarding the organization of sports activities in Belgian prisons. The authorities admit sports activities are not a priority but emphasized the numerous organizational (lack of space, lack of facilities, lack of human resources) and budgetary constraints and barriers that hinder the development of fruitful policies. Furthermore, the access to sports activities and facilities varies a lot from one prison to another, and sometimes relies (too) strongly on individual initiatives from several staff members committed to sports and prisoners' needs in this respect. The organization and regulation of sports in prison therefore has no real guiding principle nor institutional agenda at the global level (Sempé, 2016). In Belgium, this topic also suffers from the 'balkanization' of the competencies across the various state levels. Different institutions are in charge of prison infrastructures (buildings), health in prison etc. As the Belgian state reforms have gone by for almost five decades, this results in a blurred situation with dispersed means of action and competent institutions, which often ends up nowhere and makes any global and consistent sports policy in prison very unlikely.

CONCLUSION

In this chapter, we analyzed the intertwined relationship between sports (fitness) activities and the use of IPEDs (AAS) in prison. We showed that although there are AAS users among inmates, steroid use in prison seems marginal compared to that of other drugs. AAS use is also largely connected with the practice of sports activities, in particular, fitness training. This is indicative of the instrumental goal-oriented dimension of AAS by prisoners. On the one hand, AAS are used for athletic/performance purposes, i.e. increasing muscular strength, improving his condition etc. On the other hand, AAS help gain or maintain a satisfactory body (self-)image, which has implications on the own identity, prestige and power relations within the prison community. In jail, the body is major symbolic capital that is intended to reinforce status and cope with the difficulties and actual conditions of incarceration. We also observed differences in the perceived legitimacy of the various drugs that are used by inmates and regulated by prison staff members. While the latter are more tolerant towards AAS due to their supposedly less harmful properties for health and safety, prisoners are less prone to openly confess to using AAS. Steroid use is thus more hidden from other inmates because admitting to using AAS would damage the inmate's reputation, the legitimacy of his muscled body, and the subsequent goals of individual power and prestige. Finally, we addressed two main questions raised by our study, i.e. the challenges related to the organization of sports activities in prison and the prevention of AAS (mis)use. First, we showed that sports activities are the poor relation of prison policies due to the many organizational and financial constraints prisons are facing. Second, we emphasized the need for more research on the possible side effects of AAS use for inmates, including the reflection about care and treatment options. Both at the academic and policy levels, these questions have received scant attention to date. This contribution is therefore an invitation to scholars and policymakers to further analyze and elaborate on these challenging issues of the prison ecosystem.

KEY READINGS

(1) Coakley, J. (2015). Drug use and deviant overconformity. In V. Møller, I. Waddington, & J. Hoberman (Eds.), *Routledge handbook of drugs and sport* (pp. 379–392). Routledge.

   A must-read in doping research to better understand how the perceived legitimacy of drug use can be redefined within subcultural environments.

(2) Gallant, D., Sherry, E., & Nicholson, M. (2015). Recreation or rehabilitation? Managing sport for development programs with prison populations. *Sport Management Review*, 18, 45–56.

   A contribution that investigates the role of sport in enacting social change; in particular, its positive influence on inmates' health and behaviour.

(3) Kolind, T., & Duke, K. (2016). Drugs in prisons: Exploring use, control, treatment and policy. *Drugs: Education, Prevention and Policy*, 23(2), 89–92.

   The authors showed that prisons are a high-risk environment for drug initiation and use. A key reading to contextualize the use of steroids in prison.

(4) Meek, R. (2014). *Sport in prison. Exploring the role of physical activity in correctional settings*. Routledge.

   This seminal book provides a general overview of the various ways sport can impact diverse groups of prisoners and prison staff. It draws from a great number of primary and secondary data sources.

(5) Ricciardelli, R., Maier, K., & Hannah-Moffat, K. (2015). Strategic masculinities: Vulnerabilities, risk and the production of prison masculinities. *Theoretical Criminology*, *19*(4), 491–513.

This article addresses how the risk-prone environment of the prison shapes prisoners' behaviours and the production of masculinities. A key reading focusing on the role played by steroid use in the construction of inmates' body image.

REFERENCES

Andreasson, J., & Henning, A. (2021). *Performance Cultures and doped bodies: Challenging categories, gender norms, and policy responses*. Common Ground.

Andreasson, J., & Johansson, T. (2020). Re-conceptualizing doping and masculinity. In J. Andreasson & T. Johansson (Eds.), *Fitness doping. Trajectories, gender, bodies and health*. Palgrave Macmillan.

Beaver, K., Vaughn, M., DeLisi, M., & Wright, J. (2008). Anabolic-androgenic steroid use and involvement in violent behavior in a nationally representative sample of young adult males in the United States. *American Journal of Public Health*, *98*, 2185–2187.

Becker, H. (1963). *Outsiders*. Free Press.

Boys, A., Farrell, M., Bebbington, P., Brugha, T., Coid, J., Jenkins, R., Lewis, G., Marsden, J., Meltzer, H., Singleton, N., & Taylor, C. (2002). Drug use and initiation in prison: Results from a national prison survey in England and Wales. *Addiction*, *97*(12), 1551–1560.

Braun, V., & Clarke, V. (2006). Using thematic analysis in psychology. *Qualitative Research in Psychology*, *3*, 77–101.

Buckaloo, B. J., Krug, K. S., & Nelson, K. B. (2009). Exercise and the low-security inmate changes in depression, stress, and anxiety. *The Prison Journal*, *89*, 328–343.

Carpentier, C., Royuela, L., Montanari, L., & Davis, P. (2018). The global epidemiology of drug use in prison. In S. A. Kinner & J. D. Rich (Eds.), *Drug use in prisoners: Epidemiology, implications, and policy responses* (pp. 17–41). Oxford University Press.

Cashin, A., Potter, E., & Butler, T. (2008). The relationship between exercise and hopelessness in prison. *Journal of Psychiatric and Mental Health Nursing*, *15*, 66–71.

Christiansen, A. V., Schmidt Vinther, A., & Liokaftos, D. (2017). Outline of a typology of men's use of anabolic androgenic steroids in fitness and strength training environments. *Drugs: Education, Prevention & Policy*, *24*(3), 295–305.

Coakley, J. (2015). Drug use and deviant overconformity. In V. Møller, I. Waddington, & J. Hoberman (Eds.), *Routledge handbook of drugs and sport* (pp. 379–392). Routledge.

Collingwood, T., Sunderlin, J., Reynolds, R., & Kohl, H. (2000). Physical training as a substance abuse prevention intervention for youth. *Journal of Drug Education*, *30*, 435–451.

Connor, D. P., & Tewksbury, R. (2016). Inmates and prison involvement with drugs: Examining drug-related misconduct during incarceration. *Journal of Contemporary Criminal Justice*, *32*(4), 426–445.

Coomber, R., & Moyle, L. (2014). Beyond drug dealing: Developing and extending the concept of 'social supply' of illicit drugs to 'minimally commercial supply'. *Drugs: Education, Prevention & Policy*, *21*(2), 157–164.

Coquet, R., Roussel, P., & Ohl, F. (2018). Understanding the paths to appearance- and performance-enhancing drug use in bodybuilding. *Frontiers in Psychology*, *9*, 1431.

Crewe, B. (2011). Soft power in prison: Implications for staff–prisoner relationships, liberty and legitimacy. *European Journal of Criminology*, *8*(6), 455–468.

De Maere, W., Hariga, F., Bartholeyns, F., & Vanderveken, M. (2000). *Santé et usage de drogues en milieu carcéral*. Rapport de recherche. Politique Scientifique Fédérale belge.

Devis-Devis, J., Peiro-Velart, C., & Martos-Garcia, D. (2012). Sport & physical activity in European prisons: A perspective from sport personnel. www.prisonersonthemove.eu

EMCDDA. (2019). *Rapport européen sur les drogues 2019: Tendances et évolutions*. Office des publications de l'Union européenne.

Fazel, S., Yoon, I. A., & Hayes, A. J. (2017). Substance use disorders in prisoners: An updated systematic review and meta-regression analysis in recently incarcerated men and women. *Addiction, 112*, 1725–1739.

Fincoeur, B., & Rullo, J. (2021). Je pousse donc je suis: Du rôle de la musculation et des produits de la performance en prison. *Déviance et Société, 45*(2), 231–263.

Fischer, J., Butt, C., Dawes, H., Foster, C., Neale, J., Plugge, E., & Wright, N. (2012). Fitness levels and physical activity among class A drug users entering prison. *British Journal of Sports Medicine, 46*(16), 1142–1144.

Foucault, M. (1975). *Surveiller et punir*. Gallimard.

Fusch, P. I., & Ness, L. R. (2015). Are we there yet? Data saturation in qualitative research. *The Qualitative Report, 20*(9), 1408–1416.

Gallant, D., Sherry, E., & Nicholson, M. (2015). Recreation or rehabilitation? Managing sport for development programs with prison populations. *Sport Management Review, 18*, 45–56.

Goffman, E. (1961). *Asylums: Essays on the social situation of mental patients and other inmates*. Anchor Books.

Gras, L. (2003). Carrières sportives en milieu carcéral : l'apprentissage d'un nouveau rapport à soi. *Sociétés Contemporaines, 49–50*, 191–213.

Gurney, J. N. (1985). Not one of the guys: The female researcher in a male-dominated setting. *Qualitative Sociology, 8*, 42–62.

Hanson, B. L., Faulkner, S. A., Brems, C., Corey, S. L., Eldridge, G. D., & Johnson, M. E. (2015). Key stakeholders' perceptions of motivators for research participation among individuals who are incarcerated. *Journal of Empirical Research on Human Research Ethics, 10*, 360–367.

Havnes, I. A., Jørstad, M. L., & Wisløff, C. (2019). Anabolic-androgenic steroid users receiving health-related information; health problems, motivations to quit and treatment desires. *Substance Abuse Treatment, Prevention, and Policy, 14*(1), 20.

Henne, K., & Livingstone, B. (2020). More than unnatural masculinity. Gendered and queer perspectives on human enhancement drugs. In K. van de Ven, K. Mulrooney, & J. McVeigh (Eds.), *Human enhancement drugs* (pp. 13–26). Routledge.

Horwitz, H., & Christoffersen, T. (2019). A review on the health dangers of anabolic steroids. *Adverse Drug Reaction Bulletin, 317*(1), 1227–1230.

Hughes, R. (2003). Drugs, prisons, and harm reduction. *Journal of Health & Social Policy, 18*(2), 43–54.

Ireland, J. (1999). Bullying amongst prisoners: A study of adults and young offenders. *Aggressive Behavior, 25*, 162–178.

Jewkes, Y. (2005). Loss, liminality and the life sentence. Managing identity through a disrupted life course. In A. Liebling & S. Maruna (Eds.), *The effects of imprisonment* (pp. 366–388). Willan.

Kiepek, N., & Baron, J. L. (2019). Use of substances among professionals and students of professional programs: A review of the literature. *Drugs: Education, Prevention & Policy, 26*(1), 6–31.

Kimergard, A. (2015). A qualitative study of anabolic steroid use amongst gym users in the United Kingdom: Motives, beliefs and experiences. *Journal of Substance Use, 20*(4), 288–294.

Klötz, F., Petersson, A., Hoffman, O., & Thiblin, I. (2010). The significance of anabolic androgenic steroids in a Swedish prison population. *Comprehensive Psychiatry, 51*(3), 312–318.

Kolind, T., & Duke, K. (2016). Drugs in prisons: Exploring use, control, treatment and policy. *Drugs: Education, Prevention & Policy, 23*(2), 89–92.

Liebling, A., & Arnold, H. (2004). *Prisons and their moral performance: A study of values, quality, and prison life*. Oxford University Press.

Lucke, J. C., Bell, S. K., Partridge, B. J., & Hall, W. D. (2011). Academic doping or Viagra for the brain? *EMBO Reports, 12*, 197–201.

Lundholm, L., Käll, K., Wallin, S., & Thiblin, I. (2010). Use of anabolic androgenic steroids in substance abusers arrested for crime. *Drug and Alcohol Dependence, 111*(3), 222–226.

Martos-Garcia, D., Devis-Devis, J., & Sparkes, A. (2009). Sport and physical activity in a high security Spanish prison: An ethnographic study of multiple meanings. *Sport, Education and Society, 14*(1), 77–96.

McVeigh, J., & Begley, E. (2017). Anabolic steroids in the UK: An increasing issue for public health. *Drugs: Education, Prevention & Policy, 24*(3), 278–285.

Meek, R. (2014). *Sport in prison. Exploring the role of physical activity in correctional settings.* Routledge.

Meek, R., & Lewis, G. (2014). The impact of a sports initiative for young men in prison: Staff and participant perspectives. *Journal of Sport & Social Issues, 38*(2), 95–123.

Mjåland, K. (2016). Exploring prison drug use in the context of prison-based drug rehabilitation. *Drugs: Education, Prevention & Policy, 23*(2), 154–162.

Nelson, M., Specian, V., Tracy, N., & DeMello, V. (2006). The effects of moderate physical activity on offenders in rehabilitative program. *Journal of Correctional Education, 57*(4), 276–285.

O'Hagan, A., & Hardwick, R. (2017). Behind bars: The truth about drugs in prisons. *Forensic Research & Criminology International Journal, 5*(3), 158.

Pope, H., Kanayama, G., Athey, A., Ryan, E., Hudson, J., & Baggish, A. (2014). The lifetime prevalence of anabolic-androgenic steroid use and dependence in Americans: Current best estimates. *American Journal on Addictions, 23*(4), 371–377.

Ricciardelli, R., Maier, K., & Hannah-Moffat, K. (2015). Strategic masculinities: Vulnerabilities, risk and the production of prison masculinities. *Theoretical Criminology, 19*(4), 491–513.

Ross, M. (2013). *Health and health promotion in prisons.* Routledge.

Sabo, D. (2001). Doing time, doing masculinity: Sports and prison. In D. Sabo, T. Kupers, & W. London (Eds.), *Prison masculinities* (pp. 61–66). Temple University Press.

Salinas, M., Floodgate, W., & Ralphs, R. (2019). Polydrug use and polydrug markets amongst image and performance enhancing drug users: Implications for harm reduction interventions and drug policy. *International Journal of Drug Policy, 67*, 43–51.

Sander, G., Scandurra, A., Kamenska, A., MacNamara, C., Kalpaki, C., Fernandez Bessa, C., Laso, G. M., Parisi, G., Varley, L., Wolny, M., Moudatsou, M., Pontes, N. H., Mannix-McNamara, P., Libianchi, S., & Antypas, T. (2016). Overview of harm reduction in prisons in seven European countries. *Harm Reduction Journal, 13*, 28.

Schulte, H. M., Hall, M. J., & Boyer, M. (1993). Domestic violence associated with anabolic steroid abuse. *American Journal of Psychiatry, 150*(2), 348.

Sempé, G. (2016). *Sports et prisons en Europe.* Council of Europe Publishing.

Shewan, D., Gemmell, M., & Davies, J. (1994). Prison as a modifier of drug using behaviour. *Addiction, 2*, 203–215.

Thomas, C. (1977). Theoretical perspectives on prisonization: A comparison of the importation and deprivation models. *Journal of Criminal Law and Criminology, 68*, 135–145.

Tompkins, C. (2016). "There's that many people selling it": Exploring the nature, organisation and maintenance of prison drug markets in England. *Drugs: Education, Prevention & Policy, 23*(2), 144–153.

Wacquant, L. (2002). *Corps et âme. Carnets ethnographiques d'un apprenti boxeur.* Agone.

Wiegel, C., Sattler, S., Göritz, A. S., & Diewald, M. (2015). Work-related stress and cognitive enhancement among university teachers. *Anxiety, Stress & Coping, 29*(1), 100–117.

Zurhold, H., & Stöver, H. (2016). Provision of harm reduction and drug treatment services in custodial settings – Findings from the European ACCESS study. *Drugs: Education, Prevention & Policy, 23*(2), 127–134.

Chapter 8

HOW DIGITAL FITNESS FORUMS SHAPE IPED ACCESS, USE, AND COMMUNITY HARM REDUCTION BEHAVIOURS

Luke A. Turnock and Honor D. Townshend

ABSTRACT

With digital spaces an increasing feature of our everyday lives, and the internet now a primary means of sourcing IPEDs and information regarding their use, this chapter seeks to understand how digital fitness forum communities shape the dissemination of culturally embedded harm reduction advice. Findings are drawn from two netnographic studies of fitness forums, which identify several key areas in which community norms and structures served to inform harm reduction behaviours. This included embedded forum reputation systems and the ways in which these shaped IPED access, including through elevating 'expert' users and encouraging informed discussion regarding product quality, to the emergence of steroid testing services from forums as a community harm reduction tool. Second, forums were observed to often encourage users to conduct research and inform themselves regarding safe use, though limitations to this norm were also documented in relation to poor-quality medical advice, highlighting the issues with IPED users' reliance on anecdotal advice in the contexts of prohibition. Finally, the role of digital fitness forums as 'digital backstage' is considered, examining both how this can be harmful to IPED users from excluded or 'otherised' groups, but simultaneously offers cultural participants the opportunity for airing vulnerabilities in a space where their masculine identity is not threatened in doing so, thus facilitating harm reduction among cultural 'insiders'.

Doping in Sport and Fitness
Research in the Sociology of Sport, Volume 16, 155–179
Copyright © 2023 by Emerald Publishing Limited
All rights of reproduction in any form reserved
ISSN: 1476-2854/doi:10.1108/S1476-285420220000016009

Keywords: IPEDs; online supply; forums; masculinities; harm reduction; safe spaces

INTRODUCTION

As research across the world and among a range of disciplines is increasingly turning to online platforms and digital cultures (Abidin, 2013), the role of the 'digital community' is of more importance than ever. 'Communities' as a concept are characterized by Hamman (1998) as (1) a group of people who, (2) share social interaction and (3) some common ties between themselves and the other members of the group, and who (4) share an area for at least some of the time. It is taken in more recent studies that the requirement within Hamman's definition of sharing 'an area' does not necessitate a physical space but can also be applied to online spaces (Sillence & Baber, 2004).

Some of the most common formats for these online communities are social media and interest-based forums. Though there are no definitive figures for levels of participation in online forums generally, in 2011 it was estimated that forums were still 'regularly' used by approximately 20% of internet users in the United States, and 10% in the United Kingdom (Li & Bernoff, 2011). Reasons for engaging in forums varies dependent on the interest the forum is catering to, with cited reasons varying from improving professional performance (Carceller et al., 2013) to reassurance on health concerns (Tanis, 2008). But what is present throughout is the role of community and socializing in the maintenance of engagement in online spaces (Brennan et al., 2010; Pitta & Fowler, 2005; Tanis, 2008).

Digital fitness communities specifically are noted as sharing these social characteristics by Underwood (2017), who highlights the role of shared cultures and companionship as important factors in the use of these platforms. The social element of these communities is important, but also important is how their existence enables other functions of the forum. Specifically, the development of a digital safe space as defined by the characteristics of physical safety; metaphorical safety; familiarity and comfort; and the capacity to encourage risk (Hunter, 2008). The latter element of Hunter's (2008) characterization is of particular importance within these contexts, owing to fitness forums' additional role as platforms for information sharing and the social supply of IPEDs (Turnock, 2021a). Fitness forums are a significant portion of the online forum sphere, with a simple Google search for 'Fitness forums' returning tens of millions of results. While fitness forums are diverse in nature, with topics such as diet, competition and body composition frequently discussed and debated across these platforms, in many of these spaces the topic of IPEDs is also frequently discussed, with some specific forums dedicated primarily to this topic. Contemporary society is an increasingly virtual one (Dufva & Dufva, 2019), something which has only been heightened further by the reduction in physical social spaces during the COVID-19 pandemic, and resulting increase in consumption of digital fitness content (Hayes, 2022). As such, the role of these spaces in the information sharing regarding IPEDs is only of increasing importance.

This social role of fitness forums is of particular significance in the context of online platforms more broadly serving increasingly as a primary point of access to the purchase of IPEDs (Cordaro et al., 2011; Hall & Antonopoulos, 2015; van de Ven & Koenraadt, 2017). Van de Ven et al. (in press) highlight the range of online marketplaces, ranging from illegitimate online pharmacies (Hall et al., 2017), IPED-selling websites, online sellers on e-commerce markets, dark web platforms (Hall & Antonopoulos, 2015), as well as social media, online messenger platforms and forums, this latter three of which are predominantly utilized to discuss, advertize and share information relating to IPEDs (van de Ven et al., in press).

Knowledge regarding safe access and use of IPEDs is made difficult for users owing to their illegality in many jurisdictions and consequent lack of clear advice for safe and sensible use through official channels (Antonopoulos & Hall, 2016; Hanley-Santos & Coomber, 2017; Underwood, 2017). Whilst in recent years attempts have been made to improve the knowledge public health agencies have regarding advice for safe IPED use (Atkinson et al., 2021; Harvey et al., 2019), most users still choose to rely on subculturally embedded systems of advice for this information (Antonopoulos & Hall, 2016; Van de Ven & Mulrooney, 2017), often distrusting official sources where these do exist due to prior misrepresentation of IPED effects and harms, and perceiving unofficial channels as giving more honest advice (see Turnock, 2021b). Consequently, as digital spaces become an increasingly important domain for IPED access and information regarding use (Brennan et al., 2016), the contexts surrounding the delivery of this culturally embedded advice becomes significant to understanding contemporary harm, and harm reduction, within IPED-using cultures.

With forums acting as a primary point of engagement with lifting cultures (Henning & Andreasson, 2019; Turnock, 2021a), these digital spaces are significant sites to explore in assessing how culturally embedded advice helps to shape IPED-related harm reduction practices in contemporary fitness cultures. Whilst some IPED-related knowledge found on digital forums may be poor or uninformed (see Brennan et al., 2016), our research into these communities indicates a number of community-developed methods by which understanding of safe(r) use and access is facilitated and culturally embedded harm reduction enacted. This chapter shall therefore explore the ways in which forum community self-regulation mechanisms may lead to more informed practices in relation to IPED access and wellbeing-conscious use, encouraging forum visitors towards more 'wellbeing' or 'expert' approaches to use (Christiansen et al., 2017; Zahnow et al., 2018), as well as the limitations to this suggestion, before turning to an analysis of the broader role of forums as digital 'safe spaces' for posters, and the particular relevance of this to community harm reduction.

To achieve this, the chapter shall first examine the ways in which the forums studied shaped users' approach to IPED access, examining how community reputation mechanisms helped disseminate 'expert' community information on product and seller quality, before looking at a specific example of harm reduction which emerged directly from forum communities in the form of steroid testing services, and how these shape understandings of IPED quality and access in digital communities. This is followed by an exploration of the ways in which forums encourage a more informed approach to IPED use among their userbase, offering advice on safe use for those lacking experience or access to such advice elsewhere, and discouraging harmful practices. This is followed by an exploration of how broader wellbeing advice is disseminated to users on forums and how these practices may also help with harm minimization, though potentially may also propagate misinformation. Finally, the role of IPED forums as gendered spaces, where users feel free to share information that may be harmful to their 'frontstage' presentation of self (Goffman, 1959), shall also be discussed, paying attention to how this can both create hostile and misogynistic spaces which exclude some potential advice-seekers from accessing information, but may simultaneously facilitate harm reduction for their primary userbase through encouraging discussion of concerns which might threaten posters' sense of self in their offline, non-anonymous lives.

METHODS

Data utilized in this research originate in two original studies completed by the authors, both of which explored the cultures of digital fitness forums and forum users' experiences accessing and using IPEDs, Luke's commencing in 2014, and Honor's in 2020. This section offers a brief overview of the methods of the two projects, in order to contextualize our findings.

Study A: IPED Markets and Cultural Contexts to Use and Supply

Luke's study can be described as a 'connective ethnography' (Gibbs & Hall, 2021), in which he engaged in extensive netnographic study (Kozinets, 2015) of forum spaces, simultaneous to ethnographic research in the UK gym sites, with findings constructed from observations and comparative analyses across these combined fieldsites. This blending of digital and 'offline' research has been adopted in numerous recent explorations of IPED-using cultures (Andreasson & Johansson, 2014, Antonopoulos & Hall, 2016; van de Ven & de Zeeuw, 2021), reflecting the significance of overlap between these cultural sites within IPED-using communities (van de Ven & Koenraadt, 2017), and increasing importance of our digital selves in our everyday lives (Dufva & Dufva, 2019).

The offline portion of Luke's research examined IPED use in five 'hardcore' and four more 'commercial' gyms in South-West England. Data were drawn from 18 in-depth semi-structured interviews with individuals felt to be particu-larly knowledgeable regarding IPED use or supply, along with hundreds of informal discussions with gym users regarding their experiences and observations (see Turnock, 2021c for detail), all of which informed the construction of findings from the digital portion of the research. Additionally, Luke's experience as a former competitive powerlifter facilitated cultural understandings (Salinas et al., 2019), and his positionality as a cultural 'insider' must therefore be acknowledged to fully situate Luke's role in the construction of findings (Blackman, 2016; Charmaz, 2014).

For the digital portions of this research, the primary fieldsite was one of the largest fitness forums operating when research commenced (2014), from which 28,801 unique posts from 98 IPED-related threads were collected for analysis, following a period of immersion in forum culture (see Turnock, 2021a for detail). This portion of the research adopted a 'passive netnographic' approach to data collection, allowing the collection of rich, uncensored discourse whilst avoiding unnecessary disruption to the community (Brennan et al., 2018a; Enghoff & Aldridge, 2019). Further sampling of other forums, based on purposive sampling of threads related to specific themes identified from the main fieldsite, led to a further 10 forums being sampled, again adopting a passive netnographic approach.

All forums studied were open-access, with data cited from this portion of the study drawn from publicly accessible threads. Nonetheless, ethical considerations regarding anonymization and appropriate limits to data use were respected (see Turnock, 2021a, pp. 27–31), following best practice identified in the literature (Barratt, 2011; Enghoff & Aldridge, 2019; Henning & Andreasson, 2019). Findings across both digital and 'offline' portions of the research were analyzed manually using thematic and narrative analysis, with themes developed through a grounded theory approach to the discovery of theory from data, using the constant comparative method (Charmaz, 2014; Glaser & Strauss, 2017). Ethical approval was granted by the University of Plymouth.

Study B: Gender Identities and IPED Use

Honor's research was conducted in part for her Doctoral thesis, which sought to research the role of gender identities and the impact of COVID-19 on the use of IPEDs. This research utilized a netnographic methodology (Kozinets, 2015) in order to explore the nature of online interactions and socializations. Data were collected from a selection of conversation threads across four open-access fitness forums across a five-month period in 2020. The data were then subject to manual thematic and narrative content analyses. The date range of this research was during the United Kingdom's first wave of COVID-19, and as such the research was grounded within this context and search terms utilized reflect this, but nonetheless produce results which serve to highlight contemporary trends within online forums more generally.

Two Google searches for 'fitness forum' and 'bodybuilding forum' were utilized, and a selection of four of most-popular results were then chosen for analyses dependent on them matching the following criteria: Forums only; open-access (not requiring sign-up or payment to access); fitness-specific (or have a dedicated sub-forum); forums containing a 'search' function; English-language; currently active forums. The final utilized forums were: City Data (Exercise and Fitness sub-forum); The Student Room (Fitness sub-forum); UK-Muscle and underground (UG) Bodybuilding.

Upon selection of the forums, a content strategy was outlined which utilized major terminology relating to COVID-19 to find relevant material to the time period (1) COVID-19, (2) COVID 19, (3) Coronavirus, (4) Corona Virus, (5) Rona. Content was then subject to further inclusion criteria in order to be included, namely comments must have been posted between 1st March 2020 and 25th July 2020; must contain information related to or mention of COVID-19; and only the first 10 pages of multi-page threads were to be included.

A total of 115 forum threads were thematically assessed. All forum threads were sorted by date, and were compiled and analyzed for relevance to five themes developed utilizing a deductive framework whereby two researchers reviewed forum content, created an overarching list of topic themes, and those relevant to thesis were selected, two of which collected data relevant to this chapter, entitled: Motivation for use (of IPEDs), and general attitudes towards IPED use. This research was conducted with ethical approval from the University of Hertfordshire.

FINDINGS

How Forums Shape IPED Access and Use

A common concern within IPED-using communities relates to product quality, with users eager to ensure they are accessing safe, correctly dosed IPEDs (Coomber et al., 2014; van de Ven & Koenraadt, 2017). Quantitative testing has frequently shown illicit IPEDs to be underdosed, or containing different compounds to those on labels (Coomber et al., 2014; Fabresse et al., 2021; Kimergård et al., 2014a), and it is common knowledge among users that most black-market steroids are not pharmaceutical-grade, but created in underground labs (UGLs) of varying quality (Kimergård et al., 2014b; Llewellyn & Tober, 2010; Turnock, 2020). Consequently, many IPED users adopt buying strategies that attempt to minimize the risk of acquiring poor-quality product, with the advice of experienced users serving as a key means by which legitimacy is assessed (Antonopoulos & Hall, 2016; Bilgrei, 2018; Coomber & Salinas, 2019; van de Ven & Koenraadt, 2017).

A key area to understand regarding how forums shape access and use consequently relates to the ways in which advice regarding product quality and seller legitimacy is navigated and disseminated within forum cultures. This section shall examine first the ways in which forums facilitated 'bottom up' community regulation through the formation of cultural systems of 'reputation', before turning to the emergence of steroid testing services as a specific example of a harm reduction strategy that emerged directly from the forums.

Community Reputation Mechanisms and Quality Concerns

Whilst reputation mechanisms exist in gyms on a 'micro' scale, with experienced bodybuilders and gym owners advising less-informed parties regarding which products they should access (Antonopoulos & Hall, 2016; Coomber & Salinas,

2019), forums facilitate such advice on a macro scale. As open spaces where uncensored discourse occurs, forum communities encourage the sharing of experiences accessing different sellers and labs, with informed users advising which are perceived to be legitimate and which are considered less reputable. Advice in these spaces is thus drawn from a diversity of informed parties who collaboratively shape understandings, whilst enabling those without existing 'offline' subcultural connections to access such information.

These community reputation systems can be fairly advanced, with individual posters building a digital 'rep' based on how helpful their advice is, how experienced a user they are and broader community standing (see Andreasson & Johansson, 2016). Consequently, each forum will have a group of users with good 'rep' to whom others will generally defer, based on their demonstrated expertise. Such 'expert' members in Luke's research included competitive powerlifters, bodybuilders, steroid 'brewers' (see Turnock, 2020) and individuals with academic or professional chemistry backgrounds (verified by others with such backgrounds). These posters would openly discuss their experiences and advise less-experienced posters regarding what was considered good quality and what to avoid, disseminating the culturally embedded advice identified among gym-based cultural 'experts' on an international scale:

Anon: So Darklord is the guy I need to see if I want to join the bicycle race?
Nito: Well there are many sources out there, but he is pretty prevalent here because he is reliable, has not terrible prices for decent gear and is an open source.
Knob: Darklord is legit, confirmed by every single person who has ever ordered from him.

Significantly, forums displayed more 'formal' methods for making these assessments compared to gyms, with norms emerging whereby expert posters would formally 'verify' the legitimacy of sellers for the community, through buying 'sample' orders and offering reviews of product effects and service received. With numerous posters offering such reviews, community members could easily access opinions regarding lab or seller reputations when considering where to buy from:

The official Gainsbrah review: You've probably seen this new guy in recent threads advertising for pharma gear... In order to confirm his legitimacy, I decided to go through with a small order... Tl; dr GainsBrah's services while being highly price attractive (disregarding shipping entirely) are in no way ready for any sort of real volume of customers.

Consequently, posters indicated a strong perception that the price, product quality and service received through forums was generally much better than in gyms, as 'scammers' (including 'false posters' and 'sock puppets') were rapidly identified, whilst those with good product or service were elevated with positive 'rep'. With the majority of established posters having accessed IPEDs through gym-based sources previously, this perception reflected the experiences of countless users who felt they benefitted from these community reputation systems.

Notably, community reputation norms also encouraged suppliers in forum spaces to adopt more customer-oriented sales strategies, more akin to aspects of 'social supply' practices (see van de Ven & Koenraadt, 2017). Given the open discussions of experiences and importance of community reputation, suppliers were often seen responding to publicly posted queries or complaints in a manner aimed at satisfying not only affected customers but also other forum members likely to read these threads, with supplier reputation shaped by the outcome of these interactions:

> Heating may have been a bit off which is why people are getting PIP (post-injection pain), which is also why I posted in the other thread to heat them up in the oven in hopes of having them constituting better. If that doesn't help the PIP I will reimburse people.

> That's one of the things I really like about Fatman and Darklord... you can just internet shout at them if you're unhappy with the product.

The community reputation systems of forums thus allowed users to access informed advice regarding product more consistently than is possible for many in gym environments, where pre-existing connections are necessary, and may be difficult for some users to make (Antonopoulos & Hall, 2016). With culturally embedded advice systems important for harm reduction within IPED-using communities (Van de Ven & Mulrooney, 2017), forums as spaces where such advice is openly and collaboratively refined and disseminated highlight their capacity to facilitate harm reduction among their userbase.

Steroid Testing Services
A highly visible means by which forums encouraged informed access was through the presence of steroid testing services and posting of test results in these spaces. Drug testing services are increasingly advocated as a harm reduction measure in public health (Harper et al., 2017; Measham, 2019), and given the prevalence of poor-quality product in the illicit IPED market (Coomber et al., 2014), the value of testing services for these communities has been apparent for some time (Turnock, 2021a).

In Luke's research, he documented how one of the earliest commercial testers began advertizing on forums around 2014, offering to test IPEDs using HPLC/MS. Located in a Central European country with relaxed rules on IPED possession, and benefitting from purchasing power disparities in an international digital market, 'Milo' offered to test samples for a comparatively low fee (80 Euros), generating immediate interest. Once forum regulars with chemistry experience suggested results looked legitimate, many posters began accessing these services, leading to users across several forums beginning to ask for test results when looking to buy:

> Buyer: Anybody bother testing FM or DL's [product]?
> Fatman: I've had my stuff lab tested.
> Buyer: I Assume you'll prove that before doing business?
> Fatman: [Posting trenbolone results] I can provide the mass specs for most of my stuff.

Whilst there was debate regarding the legitimacy of these services, with some posters suggesting testers could take payment from UGLs to make fake reports, the community reputation mechanisms discussed earlier similarly facilitated this discussion, with debates around tester legitimacy paralleling the open debates regarding product quality and supplier reputation in these spaces:

> ...[one homebrewer] sent duplicate blind samples to [tester] and another lab. The results matched. He's not making up numbers or guessing. His results are legitimate.

Indeed, whilst a broad consensus emerged that these services were legitimate, the open discussion of concerns actually led to a further evolution in harm reduction in forum spaces. On the Thinksteroids forums, moderators promote the crowd-funded testing service anaboliclab.com, a self-described harm reduction service that secretly purchases IPEDs from well-known sources to test, and publishe results open-access online. Thinksteroids not only shares these results with their userbase but also additionally includes badges for supporters of this crowd-funded service to display on their forum profiles to show they are contributing to community harm reduction, encouraging greater participation with this service.

By encouraging product testing and disseminating results, forums thus circulate harm reduction information to countless users. With both commercial and crowd-funded testing having emerged out of forum communities, it is clear these spaces have had a significant impact on IPED access and use as a consequence. As one forum regularly commented regarding the impact of testing services, 'Everyone and their grandma tests these days, and the internet enables rapid transmission of knowledge, feedback and reviews', meaning poor-quality product is rapidly identified, and this information disseminated in a way not possible previously. Whilst poor-quality product remains prevalent in the underground market (Fabresse et al., 2021), forums clearly act as a significant space for disseminating harm reduction advice in this area. This illustrates how the cultural and structural aspects of forums encouraged more informed approaches to IPED access and use through 'bottom up' community policing and innovation, indicating their value to users as spaces for harm reduction. This builds on existing understanding of the ethnopharmacological knowledge of IPED-using subcultures (Andreasson & Johansson, 2016; Monaghan, 2001) and the ways in which this is collaboratively disseminated and (re)defined.

Encouraging Informed Use

Examining the relationship between forum communities and harm reduction more broadly, the presence of informed users openly posting guidance in forum space was observed to help correct misunderstandings among less-informed posters and shape community knowledge of use. A clear example in Luke's study came from a poster who detailed the cycle he had taken, and complained he had gotten bad side-effects, alleging the product use must have been defective.

Subsequent discussion over the issue, however, enabled informed posters to observe that, based on the information offered, it was most likely the commenter's over-use of accessory drugs Selective Estrogen Receptor Modulators (SERMs) that caused the negative effects cited, rather than the product itself:

> Sounds like you tanked your E2, nothing to do with the gear. You shouldn't have gotten into this whole thing with this amount of knowledge.

The collaborative aspects of forum discussions thus helped address misinformation, through encouraging informed users to openly address and rebut less-informed commenters, providing valuable information for those reading threads. Indeed, the forum cultures Luke observed had strong norms of encouraging their userbase to conduct reading and research before engaging in IPED use, seen in examples of posters asking for sources without first demonstrating requisite knowledge:

> Kid, lurk more. Join different forums. Do your research. If you have to ask for a source, you haven't done your due diligence.

These trends were also highlighted in Honor's research, which showed similar advice-giving mechanisms within forums, with a seemingly increased importance due to the lockdown context of the research period. One such heightened role of knowledge-sharing observed was that of long-standing forum members advising as to the impact to IPED supply chains during this worldwide period of uncertainty. This ranged from exchanging warnings regarding concerns over quality of products, to identifying fake advertisements for IPEDs, to disparaging comments regarding those intent on 'homebrewing' steroids (see Brennan et al., 2018a) without demonstrating the requisite knowledge or capacity to undertake this:

> Another gammon intent on preparing injectables in his house.

Despite the differences in research context and time period, the same peer advice network was thus highlighted in both studies. Significantly, a number of posts discouraging use were observed in Honor's study, with many long-term self-stated IPED users suggesting that individuals should not start using, sometimes due to the context of COVID-19 and lockdown, but often regardless of this:

> You're trying to overcome your lack of knowledge by using steroids.

There is often a tendency within research to critique the role of peer-to-peer information sharing, particularly in online spaces, due to the concern of misinformation potentially leading to high-risk behaviours (Tighe et al., 2017). However, the forums we observed in the majority showed evidence of a supporting environment, often utilizing anecdotal observations by necessity (Underwood, 2017), but clearly pointing peers towards harm reduction approaches. As such, it is arguable that these spaces have the potential to reduce harm as much as they do to increase it, should forum recommendations translate into actual enacted behaviours. This is of particular significance to users in countries which lack effective public harm reduction service provision for IPED users, given variation in the control of IPEDs and attitudes towards harm reduction across jurisdictions (Henning & Andreasson, 2022).

In this context, it is significant to note that Luke further observed the influence of forum recommendations on informed participants in his gym-based research, where several competitive powerlifters (i.e. 'expert' users) discussed utilizing information from forums, which consequently shaped the advice they offered others as respected figures in their gyms:

> I done a lot of research trawling bodybuilding forums, you can get a lot of information from there.

This overlap between 'online' and 'offline' access, with information on source quality and safe use shared across both spheres, illustrates how the community reputation mechanisms of digital forums shape not only forum posters' understanding, but impact on the 'offline' steroid market as well, as reputations spread beyond the confines of digital space to gym environments (see van de Ven & Koenraadt, 2017). Consequently, many 'expert' individuals in offline spaces may in fact receive much of their understanding from forums, directly or second-hand, illustrating the importance of these digital spaces even when exploring cultures where 'offline' norms of access are 'resilient' (Coomber & Salinas, 2019).

Community, Wellbeing Advice and Harm (Reduction?)

In both studies, we observed that the poster population were often long-term members, posting regularly and consistently for years, with the role of socializing evidenced throughout our research. There is evident familiarity among long-term posters, and this encourages conversation to stray to topics surrounding individuals' lives, wellness, entertainment and more. Specifically of importance though is how these social spaces enable open discussion and provision of advice relating to IPED use itself, and wellness more generally. This can be observed with long-term forum users becoming seen as authoritative sources for information, as well as often acting as translators for academic jargon-filled articles. This democratization of information observed within fitness forums is observable in many other spheres of digital social spaces (Jebril et al., 2013); however, because of the nature of wellness, substance use and health-related content observable on fitness forums, these spaces warrant further attention regarding how their 'open' advice structures may result in potential harms.

Building on the aforementioned reputation mechanisms, the community aspects of forums were observed in both studies to help facilitate communication of valuable harm reduction advice, and experienced forum posters would often respond to queries and offer advice regarding dosage, harm reduction, tapering, medical assistance and other aspects of wellbeing relevant to use. In both studies, we observed informed, long-term IPED users cautioning less-experienced posters to not start using, or to minimize dosages, exemplifying the harm reduction advice documented for 'expert' users elsewhere (Antonopoulos & Hall, 2016; Christiansen et al., 2017).

On the other hand, the openness of forums to novel and anecdotal debate also indicates potential for harm, and both authors noted examples of information being posted that could lead to problematic health outcomes if followed uncritically. Honor observed that in relation to COVID-19, there was debate involving significantly opposing views regarding the impact of IPEDs on potential infection, with misinterpreted medical information utilized to evidence both perspectives. Namely, the perspectives that use of anabolic–androgenic steroids (AAS) would either worsen or better chances of recovering from COVID-19 infection:

> If you have high blood pressure from steroids Coronavirus will kill you'

> Low testosterone in males is also being linked to more serious cases. Wouldnt fancy doing a PCT right now!

This topic, and the health and wellbeing discussions observed in general, poses one of the highest risk behaviours observed on forums, due to the potential for serious negative consequences for individuals based on un-evidenced and contradictory claims made across threads. Whilst sometimes news articles and academic studies were referenced, often discussions were anecdotal in nature, and whilst this is often by necessity (Underwood, 2017), such interactions illustrate the potential for misinformed advice to be disseminated in these spaces, as observed by other researchers in relation to 'blood-letting' (Brennan et al., 2018b) and DNP dosing (McVeigh et al., 2017).

The presence of misinformed wellness-related information, combined with the potential for active responses and trust from the community if shared by established community members, therefore presents potential issues. This is particularly relevant in the context of Honor's research occurring during the lockdown period in the United Kingdom, leading to a lack of access to healthcare (Davillas & Jones, 2021), and health-maintenance facilities and equipment such as blood-pressure testing facilities usually available in pharmacies, something observed and commented upon on the forums:

> ...normally I would just do blood and get hormones checked but now with this covid 19 floating around I want nothing to do hospitals and clinics. (sic)

As such, it is highly plausible that the move to individual self-access and self-control regarding independent health and wellness which has been observed in recent years (Nijland et al., 2008; Turnock, 2021b) was heightened during the context of lockdowns, with the contexts of wellness information on these health-related forums illustrating the potential risks of this transition. This is further evidenced by Whitfield et al.'s (2020) research which highlighted a reduced uptake of NSP (Needle and Syringe Programmes) specifically within IPED users during this time period.

Whilst Honor's findings must be understood in the context of the mainstream debate around COVID and harm similarly being confused and frequently contradictory during this period (Szakolczai, 2021), Luke also identified discourse relating to wellbeing that illustrates risks within forums' community-embedded advice norms, even preceding COVID. Whilst many experienced posters recommended those interested in IPED use monitor their health with their doctor, for example, the sharing of negative experiences with or perceptions of medical professionals was also commonplace, even among long-term community figures, with some established posters cautioning others not to reveal their AAS use to doctors, owing to their perceived incompetence or prejudice against IPED users:

Q: Can/should you tell your doctor when you go to check-ups that you're on gear? Do your doctors know?

A: My previous doctor told me I would get testosterone poisoning from using steroids. I don't tell them anymore.

Whilst 'challenging medicine' is a well-documented phenomenon among IPED-using cultures (Dunn et al., 2016; Harvey et al., 2019; Monaghan, 1999), with researchers working on ways to reduce this distrust (Atkinson et al., 2021), it is clear that the posting of such anecdotes by respected community members had the potential to deter posters from seeking appropriate help, and reinforced the previously noted cultural perception that 'official' advice was less trustworthy than that on forums, even in jurisdictions where users were able to access such advice. Despite these being a minority of voices, the potential for harm within community-embedded advice mechanisms is clearly apparent in such examples.

Issues may also arise from the irreverent nature of much forum culture, as highlighted by Underwood (2017) in relation to in-jokes and trolling among the Zyzz fandom. In Luke's research, some established posters would joke about using 'YOLO' doses of steroids because they found it funny to claim they took health-threatening amounts: '[will] see if I develop instant jaundice'. Whilst cultural insiders understood these posts were facetious, for the uninitiated such discourse could potentially translate into real-world harm if followed. Whilst the dictum of 'lurk more' if obeyed would lead posters to recognize such content as ironic, this does not preclude harm from new cultural entrants believing or following such information, as may have occurred with the influx of health enthusiasts unfamiliar with forum cultures during the COVID lockdowns.

Whilst forums act as useful tools for understanding effective IPED use and disseminating wellbeing-related advice, the very openness and community aspects which allow for these benefits also clearly have potential for propagating misinformation and harm, and their value for facilitating harm reduction must therefore be understood within this context.

Gender and the 'Backstage' Space of Forums

Building on how social aspects of forum communities shape IPED and wellbeing-related advice, it is worth examining the role of forums as gendered 'safe spaces' for posters, and how the role of forums as 'backstage' spaces (Goffman, 1959; Kilvington, 2021) may impact on discourse. Underwood (2018) highlights how the perceived 'safety' of forums and digital cultures may facilitate support and disclosures which could threaten 'front stage' presentation of self, particularly in relation to masculinities, and this is significant to understanding the ways in which advice is sought and harm reduction enacted in forum spaces. This must first, however, be understood critically in the context of anonymous (and pseudonymous) forums' capacity to encourage misogyny, homophobia, or harmful discourse, in order to fully appreciate the extent to which forums act as gendered spaces of either harm reduction, or simply harm.

Safe spaces are identified by Hunter (2008) as physical or virtual spaces that encompass four qualities: physical safety; metaphorical safety; familiarity and comfort; and the capacity to encourage risk. As such, the developed 'safe spaces' of forums are often seen to be utilized for discussing not only fitness and IPED use but also personal lives, health and politics. Though framed here broadly as 'safe spaces', it is important to acknowledge that the 'safety' developed within these online spaces is dependent on individuals' identities and is not without exclusions. Kilvington (2021) draws upon Goffman's (1959) concepts of the 'front stage' and 'backstage' to explore the differences between online and offline communication in the context of hateful messages, arguing the perceived anonymity of online spaces presents as a 'virtual backstage' which removes the commenter from the view and critique of 'front stage', leading to the sharing of content which posters would not present in their daily lives outside of these 'invisible' contexts. This section shall consequently examine first how this position of fitness forums as a 'virtual backstage' excluded groups from participating in forum culture, thus limiting their ability to access harm reduction advice (see also Andreasson & Henning, 2021), before considering the ways in which this feature of anonymous forums was potentially beneficial in reducing some harms among (principally male, heterosexual) users.

Whilst it is important to highlight that attitudes displayed on forums did vary, with discussions regarding female use of IPEDs, workout routines and biological differences between sexes, the majority of comments relating to women and/or LGBTQ + communities observed followed four general themes: (1) lack of trust of women, (2) hyper-sexualization of women, including female forum posters, (3) derogatory discussion of women's physical appearances and (4) homophobia:

(1) Yeah this is why I've never told any of my partners about my AAS use, don't care about all that honesty nonsense, it's just giving them ammo to f**k you over with eventually. Had too many bad experiences with women to trust them with that knowledge.
(2) Just sext me dirty things the whole time and I could distract you.
(3) The fat blonde f**k across the road from me comes out looking disgusting in her yoga pants.
(4) Nothing to see here, just another skinny f**got.

Regarding the former theme, Ging (2019) suggests the assertion of tropes that actively demean women, including that of being untrustworthy, is an active reassertion of male cultural dominance. Arguably then the presence of comments of this nature evidences the virtual safe space created within these forums, enabling discussions which otherwise may be considered problematic and/or offensive. Contrastingly, Marche (2016) suggests that online language is often a performance of fantasy indulgence, and as such comments observed online should not be considered representative of an individual in 'real-life', let alone representative of an entire community. However, Ging (2019) reiterates that regardless of online comments' representativeness of individual's actual beliefs, to dismiss these online behaviours is to ignore a real issue.

In relation to the second theme, similarly to how the male gaze has been traditionally observed in the (male) safe space of the physical gym (Andreasson & Johansson, 2013; Graham et al., 2013), the online forum community similarly enabled the hyper-sexualization of women, and often this was specifically directed at the minority of female forum users. Whilst such behaviours have been observed on forums for some time (Andreasson & Henning, 2021; Germain et al., 2021; Henning & Andreasson, 2019), the lockdown context to the research is also important to consider here. Due to the lack of access to physical fitness spaces, it is plausible that the prevalence of these comments may have increased, especially when considering many forum users also discussed their use of traditional gym settings for heterosexual flirtation:

> A lot of guys probably also miss being near the females at the gym. Many are coed. I miss the running events for that reason - meeting women. They tend to open up to me after the ten mile mark (sic).

Among threads that contained elements of the third theme there were opposing views voiced, signifying that the safe spaces created in these online contexts do not always present challenge-free environments. However, the predominant theme of these discussions being inherently negative is indicative of a platform within which the safe space that is created is only for a specific community of individuals.

Relating to the homophobic attitudes displayed in the observed forums, it was noted that often this language was directly linked by the forum posters to body image ideals. O'Brien et al. (2013) study highlighted a link between athleticism and homophobia, stating that 'physical identity and athletic attributes based around masculine ideals also appear to contribute to this prejudice in males' (p. 891). Whilst Luke's research indicated some contradictions here, including appropriation of terminology from gay culture seemingly incongruous with 'truly' homophobic attitudes (see Anderson & McCormack, 2018; cf Klein, 1993), most notably posters' use of 'twink' and 'bear'/'bear mode' when discussing physique ideals (the latter particularly given positive connotations), the deliberate use of offensive or othering language in these spaces nonetheless clearly serves to signify both the 'backstage' nature of this space for posters, as well as further highlighting that a seemingly unspoken criteria for inclusion within this space were present, as with the aforementioned cultural in-jokes.

Though the negative language and performative attitudes displayed due to the felt 'safe space' of the forums has been highlighted here, it is important to note that it is also these feelings of safety and reliance on other forum posters that enables users to seek advice regarding their own wellbeing and IPED use. Though the latter does pose potential issues related to the reliability of said advice (discussed above), the existence of an open community is something that can be utilised to promote harm-reducing behaviours and spread reliable information, too, and as such provides a unique opportunity for researchers and practitioners in the field seeking to understand community harm reduction.

In examining the position of forums as safe spaces, it is therefore significant to explore examples of the positive engagement this facilitated. Underwood (2018), and Underwood and Olson (2019), in exploring the (almost exclusively male) Zyzz fandom of amateur bodybuilders, discuss how the digital environment in some ways encouraged the de-gendering of traditionally feminized traits such as emotional vulnerability, intimacy and support, offering a space in which men who perceived themselves as traditionally masculine were free to engage in discourse which might threaten these identities outside the contexts of the backstage spatiality created by the (pseudo-)anonymity of forum spaces. Reflecting this, Luke documented numerous instances where posters would discuss topics they might not raise 'in real-life' owing to concerns these could harm their masculine (self-)image, regarding fears of failure, suicidal ideation, family issues, and other topics on which orthodox masculinities may not allow for honest discussion, often to men's detriment (see Coen et al., 2013). The 'virtual backstage' of forums, meanwhile, facilitated men whose identities were heavily invested in traditional masculinity to express vulnerability, and receive or offer emotional support without threatening this identity.

This links with observations Luke made in Turnock (2021d), regarding how men in rural hardcore gyms, whilst clinging to problematic ideas of masculinity in some respects, also used the gym as a means of engaging peers for support, and voicing vulnerabilities whilst participating in a shared 'masculine' endeavour, which allowed men with more orthodox understandings of masculinity to engage in shared support without threatening their masculine identity. The use of exclusionary language on forums may therefore be considered to reflect attempts to assert control over this space as a means of protection, voicing performative opposition to normative narratives regarding what one 'cannot say' as a means of solidifying for oneself the notion of the forum as a space where one can voice all thought – and thus express vulnerabilities – without repercussion. This is again particularly relevant in the COVID lockdown context, where concerns regarding mental health among IPED users were heightened (Dunn & Piatkowski, 2021).

This feeling of security in sharing vulnerabilities can also notably be seen in relation to IPEDs, in posters' willingness to discuss potentially embarrassing topics they might otherwise avoid addressing in the absence of this safe space. This could be seen in relation to help-seeking regarding: development of gynaecomastia, erectile dysfunction, issues regarding gonadal hypotrophy or testicular pain, and other topics that might otherwise go undiscussed for fears of harming one's masculine credibility. In Luke's gym-based research, he documented issues that YOLO-type users had in relation to not seeking help until after such problems had already become significant. These users, who tended to engage with digital fitness cultures through social media rather than forums, avoided the help-seeking observed among forum posters because 'No-one wants to put themselves down on social media, do they?' (Turnock, 2018, p. 111). Those whose main engagement with digital fitness communities was through forums, by contrast, were able to voice potentially embarrassing issues under the protection of pseudonymity in these spaces, and feelings of community, allowing them to receive advice without fear of harming their masculine credibility.

Community behaviours facilitated by the 'safe space' atmosphere of forums, whilst having negative impacts on some users (Andreasson & Henning, 2021), must therefore be understood to also facilitate men's engagement with support and help-seeking in a way their understanding of masculinity might otherwise hinder, with the 'protective' nature of these spaces thus offering positives in addition to negatives.

DISCUSSION AND CONCLUSION

This exploration has highlighted the ways in which forum communities shape IPED use and harm reduction behaviours, with the social aspects of forums playing a key role across these areas. Both research projects indicate the positives for community harm reduction norms that arise out of the collaborative aspects of forums, particularly regarding their facilitating culturally embedded systems of 'expert' advice observed previously (e.g. Van de Ven & Mulrooney, 2017) on a 'macro' scale. With prohibition making 'official' advice regarding safe use, as well as verified pharmaceutical product, largely inaccessible from the perspective of users (Coomber et al., 2014; Dunn et al., 2021; Underwood, 2017), the reputation systems witnessed on forums were observed to allow posters to more clearly discriminate between sources of information, and many forum users cited the beneficial effects of these community norms on product quality and advice offered in these spaces. With the emergence of steroid testing services perhaps the most visible example of how forum communities collaboratively advanced harm reduction norms and offered innovation not possible in gym or non-collaborative digital settings, it is clear that forum spaces must be understood as key sites for understanding the dissemination of culturally embedded harm reduction information, particularly given the interaction between digital and 'real world' spaces within fitness cultures (Turnock, 2018; van de Ven & Koenraadt, 2017). Nonetheless, more specific research exploring the translation of forum content to actual enacted behaviours would be required to state conclusively how impactful digital reputational norms are on behaviours and access within the broader fitness community.

Whilst the advice systems on forums often positively shaped user behaviours in the direction of harm reduction, the democratization of information must not be viewed uncritically, and whilst forums helped posters to advance community understanding of safe use and wellbeing, the presence of misinformed and poor advice in these spaces nonetheless indicates the potential for harm, particularly if accessed by those without existing cultural understandings, as likely occurred following the increase in interest in digital fitness spaces during the lockdown period (Hayes, 2022). Whilst the presence of misinformation on forums has been identified for some time, along with narratives of distrust regarding the medical community in these spaces (Brennan et al., 2016), our research highlights the specific risks which this presented to uninitiated cultural entrants, particularly heightened in the COVID lockdown context, evidencing the importance of understanding how forum posts translate into 'real world' behaviours among a diversity of user types, building on Luke's work which did this for powerlifters (Turnock, 2018).

Building on these findings, the ways in which forums might be encouraged to shape their community understandings in positive directions are therefore worth considering, particularly given some forum moderators have already demonstrated a willingness to follow the recommendations of academics for improving their service delivery, as Andreasson and Henning (2021) note for the Thinksteroids forum's introduction of a specific women only forum for discussing doping. In addition to this forum's noted efforts to promote crowd-funded product testing, and ensure this harm reduction advice is appropriately disseminated, Thinksteroids also notably host articles by experts on IPED use, encouraging their userbase to keep up-to-date on expert academic thought on topic around use and harm reduction. As an example of a forum conscious of their role as sources for culturally-embedded harm reduction advice, Thinksteroids illustrates how the positive aspects of community harm reduction advice might be enhanced by conscious policies from forum owners and moderators to better ensure expert advice is accessible and misinformation addressed, whilst maintaining the positive social aspects which draw posters to forums.

Turning to the position of forums as safe spaces, it is clear that the feeling of community and protection engendered by the identification of these spaces as such facilitates the sharing of information which may aid in harm reduction. It is equally clear, however, that the exclusionary nature of these spaces is also likely to be detrimental for many, for example, if women intending to use IPEDs find forums inaccessible and are thus unable to benefit from culturally embedded harm reduction advice; a fact made particularly pertinent as our understanding of who uses IPEDs evolves (Andreasson & Henning, 2021; Henning & Andreasson, 2019). Returning to Thinksteroids, the forum's noted creation of separate areas catering to women's training and advice needs, explored by Andreasson and Henning (2021), again offers illustration of how the negative impacts of the 'backstage space' aspect to forum cultures might be navigated in a way that nonetheless maintains the 'protective' aspects to forum spaces that potentially vulnerable men rely on in other areas of their site (Turnock, 2021d; Underwood & Olson, 2019). So far as such policies allow male users to continue to discuss potentially embarrassing topics in a way that does not threaten their masculine self-identity, whilst also allowing posters who do not fit the typical forum culture a space in which they can also feel safe and receive valuable advice, such policies offer illustration of ways in which forum structures might be shaped to increase participation with advice mechanisms across a range of populations interested in digital fitness and wellbeing content. Based on our findings, the promotion of such practices may be a beneficial direction for forums to follow in the short-tomedium term, whilst greater changes regarding the navigation of understandings of gender and masculinity, which will take a lot longer, occur at the cultural level (Turnock, 2021e). However, with the stratification of members explicit, in terms of trusted members and in terms of gender, this may present some difficulties in effectively encouraging harm reduction for users excluded by the issues highlighted here.

Finally, it is significant to consider the changing nature of digital body-oriented, IPED-consuming cultures. Although we noted similarities in the forum cultures observed despite the time period between our respective studies, the specific contexts of lockdown and shifts in accessibility to health services and IPED supply noted in Honor's work illustrate the importance of understanding the advice offered within these cultures as dynamic, and subject to broader socioeconomic, political and cultural shifts (Gibbs, 2021). Building on this, whilst forums once operated as the primary point of engagement for lifting cultures, it is significant to note that most new entrants into digital fitness cultures today are likely to engage with these cultures primarily through social media, where there are differing norms surrounding advice offered and levels of comfort sharing information, as Luke observed when comparing the experiences of powerlifters and 'lads' in his research (Turnock, 2018). The findings offered in this chapter might therefore contribute to ongoing research examining social media-based digital fitness cultures and the extent to which these replicate, or differ from, the community norms of harm reduction observed for forums.

KEY READINGS

(1) Turnock, L. A. (2021a). *Supplying steroids online: The cultural and market contexts of enhancement drug supply on one of the world's largest fitness & bodybuilding forums*. Plymouth Policy Research Institute.

A book based on study A from this chapter, exploring the cultural and market contexts to IPED supply over fitness forums. Uses netnographic findings to explore how forums shape access, supply and advice regarding IPED use, as well as detailing some of the innovations that emerged from forum communities in relation to harm reduction.

(2) Van de Ven, K., & Mulrooney, K. J. D. (2017). Social suppliers: Exploring the cultural contours of the performance and image enhancing drug (PIED) market among bodybuilders in the Netherlands and Belgium. *International Journal of Drug Policy*, *40*, 6–15. https://doi.org/10.1016/j.drugpo.2016.07.009

Article exploring the ways in which the supply of IPEDs links to social and cultural embeddedness of suppliers, with much advice regarding use shaped by social relations and sellers' cultural capital. Demonstrates how the structure of IPED markets is often intimately tied to cultural contexts and how harm reduction advice is disseminated within communities of fitness enthusiasts.

(3) van de Ven, K., & Koenraadt, R. (2017). Exploring the relationship between online buyers and sellers of image and performance enhancing drugs (IPEDs): Quality issues, trust and self-regulation. *International Journal of Drug Policy*, *50*, 48–55. https://doi.org/10.1016/j.drugpo.2017.09.004

Article examining the online supply of IPEDs which notes distinctions between online pharmacies which try to mislead buyers and sellers invested in 'social supply' practices as part of their business. Highlights strategies adopted by both consumers and suppliers to minimize risk and harms in dealing with the online market for IPEDs, paralleling strategies observed on forums.

(4) Tighe, B., Dunn, M., McKay, F. H. and Piatkowski, T. (2017). Information sought, information shared: Exploring performance and image enhancing drug user-facilitated harm reduction information in online forums. *Harm Reduction Journal*, *14*(1), 1–9. https://doi.org/10.1186/s12954-017-0176-8

Article examining the advice sought and offered on digital IPED forums, and types of evidence/data forum communities engage with in relation to safe IPED use. Illustrative of the significance of anecdotal information to these communities, as well as how they navigate misinformation or gaps in knowledge within their cultural spaces.

(5) Underwood, M., & Olson, R. (2019). 'Manly tears exploded from my eyes, lets feel together brahs': Emotion and masculinity within an online body building community. *Journal of Sociology*, *55*(1), 90–107. https://doi.org/10.1177/1440783318766610

Article which examines the gendered aspects to digital amateur body-building communities, and the ways in which these may simultaneously propagate hegemonic aspects of masculinity whilst also acting as safe spaces where vulnerabilities and emotions may be displayed by men involved in them. Relevant to the discussions of frontstage/backstage digital spaces in the present chapter.

ACKNOWLEDGEMENTS

Luke would like to thank Nick Gibbs for his advice regarding this chapter.

Honor would like to thank Anna Tippett for her input and advice regarding her original study.

FUNDING

Luke's research did not receive any specific grant from funding agencies in the public, commercial, or not-for-profit sectors.

Honor's research was undertaken as part of her University of Hertfordshire-funded PhD research. She did not receive any further specific grant from funding agencies in the public, commercial, or not-for-profit sectors.

REFERENCES

Abidin, C. (2013). 'Cya IRL': Researching digital communities online and offline. *Limina: A Journal of Historical and Cultural Studies, Special Edition: Humanising Collaboration, 18*(2), 1–17.

Anderson, E., & McCormack, M. (2018). Inclusive masculinity theory: Overview, reflection and refinement. *Journal of Gender Studies, 27*(5), 547–561. https://doi.org/10.1080/09589236.2016.1245605

Andreasson, J., & Henning, A. (2021). Challenging hegemony through narrative: Centering women's experiences and establishing a sis-science culture through a women-only doping forum. *Communication & Sport.* https://doi.org/10.1177/21674795211000657

Andreasson, J., & Johansson, T. (2013). Female fitness in the blogosphere: Gender, health, and the body. *Sage Open, 3*(3). https://doi.org/10.1177/2158244013497728

Andreasson, J., & Johansson, T. (2014). *The global gym: Gender, health and pedagogies.* Palgrave Macmillan.

Andreasson, J., & Johansson, T. (2016). Online doping: The new self-help culture of ethno-pharmacology. *Sport in Society: Cultures, Media, Politics, Commerce, 19*(7), 957–972. https://doi.org/10.1080/17430437.2015.1096246

Antonopoulos, G. A., & Hall, A. (2016). 'Gain with no pain': Anabolic-androgenic steroids trafficking in the UK. *European Journal of Criminology, 13*(6), 696–713. https://doi.org/10.1177/1477370816633261

Atkinson, A. M., van De Ven, K., Cunningham, M., de Zeeuw, T., Hibbert, E., Forlini, C., Barkoukis, V., & Sumnall, H. R. (2021). Performance and image enhancing drug interventions aimed at increasing knowledge among healthcare professionals (HCP): Reflections on the implementation of the Dopinglinkki e-module in Europe and Australia in the HCP workforce. *International Journal of Drug Policy*, 103141. https://doi.org/10.1016/j.drugpo.2021.103141

Barratt, M. J. (2011). Discussing illicit drugs in public internet forums: Visibility, stigma, and pseudonymity. In Proceedings of the 5th International Conference on Communities and Technologies (pp. 159–168). https://doi.org/10.1145/2103354.2103376

Bilgrei, O. R. (2018). Broscience: Creating trust in online drug communities. *New Media & Society, 20*(8), 2712–2727. https://doi.org/10.1177/1461444817730331

Blackman, S. (2016). The Emotional Imagination: Exploring critical ventriloquy and emotional edgework in reflexive sociological ethnography with young people. In S. Blackman & M. Kempson (Eds.), *The subcultural imagination* (pp. 77–91). Routledge.

Brennan, K., Monroy-Hernández, A., & Resnick, M. (2010). Making projects, making friends: Online community as catalyst for interactive media creation. *New Directions for Youth Development, 2010*(128), 75–83. https://doi.org/10.1002/yd.377

Brennan, R., Wells, J. S., & van Hout, M. C. (2016). The injecting use of image and performance-enhancing drugs (IPED) in the general population: A systematic review. *Health and Social Care in the Community, 25*(5), 1459–1531. https://doi.org/10.1111/hsc.12326

Brennan, R., Wells, J., & Van Hout, M. C. (2018a). "Blood letting"—Self-phlebotomy in injecting anabolic-androgenic steroids within performance and image enhancing drug (PIED) culture. *International Journal of Drug Policy, 55*, 47–50. https://doi.org/10.1016/j.drugpo.2018.02.011

Brennan, R., Wells, J. S., & van Hout, M. C. (2018b). 'Raw juicing'–An online study of the home manufacture of anabolic androgenic steroids (AAS) for injection in contemporary performance and image enhancement (PIED) culture. *Performance Enhancement & Health, 6*(1), 21–27. https://doi.org/10.1016/j.peh.2017.11.001

Carceller, C., Dawson, S., & Lockyer, L. (2013). Improving academic outcomes: Does participating in online discussion forums payoff? *International Journal of Technology Enhanced Learning, 5*(2), 117–132. https://doi.org/10.1504/IJTEL.2013.059087

Charmaz, K. (2014). *Constructing grounded theory: A practical guide through qualitative analysis* (2nd ed.). Sage.

Christiansen, A. V., Vinther, A. S., & Liokaftos, D. (2017). Outline of a typology of men's use of anabolic androgenic steroids in fitness and strength training environments. *Drugs: Education, Prevention & Policy, 24*(3), 295–305. https://doi.org/10.1080/09687637.2016.1231173

Coen, S. E., Oliffe, J. L., Johnson, J. L., & Kelly, M. T. (2013). Looking for Mr. PG: Masculinities and men's depression in a northern resource-based Canadian community. *Health & Place, 21*, 94–101. https://doi.org/10.1016/j.healthplace.2013.01.011

Coomber, R., Pavlidis, A., Santos, G. H., Wilde, M., Schmidt, W., & Redshaw, C. (2014). The supply of steroids and other performance and image enhancing drugs (PIEDs) in one English city: Fakes, counterfeits, supplier trust, common beliefs and access. *Performance Enhancement & Health, 3*(3–4), 135–144. https://doi.org/10.1016/j.peh.2015.10.004

Coomber, R., & Salinas, M. (2019). The supply of image and performance enhancing drugs (IPED) to local non-elite users in England: Resilient traditional and newly emergent methods. In K. Van de Ven, K. Mulrooney, & J. McVeigh (Eds.), *Human enhancement drugs* (pp. 230–246). Routledge.

Cordaro, F. G., Lombardo, S., & Cosentino, M. (2011). Selling androgenic anabolic steroids by the pound: Identification and analysis of popular websites on the Internet. *Scandinavian Journal of Medicine & Science in Sports, 21*(6), 247–259. https://doi.org/10.1111/j.1600-0838.2010.01263.x

Davillas, A., & Jones, A. M. (2021). Unmet health care need and income-related horizontal equity in use of health care during the COVID-19 pandemic. *Health Economics, 30*(7), 1711–1716. https://doi.org/10.1002/hec.4282

Dufva, T., & Dufva, M. (2019, March). Grasping the future of the digital society. *Futures, 107*, 17–28. https://doi.org/10.1016/j.futures.2018.11.001

Dunn, M., Henshaw, R., & McKay, F. H. (2016). Do performance and image enhancing drug users in regional Queensland experience difficulty accessing health services? *Drug and Alcohol Review, 35*(4), 377–382. https://doi.org/10.1111/dar.12363

Dunn, M., Mulrooney, K. J., Forlini, C., van de Ven, K., and Underwood, M. (2021). The pharmaceuticalisation of 'healthy' ageing: Testosterone enhancement for longevity. *International Journal of Drug Policy, 95*(2021), 103159. https://doi.org/10.1016/j.drugpo.2021.103159

Dunn, M., & Piatkowski, T. (2021). Investigating the impact of COVID-19 on performance and image enhancing drug use. *Harm Reduction Journal, 18*(1), 124. https://doi.org/10.21203/rs.3.rs-753322/v1

Enghoff, O., & Aldridge, J. (2019). The value of unsolicited online data in drug policy research. *International Journal of Drug Policy, 73*, 210–218. https://doi.org/10.1016/j.drugpo.2019.01.023

Fabresse, N., Gheddar, L., Kintz, P., Knapp, A., Larabi, I. A., & Alvarez, J. C. (2021). Analysis of pharmaceutical products and dietary supplements seized from the black market among bodybuilders. *Forensic Science International, 322*, 110771. https://doi.org/10.1016/j.forsciint.2021.110771

Germain, J., Leavey, C., Van Hout, M. C., & McVeigh, J. (2021). 2, 4 dinitrophenol: It's not just for men. *International Journal of Drug Policy, 95*, 102987. https://doi.org/10.1016/j.drugpo.2020.102987

Gibbs, N. (2021). 'No one's going to buy steroids for a home workout': The impact of the national lockdown on hardcore gym users, anabolic steroid consumption and the image and performance enhancing drugs market. *Journal of Contemporary Crime, Harm, and Ethics, 1*(1), 45–62. https://doi.org/10.19164/jcche.v1i1.1120

Gibbs, N., & Hall, A. (2021). Digital ethnography in criminology: Some notes from the virtual field. In A. Lavorgna & T. Holt (Eds.), *Researching cybercrimes: Methodologies, ethics, and critical approaches* (pp. 283–299). Palgrave Macmillan.

Ging, D. (2019). Alphas, betas, and incels: Theorizing the masculinities of the manosphere. *Men and Masculinities, 22*(4), 638–657. https://doi.org/10.1177/1097184X17706401

Glaser, B. G., & Strauss, A. L. (2017). *Discovery of grounded theory: Strategies for qualitative research*. Routledge.

Goffman, E. (1959). *The presentation of self in everyday life*. Anchor Books.

Graham, L., McKenna, M., & Fleming, S. (2013, July). "What d'you know, you're a girl!" Gendered experiences of sport coach education. *Journal of Hospitality, Leisure, Sports and Tourism Education, 13*, 70–77. https://doi.org/10.1016/j.jhlste.2013.05.002

Hall, A., & Antonopoulos, G. A. (2015). License to pill: Illegal entrepreneurs' tactics in the online trade of medicines. In P. C. Van Duyne, A. Maljevic, G. A. Antonopoulos, J. Harvey,

& K. Von Lampe (Eds.), *The relativity of wrongdoing: Corruption, organised crime, fraud and money laundering in perspective.* Wolf Legal Publishers.

Hall, A., Koenraadt, R., & Antonopoulos, G. A. (2017). Illicit pharmaceutical networks in Europe: Organising the illicit medicine market in the United Kingdom and the Netherlands. *Trends in Organized Crime, 20*(3), 296–315. https://doi.org/10.1007/s12117-017-9304-9

Hamman, R. (1998). *The online/offline dichotomy: Debunking some myths about AOL users and effects of their being online upon offline friendships and offline community.* MPhil thesis, University of Liverpool.

Hanley-Santos, G., & Coomber, R. (2017). The risk environment of anabolic–androgenic steroid users in the UK: Examining motivations, practices and accounts of use. *International Journal of Drug Policy, 40*, 35–43. https://doi.org/10.1016/j.drugpo.2016.11.005

Harper, L., Powell, J., & Pijl, E. M. (2017). An overview of forensic drug testing methods and their suitability for harm reduction point-of-care services. *Harm Reduction Journal, 14*(1), 1–13. https://doi.org/10.1186/s12954-017-0179-5

Harvey, O., Keen, S., Parrish, M., & Van Teijlingen, E. (2019). Support for people who use anabolic androgenic steroids: A systematic scoping review into what they want and what they access. *BMC Public Health, 19*(1), 1–13. https://doi.org/10.1186/s12889-019-7288-x

Hayes, M. (2022). Social media and inspiring physical activity during COVID-19 and beyond. *Managing Sport and Leisure, 1–2*, 14–21. https://doi.org/10.1080/23750472.2020.1794939

Henning, A., & Andreasson, J. (2019). "Yay, another lady starting a log!": Women's fitness doping and the gendered space of an online doping forum. *Communication & Sport, 9*(6), 988–1007. https://doi.org/10.1177/2167479519896326

Henning, A., & Andreasson, J. (2022). Preventing, producing, or reducing harm? Fitness doping risk and enabling environments. *Drugs: Education, Prevention & Policy, 29*(1), 95–104. https://doi.org/10.1080/09687637.2020.1865273

Hunter, M. A. (2008). Cultivating the art of safe space. *Research in Drama Education, 13*(1), 5–21. https://doi.org/10.1080/13569780701825195

Jebril, N., Stetka, V., & Loveless, M. (2013). *Media and democratisation.* Reuters Institute for the Study of Journalism.

Kilvington, D. (2021). The virtual stages of hate: Using Goffman's work to conceptualise the motivations for online hate. *Media, Culture & Society, 43*(2), 256–272. https://doi.org/10.1177/0163443720972318

Kimergård, A., Breindahl, T., Hindersson, P., & McVeigh, J. (2014a). The composition of anabolic steroids from the illicit market is largely unknown: Implications for clinical case reports. *QJM: International Journal of Medicine, 107*(7), 597–598. https://doi.org/10.1093/qjmed/hcu101

Kimergård, A., McVeigh, J., Knutsson, S., Breindahl, T., & Stensbelle, A. (2014b). Online marketing of synthetic peptide hormones: Poor manufacturing, user safety, and challenges to public health. *Drug Testing and Analysis, 6*(4), 396–398. https://doi.org/10.1002/dta.1636

Klein, A. (1993). *Little big men: Bodybuilding subculture and gender construction.* State University of New York Press.

Kozinets, R. V. (2015). *Netnography: Redefined.* Sage.

Li, C., & Bernoff, J. (2011). *Groundswell: Winning in a world transformed by social technologies.* Harvard Business Review Press.

Llewellyn, W., & Tober, R. (2010). *Underground anabolics.* Molecular Nutrition, LLC.

Marche, S. (2016) "Swallowing the Red Pill: A journey to the heart of modern misogyny". *The Guardian.* https://www.theguardian.com/technology/2016/apr/14/the-red-pill-reddit-modern-misogyny-manosphere-men. Accessed on March 14, 2021

McVeigh, J., Germain, J., & Van Hout, M. C. (2017). 2, 4-dinitrophenol, the inferno drug: A netnographic study of user experiences in the quest for leanness. *Journal of Substance Use, 22*(2), 131–138. https://doi.org/10.3109/14659891.2016.1149238

Measham, F. C. (2019). Drug safety testing, disposals and dealing in an English field: Exploring the operational and behavioural outcomes of the UK's first onsite 'drug checking' service. *International Journal of Drug Policy, 67*, 102–107. https://doi.org/10.1016/j.drugpo.2018.11.001

Monaghan, L. (1999). Challenging medicine? Bodybuilding, drugs and risk. *Sociology of Health & Illness, 21*(6), 707–734. https://doi.org/10.1111/1467-9566.00180

Monaghan, L. (2001). *Bodybuilding, drugs and risk*. Routledge.

Nijland, N., van Gemert-Pijnen, J., Boer, H., Steehouder, M., & Seydel, E. (2008). Evaluation of internet-based technology for supporting self-care: Problems encountered by patients and caregivers when using self-care applications. *Journal of Medical Internet Research, 10*(2), e13. https://doi.org/10.2196/jmir.957

O'Brien, K. S., Shovelton, H., & Latner, J. D. (2013). Homophobia in physical education and sport: The role of physical/sporting identity and attributes, authoritarian aggression, and social dominance orientation. *International Journal of Psychology, 48*(5), 891–899. https://doi.org/10.1080/00207594.2012.713107

Pitta, D. A., & Fowler, D. (2005). Internet community forums: An untapped resource for consumer marketers. *Journal of Consumer Marketing, 22*(5), 265–274. https://doi.org/10.1108/07363760510611699

Salinas, M., Floodgate, W., & Ralphs, R. (2019). Polydrug use and polydrug markets among image and performance enhancing drug users: Implications for harm reduction interventions and drug policy. *International Journal of Drug Policy, 67*, 43–51. https://doi.org/10.1016/j.drugpo.2019.01.019

Sillence, E., & Baber, C. (2004). Integrated digital communities: Combining web-based interaction with text messaging to develop a system for encouraging group communication and competition. *Interacting with Computers, 16*(1), 93–113. https://doi.org/10.1016/j.intcom.2003.11.007

Szakolczai, J. M. (2021). Everyday deviants: How the pandemic has rendered normality transgressive and the 'normals' transgressors. In *British society of criminology, crime and harm: Challenges of social and global justice? Open University*, 7th July. Open University. [conference presentation].

Tanis, M. (2008). Health-related on-line forums: What's the big attraction? *Journal of Health Communication, 13*(7), 698–714. https://doi.org/10.1080/10810730802415316

Tighe, B., Dunn, M., McKay, F. H., & Piatkowski, T. (2017). Information sought, information shared: Exploring performance and image enhancing drug user-facilitated harm reduction information in online forums. *Harm Reduction Journal, 14*(1), 1–9. https://doi.org/10.1186/s12954-017-0176-8

Turnock, L. A. (2018). *'Gear is the next weed': A qualitative exploration of the beliefs, attitudes and behaviours of performance and image enhancing drug using subcultures in the South-West of England*. Doctoral dissertation. University of Winchester.

Turnock, L. A. (2020). Inside a steroid 'brewing' and supply operation in South-West England: An ethnographic narrative case study. *Performance Enhancement & Health, 7*(3–4), 100152. https://doi.org/10.1016/j.peh.2019.100152

Turnock, L. A. (2021a). *Supplying steroids online: The cultural and market contexts of enhancement drug supply on one of the world's largest fitness & bodybuilding forums*. Plymouth Policy Research Institute.

Turnock, L. A. (2021b). Exploring user narratives of self-medicated black market IPED use for therapeutic & wellbeing purposes. *Performance Enhancement & Health*, 100207. https://doi.org/10.1016/j.peh.2021.100207

Turnock, L. A. (2021c). Polydrug use and drug market intersections within powerlifting cultures in remote South-West England. *Performance Enhancement & Health, 8*(4), 100186. https://doi.org/10.1016/j.peh.2021.100186

Turnock, L. A. (2021d). Rural gym spaces and masculine physical cultures in an 'age of change': Rurality, masculinity, inequalities and harm in 'the gym'. *Journal of Rural Studies, 86*, 106–116. https://doi.org/10.1016/j.jrurstud.2021.05.013

Turnock, L. A. (2021e). 'There's a difference between tolerance and acceptance': Exploring women's experiences of barriers to access in UK gyms. *Wellbeing, Space and Society, 2*, 100049. https://doi.org/10.1016/j.wss.2021.100049

Underwood, M. (2017). Exploring the social lives of image and performance enhancing drugs: An online ethnography of the Zyzz Fandom of recreational bodybuilders. *International Journal of Drug Policy, 39*, 78–85. https://doi.org/10.1016/j.drugpo.2016.08.012

Underwood, M. (2018). 'We're all gonna make it brah': Homosocial relations, vulnerability and intimacy in an online bodybuilding community. In A. Shields Dobson, B. Robards, & N. Carah (Eds.), *Digital intimate publics and social media* (pp. 161–176). Palgrave Macmillan.

Underwood, M., & Olson, R. (2019). 'Manly tears exploded from my eyes, lets feel together brahs': Emotion and masculinity within an online body building community. *Journal of Sociology*, *55*(1), 90–107. https://doi.org/10.1177/1440783318766610

Van de Ven, K., & Mulrooney, K. J. D. (2017). Social suppliers: Exploring the cultural contours of the performance and image enhancing drug (PIED) market among bodybuilders in the Netherlands and Belgium. *International Journal of Drug Policy*, *40*, 6–15. https://doi.org/10.1016/j.drugpo.2016.07.009

van de Ven, K., & de Zeeuw, T. (2021). Illicit performance and image enhancing drug markets in the Netherlands and Belgium. In H. Nelen & D. Siegel (Eds.), *Contemporary organized crime: Developments, challenges and responses* (pp. 25–44). Springer.

van de Ven, K., & Koenraadt, R. (2017). Exploring the relationship between online buyers and sellers of image and performance enhancing drugs (IPEDs): Quality issues, trust and self-regulation. *International Journal of Drug Policy*, *50*, 48–55. https://doi.org/10.1016/j.drugpo.2017.09.004

van de Ven, K., Mulrooney, K. J. D., & Townshend, H. D. (in press). Image and performance enhancing drug (IPED) suppliers and their motives: Following the evidence. In T. Ayres & A. Craig (Eds.), *Understanding drug dealing and illicit drug markets in the 21st century: National and international perspectives*. Routledge.

Whitfield, M., Reed, H., Webster, J., & Hope, V. (2020). The impact of COVID-19 restrictions on needle and syringe programme provision and coverage in England. *International Journal of Drug Policy*, *83*, 102851. https://doi.org/10.1016/j.drugpo.2020.102851

Zahnow, R., McVeigh, J., Bates, G., Hope, V., Kean, J., Campbell, J., & Smith, J. (2018). Identifying a typology of men who use anabolic androgenic steroids (AAS). *International Journal of Drug Policy*, *55*, 105–112. https://doi.org/10.1016/j.drugpo.2018.02.022

Chapter 9

THE 2021 WADA CODE, RECREATIONAL ATHLETES AND ETHICAL CONCERNS

Luke Thomas Joseph Cox, Andrew Bloodworth and Mike Mcnamee

ABSTRACT

In response to widespread concerns about health and fairness within elite sport, the World Anti-Doping Agency (WADA) was established as an organization to tackle the use of performance enhancing drugs in sport. Whilst significant efforts have been made to regulate performance enhancement in the context of elite sport, the use of prohibited substances continues to persist. Doping rules are now potentially applicable across sporting levels, not just within elite sport. The WADA has further formalized its jurisdiction in recreational sport by defining the term 'recreational athlete' for the purposes of their regulation within and by the 2021 WADA Code. The extension of Anti-Doping Policy into recreational sport broadens the scope of anti-doping's regulatory framework but is consistent in its health protection rationale, and its attempt to preserve sporting integrity. There are, however, a number of ethical concerns associated with the application of Anti-Doping Policy within recreational sport. Anti-doping policy was originally designed exclusively for elite athletes and although amendments have been made within the revised 2021 World Anti-Doping Code, it is unclear whether this extension is justifiable or operationalizable on a global scale. This chapter pays particular attention to the 2021 WADA Code revisions and draws attention to the role of anti-doping policy within recreational sport. Here we raise some ethical concerns associated with the 2021 WADA Code and critically examine the implications for recreational athletes.

Doping in Sport and Fitness
Research in the Sociology of Sport, Volume 16, 181–192
Copyright © 2023 by Emerald Publishing Limited
All rights of reproduction in any form reserved
ISSN: 1476-2854/doi:10.1108/S1476-285420220000016010

Keywords: Doping; recreational sport; Anti-Doping Policy; ethics; WADA; WADA Code

The World Anti-Doping Agency (WADA) was established in 1999 as a response to disjointed and unharmonized efforts to tackle drug use in elite sport (WADA, 2021a, 2021b, 2021c). WADA produces the WADA Code, a standalone document that specifies the rules that must be adopted and implemented by National Anti-Doping Organizations (NADOs) and Sports Federations within their respective countries (WADA, 2021c). The WADA Code is updated every five years and the latest version of the WADA Code went into effect in January 2021.

Whilst WADA has made very significant efforts in its attempt to protect and promote 'clean sport', doping remains a global problem. A number of prevalence studies have been conducted without the scientific community ever arriving at a consensus over methods and criteria, let alone the data. One relatively recent report, analyzing data from two international elite athletic competitions, reported estimates of 43.6% and 57.1% of elite athletes currently use doping substances (Ulrich et al., 2018). This is an abnormally high estimate, and it is in stark contrast to WADA's testing figures that outline that just 2% doping control tests report adverse analytical findings (WADA, 2020). Due to these and other apparent discrepancies, Anti-Doping Policy (ADP) and its legitimacy has been challenged by medical and social scientific researchers and scholars (Kayser et al., 2020; Møller, 2016; Murray, 2017).

Although WADA was established in response to concerns within elite sport, it has in recent times extended its scope to include recreational athletes. The revised 2021 WADA Code offers a structure for the sanctioning of recreational athletes (WADA, 2021c, p.71), provides a definition for *recreational athletes* (WADA, 2021c, p. 174) and offers NADOs the flexibility to retract names of athletes with positive doping tests (WADA, 2021c, p. 102). Notably, its framework allows for differences in sanctioning in recognition of issues surrounding proportionality. Whilst these are important steps for WADA to have made, ADP still retains much of the same policy apparatus (e.g. Code, International Standards documents etc.) for elite and recreational athletes and this raises some ethical concerns. In this chapter, we identify and explore some of these ethical concerns and critically examine their implications for recreational athletes involved.

2021 WADA CODE, RECREATIONAL SPORT AND ETHICAL CONCERNS

Until the 2021 WADA Code, athletes, both elite and recreational, were captured under one common definition (WADA, 2003, 2009, 2015). The lack of definition within the WADA Code was thought initially to be unproblematic but has led to disjointed and unharmonized applications of ADP by different NADOs. Within one European study, this specific concern was identified (Christiansen et al., 2020, pp. 24–73). Different NADOs were shown to have operationalized a range of definitions of 'athlete' within their respective countries. Some NADOs included gym users within their definition, whilst other NADOs included only individuals competing in organized competitive sport (Christiansen et al., 2020, pp. 24–73). The lack of a consensus over the definition within the WADA Code led to inequalities in treatment of different athletes between different countries, with some NADOs accused of excessively sanctioning recreational athletes. For the purposes of this chapter, we focus on organized, competitive, recreational sport but exclude, for example, 'mere' gym users or non-competitive runners.

Recent examples of the effect of definitional laxity can be found in New Zealand (Garlick, 2020; Johannsen, 2018) and Australia (Jamieson & Ordway, 2021). Due to the absence of an agreed definition concerning recreational athletes, Drug Free Sport New Zealand (DFSNZ) (the New Zealand National Anti-Doping Organization [NADO]) was accused of over-sanctioning recreational athletes. For example, individuals given clenbuterol by a personal trainer were heavily sanctioned by DFSNZ, even where the individuals concerned had retired from sport altogether (Johannsen, 2018). They were sanctioned in accordance with the 2015 WADA Code, which made no distinction between elite and recreational athletes.

The excessive sanctioning of some recreational athletes is problematic when considered from the perspective of fairness. If athletes in particular countries face greater anti-doping scrutiny and punishment than athletes in another country, then this points to inequalities between athletes. These inequalities thus act as greater or lesser disincentives to dope for some competitors rather than all. Equally, we may reasonably foresee that those athletes under the scope of a stringent NADO are likely to suffer a greater array of harms than those who are not. Hong et al. (2020) outlined that anti-doping sanctions are associated with several harms, with some athletes suggesting they were left feeling emotionally vulnerable after receiving an anti-doping sanction. The same study also suggests anti-doping sanctions were linked to feelings of depression and suicide. Due to the concerns associated with anti-doping sanctions and the lack of a common definition between NADOs leading to a range of inequalities between athletes, the 2021 WADA Code includes a definition of recreational athletes.

The WADC 2021 states:

> A natural Person who is so defined by the relevant National Anti-Doping Organization; provided, however, the term shall not include any Person who, within the five years (5) prior to committing any anti-doping rule violation, has been an International-Level Athlete (as defined by each International Federation consistent with the International Standard for Testing and Investigations) or National-Level Athlete (as defined by each National Anti-Doping Organization consistent with the International Standard for Testing and Investigations), has represented any country in an International Event in an open category or has been included within any Registered Testing Pool or other whereabouts information pool maintained by any International Federation or National Anti-Doping Organization. (WADA, 2021c, p. 174)

The definition of 'recreational athletes' within the 2021 WADA Code better establishes boundaries between 'elite' and 'recreational' populations. The inclusion of the definition allows WADA to better respond to concerns associated with potential inequalities (in particular, sanctioning inequalities) between different athletes, in different countries. Moreover, WADA better equips NADOs with the tools to harmonize their anti-doping efforts and in doing so, ensures ADP better aligns with WADA's fundamental aims. Indeed, this challenges the previously identified and divergent ways the WADA Code has been implemented. Thus, the inclusion of the definition of recreational athletes ought to be welcomed throughout the sporting world.

A second revision within the 2021 WADA Code outlines the scope for greater sanctioning leniency for recreational athletes. Previous versions of the Code saw athletes, both elite and recreational, largely treated under the same sanctioning terms. In contrast, however, the 2021 Code allows NADOs to reduce anti-doping sanctions from four years to two years or less for recreational athletes:

> 10.3.1 For violations of Article 2.3 or 2.5, the period of *Ineligibility* shall be four-years except: (1) in the case of failing to submit to *Sample* collection, if the *Athlete* can establish that the commission of the anti-doping rule violation was not intentional, the period of *Ineligibility* shall be two-years; (2) in all other cases, if the *Athlete* or other *Person* can establish exceptional circumstances that justify a reduction of the period of *Ineligibility*, the period of *Ineligibility* shall be in a range from two-years to four-years depending on the *Athlete* or other *Person's* degree of *Fault*; or (3) in a case involving a *Protected Person* or *Recreational Athlete*, the period of *Ineligibility* shall be in a range between a maximum of two-years and, at a minimum, a reprimand and no period of *Ineligibility*, depending on the *Protected Person* or *Recreational Athlete's* degree of *Fault*. (WADA, 2021c, p. 67)

The reduction in sanction length is a welcome and important revision within the 2021 WADA Code. It establishes a more proportionate response to the reality of lower-level sport (in economic, social, or political terms) to the range of harms associated with anti-doping sanctions (Hong et al., 2020). This is especially important within the WADA framework that operates on the strict liability principle; NADOs do not have to prove intent in order to sanction an athlete for an anti-doping rule violation. It is the duty of an athlete to train and perform clean. In legal terms, this is a heavy and infrequently used burden. Why ought recreational athletes who, for example, inadvertently use a product that includes a doping substance within it, be sanctioned in the same way as an elite athlete? Generally speaking, the range of motivations for recreational athletes to compete is to take exercise, have fun, enjoy a sense of belonging and secure some health benefits. Do these motivations merit significant regulation? It is far from clear. Admittedly, the borders are somewhat porous: today's recreational athletes may be tomorrow's sub-elite ones. The lack of nuanced conceptual work or policy recognition for this fact is notable.

Moreover, at the elite level, anti-doping education is provided by teams, clubs, squads and so on in order to mitigate the burden of strict liability. Within recreational sport, however, these supports are rarely, if ever, available. This point is supported within a research investigation of recreational Welsh Rugby Union players, in which over half of the participants included reported that they had not received any formal anti-doping education (Cox et al., 2021). Moreover, Christiansen et al. (2020) also noted anti-doping education for recreational athletes where it exists is a new and largely under-resourced development in comparison to elite sport. These data were retrieved from the NADOs of 28 EU Member states and further evidences the inequalities between elite and recreational athletes. By offering scope for greater sanctioning leniency, NADOs are given the flexibility to account for the potential lack of anti-doping knowledge and understanding within the recreational athlete population.

Within a third revision of the 2021 WADA Code, WADA states that NADOs can redact the names of recreational athletes who have committed anti-doping violations:

> The mandatory *Public Disclosure* required in 14.3.2 shall not be required where the *Athlete* or other *Person* who has been found to have committed an anti-doping rule violation is a *Minor*, *Protected Person* or *Recreational Athlete*. Any optional *Public Disclosure* in a case involving a *Minor*, *Protected Person* or *Recreational Athlete* shall be proportionate to the facts and circumstances of the case. (WADA, 2021c, p. 102)

This too is an important proportionality-based revision for WADA to include, considering the diverse range of motivations associated with doping in recreational sport and the perceived benefits (Cox et al., 2021). Beyond the borders of competitive organized sport, individuals using Anabolic Androgenic Steroids (AAS) report a range of perceived benefits that reach far beyond sports performance (Kotzé & Antonopoulos, 2019; Latham et al., 2019; Vassallo & Olrich, 2010). These benefits include, but are not limited to, elevated self-confidence, greater body image satisfaction, greater perceptions of sexual attraction and masculinity etc. (Christiansen, 2015, 2020). Accepting that some recreational athletes share these perceived benefits (Cox et al., 2021), it appears problematic to consider and treat these individuals in the same manner as elite athletes who intentionally cheat and aim to mislead and deceive competitors in order to achieve a performance advantage. Moreover, there are several examples of ADRVs having been committed without the intent to attain performance enhancement. Examples include the unwitting ingestion of contaminated nutritional supplements, the use of over-the-counter medications and the simple lack of anti-doping knowledge. All these scenarios can lead to unintentional breaches of the WADA Code. In any of these cases, it appears disproportionate to publicly expose recreational athletes and potentially tarnish personal and professional reputations.

Doping is associated with a range of negative social connotations: For example, shame and stigma (Bloodworth & McNamee, 2010). These negative connotations appear somewhat supported by WADA when considering the deterrence theory (Dunn et al., 2010; Moston et al., 2015; Overbye et al., 2015). It has been argued that, for WADA to better ensure doping-free sport, the potential to shame and stigmatize athletes via anti-doping rule violations is a powerful disincentive to prevent or deter cheating athletes. Notably, however, within recreational sport, where doping is sometimes unrelated to performance enhancement and cheating (e.g. where motivations are related exclusively to image enhancement), the option to redact the names of recreational athletes is a more proportionate response, while still aiming to protect health and well-being (as befits the rationale for the Code itself).

Having identified and examined some of the key changes within the 2021 WADA Code, concerning recreational athletes, we next consider the notion of consent within the WADA Code.

ANTI-DOPING, RECREATIONAL SPORT AND CONSENT

In this section, we draw attention to a specific aspect of ADP, which examines whether athlete consent and understanding is a necessary condition for ADP to be ethically defensible. It is assumed that by virtue of their participation alone, an athlete accepts the rules of that sport and with that, ADP and the rules outlined within the WADA Code and adopted and implemented by different NADOs and National Governing Bodies (NGB) around the globe. The WADA write:

> Anti-doping rules, like competition rules, are sport rules governing the conditions under which sport is played. *Athletes, Athlete Support Personnel* or other *Persons* (including board members, directors, officers, and specified employees and *Delegated Third Parties* and their employees) accept these rules as a condition of participation or involvement in sport and shall be bound by these rules. Each *Signatory* shall establish rules and procedures to ensure that all *Athletes, Athlete Support Personnel* or other *Persons* under the authority of the *Signatory* and its member organizations are informed of and agree to be bound by anti-doping rules in force of the relevant *Anti-Doping Organizations* (WADA, 2021c, p. 17).

Through the inclusion of this clause, athletes seemingly consent to, and are bound by, the WADA Code. This may be of concern when we consider that there is a potential lack of athlete understanding of these tacit agreements. Clearly, some athletes are likely to be unaware of the detail of their obligations and responsibilities under the WADA Code. Moreover, ADP has always attracted significant ethical dialogue and criticism, as has every substance use policy or law. It is a subject that deeply divides scholars, scientists and the general public. For example, previous literature has identified privacy concerns during doping control tests and raised the issue of child athletes (Christiansen, 2011). Such ethical concerns may be amplified under conditions where athletes are unaware of these rules that govern their participation in sport. Below, we examine these concerns further.

Simply by participating, athletes – both elite and recreational – are bound to ADP by the rules of their sport following their national and international federations's acceptance of the Code. Failure to comply with the rules stipulated within the Code, may result in anti-doping reprisals. Not only are anti-doping sanctions a reasonable prospect here, but one must also consider the extension of doping control tests into the recreational sport domain on which they are predicated. Doping control tests require an athlete to reveal themselves, knee to belly-button, to a doping control officer. The doping control officer must have an uninterrupted view of the genitals and observe the full passing of urine until the sample collection is complete (WADA, 2021a). Previous research has raised several ethical concerns associated with doping control tests (Christiansen, 2011), with some athletes feeling as though their personal integrity had been violated and leaving some individuals feeling vulnerable during doping control tests (Elbe & Brand, 2014; Elbe & Overbye, 2013; Elbe et al., 2012). What is more, some athletes described difficulties during urination, and this exposed these individuals to higher level of distress and discomfort, causing both short- and long-term health implications (Elbe & Brand, 2014; Elbe et al., 2012). Further complications would arise with the testing of minors. Though this is unlikely to be extended to recreational athletes, it is not explicitly ruled out either.

Although these studies were conducted with elite athletes, this insight allows us to begin to think what it is like for an athlete in these situations. Arguably, when it comes to ADP and doping control tests, elite athletes will be more aware than recreational athletes of their responsibilities, the possibility of being subject to doping control tests, and the range and severity of anti-doping sanctions they might face if anti-doping rules are violated. In recreational sport, where participation is far less formal, these athletes might have limited understanding of the WADA Code and all that it entails. If a recreational athlete is selected for a doping control test, it might therefore come as a shock to the individual, and thus the negative feelings as described within literature presented above might be exacerbated within the population of recreational athletes. This is concerning and ought not be overlooked when we consider the WADA Code and the fact that consent is assumed *ipso facto* by participation alone. If recreational athletes are unaware of what they are signing up to when they participate in sport, then this is evidently problematic and ethically questionable. Moreover, when we consider that minors could be subject to similar doping controls and experience feelings such as humiliation during the doping control process, this further supports our concerns here (Teetzel & Mazzucco, 2014).

In the case of unintentional use of doping substances, there is the possibility that lower-level athletes are unaware of the risks of supplement use. Anti-doping literature reports that up to 40% of ADRVs are committed unintentionally (de Hon & van Bottenburg, 2017). This may be particularly problematic when we consider that these individuals might be recreational athletes who lack the relevant level of understanding of ADP. One specific study examined anti-doping sanctions issued to Rugby Union players and identified that there are a disproportional number of recreational Welsh rugby players who commit ADRVs and receive anti-doping sanctions. Amongst some of the reasons for these ADRVs, athletes claimed the naïve use of nutritional supplements and a lack of anti-doping education (Whitaker & Backhouse, 2017). This suggests that the lack of comprehension of ADP is s likely to have arisen om a lack of anti-doping education. Since anti-doping education is limited within recreational sport, it is unsurprising that recreational athletes unintentionally commit ADRVs. Without a reasonable understanding of ADP, athletes will be less aware on their responsibilities. As Christiansen et al. (2020, pp. 24–73) show, ADP is currently delivered in an inconsistent manner in recreational contexts, if at all. Some NADOs note that while they have hypothetical jurisdiction outside of elite sport, they rarely intervene into such milieux. It is clear, however, that testing has been conducted in non-elite populations. A prime example is offered by numerous sub-elite Welsh rugby players who have fallen foul of doping rules (Whitaker & Backhouse, 2017; UKAD, 2021). Clearly, it is important that athletes' first interaction with anti-doping is not a test, but some form of education that may indeed detail the requirements of the testing process. This education, as is the case in many instances of good practice, may well seek to foster the sort of anti-doping values in the young that would protect against the misuse of prohibited substances in sport. This representative from the UK Anti-Doping Agency told the Forum for Doping in Recreational Sport (FAIR Project)[1]:

> Testing recreational athletes and banning them is doing little to stop the problem. So I think the programmes targeting younger sports people is a good example of a proactive, preventative approach which is trying to get these kids into the right habits right from the beginning in a healthy way. And so that when they get a little older they are not obsessed with social media and the gym IPED (Image and Performance Enhancing Drug) thing will become less of an attraction. (Christiansen et al., 2020, p. 53)

In elite sport, consent through participation is less problematic due to the notion that elite athletes enjoy greater opportunities to access anti-doping education than recreational athletes. We acknowledge that there is no global standard of provision here. Clearly, athletes from nations whose governments support anti-doping measures strongly are likely to be better informed as to their obligations. Within elite sport, clubs and NADOs provide educational sessions to athletes, however, due to the less formal structure of some recreational clubs, it is inevitable that recreational athletes will not receive the same opportunities to access anti-doping education as elite athletes. This stems from the high volume of recreational athletes and the cost of delivering education. It is also likely that elite athletes will have been required to agree and sign up to formal and explicit contracts with their respective clubs and sponsors. These contractual agreements typically refer to anti-doping commitments that further reinforce elite athletes' responsibilities when it comes to the WADA Code. Teams and sponsors will be aware that players and staff affiliated to their club or brand could damage their reputations, attract bad press and tarnish their brand image. Thus, elite athletes have greater reasons to ensure they comply with anti-doping rules and, consequently, receive greater opportunities where anti-doping education is concerned. Notably, however, the same cannot be said within recreational sport. Given the standard motivations to participate in recreational sport, there will be less pressure from clubs and sponsors to ensure recreational athletes comply with ADP. This is problematic when we consider that the WADA Code has explicitly extended ADP scope to recreational athletes. Nevertheless, the Code is still applicable at all levels of sport. If athletes, both at elite and recreational levels, are not granted fair and equal opportunities where anti-doping education is considered, it appears questionable how they could ought to be expected to commit to the same levels of anti-doping behaviours.

How best to move forward with ADP and practice in recreational sport contexts is a pressing question. While there seems a growing awareness of a potentially large-scale doping problem in recreational sport, anti-doping still has at its core a concern with a level playing field in the elite sports context. That was certainly the focus of earlier policy. Even now, there are limited resources to press anti-doping policy into universal service. Competition for public resources is always high. It might reasonably be thought that pressing ADP into recreational level athletics was neither warranted nor cost effective as a public health intervention. Currently, it seems that organizations test infrequently at this lower level, but may target certain clubs or contexts should intelligence suggest an issue there. This may raise some concerns with elite athletes, subject to stricter application of anti-doping rules, while their recreational counterparts seem, in practice, less likely to be subject to such rules. Yet it ought not to. The range of benefits to elite and sub-elite athletes may justify greater compliance and sanctioning potential than in recreational athletes and sports. It is also worth noting that in some countries the very distinction between elite and recreational sport is less significant. Consider this description offered by the Cyprus Anti-Doping Agency:

> For us there is no clear distinction between recreational and competitive sport activities. Especially in countries like Cyprus, a small country where sport is not really at a high level, so someone might be running for recreation but can easily enter the competitions at a national level. So, it easily becomes both recreational and competitive athletes. I know in the UK the national level you'd have to go through different stages, divisions. But for us there is no clear distinction. In some sports like triathlon and marathon, it is very easy to cross this thin line and become a recreational runner or triathlete and compete in an event organized by the national federation and under our rules you become a competitive athlete. (Christiansen et al., 2020)

The possibility of athletes progressing more easily to elite sport levels in some countries because of their demographic nature, exacerbated by doping behaviours, raises a further justification for anti-doping's applicability at recreational levels. If the boundaries between recreational, sub-elite and elite athletes are so permeable as to be reasonably foreseeable, this might justify a more robust attitude towards implementation and sanctioning. Thus, for example, if country X has 100 athletes who can run a sub 2:10 marathon, should implementation of ADP to recreational athletes be more rigorous? If a country has a rugby-playing population that vastly outstrips the needs of a small professional milieu, should their sub-elite population (who may easily cross performance and national borders or boundaries) not also be subjected to rigorous policy enforcement? What is clear is that growing educational initiatives targeted at the young and recreational populations may help to foster greater support for and knowledge of anti-doping in general, but changes at NADOs should also be seriously considered.

CONCLUSION

ADP plays a significant role helping to protect sport and the individuals who engage in its activities from the use of potentially harmful substances. The revisions to the 2021 WADA Code respond to concerns previously raised regarding proportionality and address the previously identified concerns associated with definitional inconsistencies and the potential harms associated with anti-doping sanctions. Notably, however, the application of the WADA Code within recreational sport does not come without its challenges. The assumption of reasonable understanding of ADP by such populations could well be problematic. What is more, due to the size of the recreational sport population, and the heterogeneity of that population, implementing fair and consistent rules and regulations will remain a significant challenge. It is also notable that anti-doping educational opportunities are significantly limited within recreational sport when compared with elite sport. It seems, thus, unreasonable to expect similar levels of ADP commitment and compliance within both elite and recreational populations. While there are no easy answers to this problem, particularly in light of a shortage of resources, educational initiatives designed to better inform recreational athletes of anti-doping rules would address some concerns about athletes being subject to rules with which they are unfamiliar. In addition, WADA should continue to develop ADP and engage with recreational athletes to ensure this population is fairly represented and considered within future policy revisions.

KEY READINGS

(1) Christiansen, A. V., Bloodworth, A., Ham, E., & Cox, L. (2020). Doping prevention in recreational sport in Europe – A study on emerging practices among European stakeholders, Chapter 3 FAIR Final report. In *Fair-forum for anti-doping in recreational sport 2019*. Final Report (pp. 24–73). Europe Active.

Report that examines European National Anti-Doping Organizations' scope and focus within recreational sport.

(2) Cox, L. T. J., Bloodworth, A., & McNamee, M. (2021). Doping in recreational Welsh Rugby Union; Athletes' beliefs and perceptions related to Anti-Doping policy and practice. *Performance Enhancement & Health*, 100211.

Research into recreational athletes' (Welsh Rugby Union) perceptions of Anti-Doping Policy and Practice. Results raise serious concerns for the integrity of sport: (1) perceived lack of testing frequency; perceived lack of testing efficacy; and (2) advanced warning of doping control tests.

(3) WADA. (2003). The WADA Code. https://www.wada-ama.org/en/resources/the-code/world-anti-doping-code. Accessed on 3 March 2021.

The 2021 World Anti-Doping Agency Code. A standalone document that specifies the rules that must be adopted and implemented by National Anti-Doping Organizations (NADOs) and Sports Federations within their respective countries.

(4) WADA. (2003). The WADA Code. https://www.wada-ama.org/sites/default/files/resources/files/wada-2015-world-anti-doping-code.pdf. Accessed on 3 March 2021.

The 2015 WADA Code. A standalone document that specifies the rules that must be adopted and implemented by NADOs and Sports Federations within their respective countries.

(5) Johannsen, D. (2018). Drug Free Sport NZ accused of overprosecuting club athletes. https://www.stuff.co.nz/sport/other-sports/106805084/drug-free-sport-nz-accused-of-overprosecuting-club-athletes. Accessed on 3 March 2021.

News article that brings to light the over-prosecution of recreational athletes by the New Zealand National Anti-Doping Organization (Drug Free Sport New Zealand).

NOTE

1. A group of academics and people working in anti-doping exploring doping in recreational sport and effective policy responses.

REFERENCES

Bloodworth, A., & McNamee, M. (2010). Clean Olympians? Doping and anti-doping: The views of talented young British athletes. *International Journal of Drug Policy*, *21*(4), 276–282.

Christiansen, A. V. (2011). Bodily violations: Testing citizens training recreationally in gyms. In M. McNamee & V. Møller (Eds.), *Doping and anti-doping policy in sport: Ethical, legal and social perspectives* (p. 126). Routledge.

Christiansen, A. V. (2015). Drug use in gyms. In *Routledge handbook of drugs and sport* (pp. 421–438). Routledge.

Christiansen, A. V. (2020). *Gym culture, identity and performance-enhancing drugs: Tracing a typology of steroid use.* Routledge.

Christiansen, A. V., Bloodworth, A., Ham, E., & Cox, L. (2020). Doping prevention in recreational sport in Europe – A study on emerging practices among European stakeholders, Chapter 3 FAIR Final report. In *fair-forum for anti-doping in recreational sport 2019* (pp. 24–73). Europe Active. Final Report.

Cox, L. T. J., Bloodworth, A., & McNamee, M. (2021). Doping in recreational Welsh Rugby Union; Athletes' beliefs and perceptions related to anti-doping policy and practice. *Performance Enhancement & Health*, *10*, 100211.

Dunn, M., Thomas, J. O., Swift, W., Burns, L., & Mattick, R. P. (2010). Drug testing in sport: The attitudes and experiences of elite athletes. *International Journal of Drug Policy*, *21*(4), 330–332.

Elbe, A. M., & Brand, R. (2014). Urination difficulties during doping controls: An act of rebellion? *Journal of Clinical Sport Psychology*, *8*(2), 204–214.

Elbe, A. M., & Overbye, M. (2013). Urine doping controls: The athletes' perspective. *International Journal of Sport Policy and Politics*, *6*(2), 227–240.

Elbe, A. M., Schlegel, M. M., & Brand, R. (2012). Psychogenic urine retention during doping controls: Consequences for elite athletes. *Performance Enhancement & Health*, *1*(2), 66–74.

Garlick, M. (2020). Stepping out of bounds: The over-prosecution of recreational athletes in light of DFSNZ v XYZ. *Victoria University of Wellington Law Review*, *51*, 53.

Hong, H. J., Henning, A., & Dimeo, P. (2020). Life after doping—A cross-country analysis of organisational support for sanctioned athletes. *Performance Enhancement & Health*, *8*(1), 100161.

de Hon, O., & van Bottenburg, M. (2017). True dopers or negligent athletes? An analysis of anti-doping rule violations reported to the world anti-doping agency 2010–2012. *Substance Use & Misuse*, *52*(14), 1932–1936.

Jamieson, V., & Ordway, C. (2021). Exercising discretion for social/recreational athletes: Case study Athlete XYZ. In C. Ordway & R. Lucus (Eds.), *Restoring trust in sport* (pp. 64–92). Routledge.

Johannsen, D. (2018). Drug Free Sport NZ accused of overprotecting club athletes. https://www.stuff.co.nz/sport/other-sports/106805084/drug-free-sport-nz-accused-of-overprosecuting-club-athletes. Accessed on March 03, 2021.

Kayser, B., Mauron, A., & Miah, A. (2020). Current anti-doping policy: A critical appraisal. In *The ethics of sports technologies and human enhancement* (pp. 29–38). Routledge.

Kotzé, J., & Antonopoulos, G. A. (2019). Boosting bodily capital: Maintaining masculinity, aesthetic pleasure and instrumental utility through the consumption of steroids. *Journal of Consumer Culture, 21*(3), 683–700.

Latham, J. R., Fraser, S., Fomiatti, R., Moore, D., Seear, K., & Aitken, C. (2019). Men's performance and image-enhancing drug use as self-transformation: Working out in makeover culture. *Australian Feminist Studies, 34*(100), 149–164.

Møller, V. (2016). The road to hell is paved with good intentions—A critical evaluation of WADA's anti-doping campaign. *Performance Enhancement & Health, 4*(3–4), 111–115.

Moston, S., Engelberg, T., & Skinner, J. (2015). Self-fulfilling prophecy and the future of doping. *Psychology of Sport and Exercise, 16*, 201–207.

Murray, T. H. (2017). A moral foundation for anti-doping: How far have we progressed? Where are the limits? In O. Rabin, & Y. Pitsiladis (Eds.), *Acute topics in anti-doping* (Vol. 62, pp. 186–193). Karger Publishers.

Overbye, M., Elbe, A. M., Knudsen, M. L., & Pfister, G. (2015). Athletes' perceptions of anti-doping sanctions: The ban from sport versus social, financial and self-imposed sanctions. *Sport in Society, 18*(3), 364–384.

Teetzel, S., & Mazzucco, M. (2014). Minor problems: The recognition of young athletes in the development of international anti-doping policies. *International Journal of the History of Sport, 31*(8), 914–933.

UKAD. (2021). Sanctions. https://www.ukad.org.uk/sanctions. Accessed on March 05, 2021.

Ulrich, R., Pope, H. G., Cléret, L., Petróczi, A., Nepusz, T., Schaffer, J., Kanayama, G., Comstock, R., & Simon, P. (2018). Doping in two elite athletics competitions assessed by randomized-response surveys. *Sports Medicine, 48*(1), 211–219.

Vassallo, M. J., & Olrich, T. W. (2010). Confidence by injection: Male users of anabolic steroids speak of increases in perceived confidence through anabolic steroid use. *International Journal of Sport and Exercise Psychology, 8*(1), 70–80.

WADA. (2003). The WADA Code. https://www.wada-ama.org/sites/default/files/resources/files/wada_code_2003_en.pdf. Accessed on March 03, 2021.

WADA. (2009). The WADA Code. https://www.wada-ama.org/sites/default/files/resources/files/wada_anti-doping_code_2009_en_0.pdf. Accessed on March 03, 2021.

WADA. (2015). The WADA Code. https://www.wada-ama.org/sites/default/files/resources/files/wada-2015-world-anti-doping-code.pdf. Accessed on March 03, 2021.

WADA. (2020). *Anti-doping testing figures report*. https://www.wada-ama.org/en/resources/laboratories/anti-doping-testing-figures-report. Accessed on March 03, 2021.

WADA. (2021a). International standards for testing and investigations. https://www.wada-ama.org/en/resources/world-anti-doping-program/international-standard-for-testing-and-investigations-isti. Accessed on March 03, 2021.

WADA. (2021b). Substances of abuse under the 2021 World Anti-Doping Code. https://www.wada-ama.org/sites/default/files/resources/files/2020-01-11_guidance_note_on_substances_of_abuse_en_0.pdf. Accessed on January 04, 2022.

WADA. (2021c). The WADA Code. https://www.wada-ama.org/en/resources/the-code/world-anti-doping-code. Accessed on March 03, 2021.

Whitaker, L., & Backhouse, S. (2017). Doping in sport: An analysis of sanctioned UK rugby union players between 2009 and 2015. *Journal of Sports Sciences, 35*(16), 1607–1613.

PART 4

GENDERING DOPING

Chapter 10

CULTURAL MANSPREADING IN DOPING ENVIRONMENTS: THEORIZING THE GENDERING OF DOPING SPACES, SEXUALITIES, AND THE SOCIAL

April Henning and Jesper Andreasson

ABSTRACT

This chapter introduces the sociologically informed concept of cultural man-spreading, *which is used to critically examine how gender and power operate in relation to doping and image and performance enhancing drug (IPED) use. Though not exclusively, the chapter centres on the online doping context and how men and women in different forums navigate their doping lifestyles and identities. By focusing on the online doping context, the chapter brackets not only the focus on sport and fitness that has dominated much research, but also the physical dimension that have been at the heart of manspreading in public discourse. Thereby the concept is theorized for wider interpretations, including analysis of men dominating spatial, social and sexual aspects/domains of doping subcultures to the detriment of women or subordinate men. Though doping subcultures are steeped in a masculinity that prioritizes muscular masculinities and construct men as experts and sources of knowledge about doping, the chapter also illustrates how both men and women sometimes play into and challenge such patterns and gender dynamics. Indeed, at times, women's presence in different doping spaces can be a challenge to the default male position. Further, by introducing women-only doping forums the chapter argues that women can begin to debate and share their experiences uninter-rupted, developing their own store of knowledge, and setting the female body*

Doping in Sport and Fitness
Research in the Sociology of Sport, Volume 16, 195–214
Copyright © 2023 by Emerald Publishing Limited
All rights of reproduction in any form reserved
ISSN: 1476-2854/doi:10.1108/S1476-285420220000016011

and experience as default. This supports the idea of a gradual formation of a sis-science doping culture.

Keywords: Doping; masculinity; gender; sport; fitness; sexuality

INTRODUCTION

The term *manspreading* is a recent addition to both formal and informal language, referring to men who sit on public transportation with legs spread widely enough to encroach on other seats, thus claiming physical space at the expense of others. Further, the term has also been used sociologically to illustrate societal structures, focusing on how men throughout history have granted themselves (or been given permission) to take up a disproportionate share of physical space in society and culture, and in doing so, also signalling male dominance. Though the word *manspreading* is relatively new – added to the *Oxford Online Dictionary* in 2015 (BBC, 2015) – the behaviour of men taking up space at the expense of others is not. Jane (2017), for example, traced the history of men sitting and standing with legs spread found in classical art representations of men and surveys of postures. Such physical positions convey the status and power of men, which reinforces the notion of their dominance over women and lower-status men. Historically and in contrast, women as far back as the late fourteenth century have been taught from childhood to avoid any such masculine connoted and unladylike positions that put emphasis on their crotch, and instead directed themselves to more contracted comportments (Jane, 2017). Men have also dominated physical spaces within organizations and workplaces, including 'spilling' into women's workspaces and resulting in women struggling to feel as if they fit into the 'masculine' workplace (Tyler & Cohen, 2010).

Though the use of manspreading as a concept for understanding daily life has shown to be useful in both formal and informal language, it has largely focused on physical space, and men's ways of 'colonizing' their physical surroundings. This focus has, however, limited its utility to understand also other ways men 'spread out' and cause women and other subordinate men to shrink back. There are other terms/concepts that have been used to capture some aspects of this – 'mansplaining' to refer to men who patronizingly explain things to women and thus colonize the social – but rarely these are able to really capture the mechanisms through which a broad range of subtle, symbolic and perhaps unconscious ways men tend to replicate and reify the dominance of masculinity in culture and society.

In this chapter, we will elaborate on the concept of *cultural manspreading* related to doping. We will use this not so much as a concept used in daily life interaction but rather as a sociologically informed theoretical tool. We use illustrative examples from research on gender dynamics in various sport and fitness settings to show the transferability of the concept between different sporting contexts, but as research on doping subcultures has identified the online environment as playing an important role in sharing experiences and disseminating knowledge about doping (Andreasson & Johansson, 2016; Harvey et al.,

2019), this doping arena will be a recurrent focus of attention for exemplifying the utility of the cultural manspreading concept. Centring the online doping experience also, in a way, serves to bracket the physical dimension that has been the focus of manspreading, opening up the concept for a wider interpretation, including the virtual, sexual and social features of manspreading. By considering the intersections of different spaces – physical, virtual, social and sexual – and how men dominate them, the aim of the chapter is to present a theoretically informed analysis of the concept of *cultural manspreading*, and illustrate how hegemonic patterns are shaped, maintained and possibly challenged within doping subcultures and across sporting contexts.

The chapter is structured as follows: First is a background section in which we explain the surfacing of the idea for this chapter and how the concept of cultural manspreading emerged in some of our previous work. Then follows a section in which we theoretically explain the notion of cultural manspreading, and how this concept can be understood as a mechanism that serves to uphold hegemonic masculinity. Thereafter follows two sections in which we sequentially discuss and illustrate how cultural manspreading may serve to reinforce and uphold hegemony, as well as how it may be challenged or resisted. In the conclusion section, we bring the threads together in a summative and theoretically informed discussion on the intersection of the physical, virtual, sexual and social aspects or domains of cultural manspreading.

BACKGROUND

We first created and introduced the concept of *cultural manspreading* in a study of women's experiences on an online doping forum (Henning & Andreasson, 2019). In this study, we used a netnographic and case-study based approach to the research (Kozinets, 2010; Yin, 2014). We followed ongoing discussions, over time, as community members shared experiences and ideas concerning doping on a website called *ThinkSteroids*. This website consists of a multitude of different thematized forums where users and potential users can engage in discussions focused on their particular area of interest. For example, there are forums that deal with health issues, legal questions, different forms of image and performance enhancing drugs (IPEDs) and more. Looking specifically at a forum called 'Women & Steroids,' we noticed that women were facing blockages in their attempts to engage with other women users, though this forum (open for everyone) was directed at women. In fact, we observed that many interactions and conversations about women's use, bodies and experiences came to be dominated by – and filtered through the experiences of – men.

Though many men on the forum were supportive of women and sought to give good advice or relay experiences of their female partners, this encroachment reflected men's sense of entitlement to doping and fitness spaces and their roles as experts within this community. While women could and did still participate, this made finding women's own experiences and accounts difficult and potentially hindered the development of a woman-centred *ethnopharmacological subculture* in which women could share their experiences and debate issues around dosing, side-effect management and harm reduction. Ethnopharmacology is important for doping communities, as many people who use IPEDs rely on community knowledge and experience of other users to plan and manage their use (Andreasson & Johansson, 2016; Monaghan, 2001). In relation to gender, the ethnopharmacological subculture of online doping could be described as sort of a broscience community (Bilgrei, 2018). Our follow-up study (Andreasson & Henning, 2021a) analyzed how reserving exclusive space for women changed the dynamic. When male members were not allowed to engage in discussions, women had space to share their own experiences, ideas and knowledge centred around the female body, laying the foundation for a woman-centred ethno-pharmacological subculture – a new *sis-science* in which the female experience and body was set as the norm (Sverkersson et al., 2020) – and allow women to become and be accepted as experts in their own right. By stopping men from spreading into this space, women were free to fill it up as they chose and to communicate with one another without interference from men forum members, though in a sort of ghettoized way.

Our conceptualizations in earlier studies were, however, theoretically rudi-mentary. We considered only parts of the ways cultural manspreading can be enacted and play out in daily life, focusing on how virtual space was negotiated by men and women, empirically. However, men's dominance of doping and fitness culture is not limited to spatial or physical concerns. Indeed, it largely mirrors or is to be understood as a mechanism that serves to uphold broader patterns that position certain types of masculinities in a dominant position relative to women and other subordinate masculinities (Connell, 1987, 1995). Within academic literature and in broader social views, doping is often linked to men via muscles associated with hegemonic conceptions of masculinity (Zahnow et al., 2018). These links have also helped determine which bodies are valued and celebrated within this subculture, most often those male bodies that are massive, muscular and lean. Indeed, much of fitness culture is built around and continues to be saturated with masculinity. Academic research into doping has also engaged in its own form of cultural manspreading, largely by focusing solely on male bodybuilders and athletes while actively ignoring women. From the now-classic studies of men and internal motivations for steroid use (Klein, 1993) to studies focused on social environments (Monaghan, 2001), occupational and ageing anxiety (Hoberman, 2005), types of (male) users (Andreasson, 2015; Christiansen et al., 2017; Zahnow et al., 2018), body image and eating disorders (Griffiths et al., 2017), and predictions (Dunn et al., 2009), academic research has highlighted, and to some extent, helped reinforce the muscles-men-doping-mas-culinity relationship and the centrality of men and masculinity in questions of doping and steroid use in particular. As Christiansen (2020, p. 5) noted,

> Even when we look specifically at female members of gyms and health clubs, most studies show that women make only very limited use of anabolic steroids. It is true that although recent years

have seen significantly more girls and women involved in bikini-fitness competitions and the like, some of whom may use steroids, few studies have been done on this topic.

Prevalence studies have found low levels of use among women, though many have also focused on male users or samples drawn from gyms where women may not choose to workout. This body of research has largely treated women as an insignificant user group (Bunsell, 2013), relegating them to the background in studies of steroids and muscle-building in favour of the more centrally located and visible male users. At the same time, it has been noted that women are more likely to use supplements considered 'less masculine,' such as human growth hormones (hGH), ephedrine and clenbuterol, as opposed to muscle-enhancing supplements such as steroids (Jespersen, 2012). This also corresponds to the (gendered) side effects associated with various substances, which is why a focus on steroid use in doping studies might be unable to grasp a bigger picture. Therefore, it is important to understand how these patterns endure even as women have emerged as a growing doping population (Andreasson & Johansson, 2020; Sverkersson et al., 2020).

HEGEMONIC MASCULINITY AND THE MECHANISM OF CULTURAL MANSPREADING

Doping – IPED use, especially that involving androgenic anabolic steroids (AAS) – for muscle building has largely developed alongside patterns and conceptualizations of hegemonic masculinity (Connell, 1995). We understand hegemony to be the dynamic legitimization processes through which men's dominance over women and other subordinate forms of masculinity is upheld in various socio-cultural contexts. As Connell (1987) explains, 'hegemonic masculinity is constructed in relation to women and to subordinated masculinities. These other masculinities need not be as clearly defined – indeed, achieving hegemony may consist precisely in preventing alternatives gaining cultural definition and recognition as alternatives, confining them to ghettos, to privacy, to unconsciousness' (p. 186). Hegemonic conceptualizations are dynamic structures and related to how we understand stability and change (Haywood et al., 2018; Hearn, 2004; Howson, 2006). In this way, dynamics and relationships between various groups of men and women are contestable and always situated in arenas of tension and conflict (Connell & Messerschmidt, 2005). This means that gender is not fixed, but conceptualizations of gender are constantly being (re)made and, at times, redefined. Fitness culture, especially those parts heavily associated with doping, has also been linked with hyper-masculine bodies and attitudes. Massively muscular bodies and sexually aggressive, heteronormative attitudes normalized within this subculture are a more extreme version of more mainstream masculinities, but these extremes also reinforce hegemonic masculinity by setting an outer limit. In some ways, men performing more hegemonic forms of masculinity benefit from others operating at the extreme, as hegemonic masculinity looks like the preferable, normal and more socially acceptable standard by comparison. This reinforces hegemonic masculinity at the top of the social gender hierarchy. Historically, men have been able to reap social status and recognition for their muscular bodies within the gym and fitness context. Women who are similarly muscular relative to their peers, however, have faced stigmatization (Dworkin, 2001; Dworkin & Wachs, 2009; McGrath & Chananie-Hill, 2009). Yet, women are not totally oppressed or powerless in this hegemonic configuration. Indeed, some may view this relationship as natural, at times resulting in *emphasized femininity* – how women willingly accommodate men's interests, views, and desires – as the 'natural' and subordinate counter to hegemonic masculinity. One of these accommodations includes women shrinking (physically and/or metaphorically) and ceding space to men. Consequently, the term cultural manspreading can be a useful tool for describing the dynamic and mechanisms through which hegemonic masculinity is maintained in society and culture.

In this chapter, we consider cultural manspreading in terms of men dominating *spatial*, *social* and *sexual* aspects/domains of doping subcultures to the detriment of women or other men – as a mechanism through which hegemonic masculinity operates. Though we can see clear separations between these domains, there are, of course, overlaps between these three. We understand spatial to encompass the physical or virtual space taken up by men. We can consider this in terms of measurement, such as how many centimetres or typed characters men take up in a given space. In terms of social aspects, we refer to how men tend to control the narrative around doping in ways that keep men, masculinity and the male body as the centre and default focus of the subculture, in a way the 'silent' norm that is taken for granted in daily interaction. This is where tensions over whose 'voice' is heard and who is accepted within doping subculture are played out. Controlling the social narrative in this way often includes simply taking up space – more posts by men in a forum work to centre the male experience in these social interactions, the same way that men taking up physical space in the weight room works to keep them and their bodies at the social centre of conversations about muscle building and muscularity. Similarly, the sexual domain focuses on how men's desires, fantasies and pleasure have been centred within the doping community with little attention given to women's sexual views. This positions men's sexual interests and pleasure as more important than women's.

Of course, there are other dimensions and dynamics at play with regards to space that we cannot fully consider here, such as the significance of race and ethnicity in determinations of who is entitled to or accepted in a given space. Despite these limitations, we see cultural manspreading as a worthwhile concept to develop as a way of better understanding hegemonic masculinity. Additionally, the structure of the findings may appear to suggest that we are positioning men as being solely responsible for upholding and perpetuating hegemonic masculinity, while holding women as the solution. This is not our intent, as we also found that some men disrupt these hegemonic patterns in their own behaviour and some women uphold these gender patterns in their engagement with men and other women. While it is necessary to draw clear distinctions and highlight the main findings from the data, the gender dynamics at play are far messier than they may appear.

CULTURAL MANSPREADING AS HEGEMONIC STABILITY

In this section, we begin by looking at how the spatial, social and sexual domains/ aspects of doping cultures operate in sport and fitness, and how these, in turn, serve to reinforce a doping culture saturated in hegemonic notions of masculinity. This section serves to illustrate the diverse ways hegemonic stability is upheld and reinforced. In the section that follows, we then consider how such patterns can be challenged and potentially destabilized.

The Male Norm, and Physical and Virtual Spaces

Historically, most public space has been male-dominated. As women have been traditionally relegated to the domestic and private spheres, men occupied physical public spaces largely unchallenged. Sports and fitness are no exceptions and have operated similarly. Women have historically been left out of sport or marginalized in both overt and more subtle ways (see Kidd, 2013). Single-sex sports teams and competitions are the norm in many competitive sports, as women and men often train and compete separately even at the recreational level. Women have also developed their own sports and sport spaces, though some of these have seen the controversial introduction of men, such as netball (Tagg, 2016) and roller derby (Pavlidis & Connor, 2016). Much of sport and the space devoted to it are focused on men and their sporting displays of masculinity. Sports stadiums, for example, may house men-only sports such as baseball or American football, leaving little to no space for women (Kidd, 2013). Even where women are successful, space remains an issue. Women's access to sports facilities has been limited and spaces they were afforded often sub-standard in comparison with men's – a pattern that still endures even at elite levels of women's sport (Archer & Prange, 2019; Mocio, 2018).

Women's exclusion within the realm of gym and fitness culture may even be starker, as gyms for muscle- and bodybuilding were almost exclusively male preserves until the late 1970s (Fair, 1999). For a long time, men could gather in greasy basement facilities to lift weights, build muscles, socialize with other men (and a few women) and construct masculine connoted bodies unquestioningly and without interruption. Men owned this space for a long time. This all changed of course, and due to *the Fitness Revolution* (Andreasson & Johansson, 2014), women have gradually and increasingly gained ground on the fitness scene and enterprise. Gym and fitness culture is, in this sense, no longer a unisex preserve. This does not mean, however, that what we are witnessing is the emergence of a cultural and physical space of gender equity. Quite the contrary, men still tend to dominate gym and fitness spaces that are largely soaked in masculine connoted ideals and accomplishments. This becomes abundantly clear if we move towards the more professional aspects or spaces of this culture, as well as to doping. Gym and fitness culture have, for example, operated as a space where doping practices have been pioneered and proliferated since the 1950s. Early synthetic testosterone substances, such as Dianabol, became go-to technologies for attaining the newly popular male form based on muscle mass and definition rather than the natural, symmetrical forms favoured in earlier decades (Andreasson & Johansson, 2020). This worked to solidify the link between muscles, doping and masculinity that underpinned fitness culture and shaped the spaces in which these bodies were built. As women began joining the bodybuilding world in the 1980s, paving the way for the fitness revolution, they also began entering physical spaces that were previously closed off to them, including gyms for training and bodybuilding competition stages (Fair, 1999). However, women's presence was not immediately accepted and they were often a sideshow – they were regarded as 'freakish' (McGrath & Chananie-Hill, 2009) – to the main event centred around men and their muscular bodies.

Largely, men and masculinities have continued to dominate muscle-building spaces and lifting platforms in gyms and fitness centres, making this 'for all' space a de facto masculine space. This has had the effect of sometimes pushing women out or relegating them to group fitness or other non-serious lifting areas (Bladh, 2020). In their study of gender dynamics in Canadian gyms, Coen et al. (2018) found that women, and to a lesser extent some men, felt compelled to shorten their time and modify or avoid using weightlifting areas due to feeling pushed out by hyper-masculine men. They note:

> Men described avoiding or leaving spaces where hegemonic masculinity was at play, while women described experiences of being crowded out of spaces by masculine performances as well as actions they undertook to minimize their consumption of time and space in the gym. The net effect of these spatial practices was to cede spatial privilege to hegemonic masculinity in a way that had an exclusionary effect on some gym users. (Coen et al., 2018, p. 33)

Despite the gyms in this research being nominally mixed gender and all areas open to everyone, weightlifting spaces were effectively masculine spaces in which women were perceived as and felt like unwelcome guests. This then reinforced the idea among both men and women that weightlifting is inherently masculine, and men therefore are entitled to the space to the detriment of women.

This is a pattern we also observed while researching online doping forums (Henning & Andreasson, 2019) and has been observed to some extent by others (Sverkersson et al., 2020). *Thinksteroids* hosts a number of forums on a wide range of topics, many related to steroid use and most focused on men. Until recently there was only one forum dedicated to women and women's doping called 'Women and Steroids,' implying that the other forums largely and normatively focused on men, men's bodies and masculinity. Despite the 'Women and Steroids' forum being nominally about and for women, threads were dominated, or even monopolized, by men and their posts (Henning & Andreasson, 2019). Men responded in greater numbers to posts by women. Men posted about or on behalf of women, and some men posted misogynistic or sexually aggressive comments towards women on the forum. No matter the intent or content of their posts, men thus flooded many threads with their views, advice, experiences and comments. By co-opting this virtual space in large numbers, men created a more or less masculine space in which they discussed women, women's bodies and women's steroid use from a male perspective. While there was no rule against it, this manspreading/spillover from the main/men's forums had several implications for women IPED users on *ThinkSteroids*. For example, some women community members sought advice and guidance on how to use IPEDs, including how to dose correctly and how to manage side effects. However, women's first-hand accounts and experiences of steroid use became harder to find due to this virtual and spatial manspreading, as women seeking them out had to navigate through and around posts from men. As men spread their comments into various threads on the 'Women and Steroids' forum, this effectively pushed women's posts and threads to the margins. Shrinking their relative space on the forum also shrank the potential for social interaction, as we will discuss in the next section. However, this also pushed some women members off the site completely, as they felt unwelcome or harassed by men. Similar to how women felt the need to minimize their presence in male-dominated gyms, some women noted that other women had left the forums or only engaged sporadically due to men's repeated interference (Henning & Andreasson, 2019). Male members, however, did not seem to grasp the effect of their presence until a new women-only forum was set up by the site moderators (Andreasson & Henning, 2021a).

Socio-Spatial Dominance

The first domain of cultural manspreading, which concerns physical and virtual space, predominantly sets the focus on the range and quantity of men's ways of dominating space. This domain is thus perhaps the one that most explicitly resonates with how the concept has been applied in daily life and public discourse. A second aspect/domain of cultural manspreading is that related to what happens in social life, and perhaps as a consequence of the first domain. Though this is clearly linked to physical or virtual space in important ways, social manspreading happens when men take over and dominate social interactions, not only in numbers but also in terms of setting the tone and focus of how things are discussed and debated. There are, of course, a variety of ways men can spread out in social interactions in daily life, such as by verbally dominating conversation, interrupting or speaking over others, ignoring challenging views, patronizingly explaining things etc. Some of these behaviours have been named – 'man-terrupting' or 'mansplaining' (Jane, 2017) – but we argue that these are effectively ways of socially manspreading. In each example, men simply push into narrative space at the expense of other perspectives and others' voices, experiences and knowledge. Men performing a hegemonic form of masculinity use these tactics to assert their dominance and the relative importance of their views, bodies and more. In much the same way as in a physical space, women's voices are pushed aside to make room for men. Drowning out women's voices not only reinforces male hegemony, it also prevents women from fully engaging in various aspects of social life.

Given their later arrival and acceptance in public and some private spaces, women have often had to push their way into social life and demand to be included. These battles for inclusion were often hard-fought as men were reluctant to cede space and power to women. As politician and author Shirley Chisholm famously noted about her run for president as a Black woman, 'if they won't give you a seat at the table, bring a folding chair.' In some ways, including women's voices, views and experiences in masculine arenas challenges hegemonic masculinity (and whiteness) simply through the act of claiming physical and social space. Often, however, this 'seat at the table' is not a real seat in terms of being on equal footing with men in social life and decision-making – it is temporary and tenuous and always at risk of being folded back up if the woman who initially brought the chair then vacates it. This is especially true in the absence of some sort of policy or broader cultural shift that gives women more permanence in male-dominated social spaces. Claiming social space is not sufficient for upsetting hegemonic patterns of masculinity if men can simply reclaim it in the physical absence of a woman fighting to keep it. When this happens, women remain interlopers. They are not fully accepted, are afforded a lower status and always at risk of being pushed back out. This reinforces the idea that they are intruding on men's social space, rather than men simply refusing to cede public or social space.

Social space can be related to physical or virtual spatial divisions, and progress in one does not guarantee progress in the other. For example, a traditionally male dominated sports club took steps to alter the way space was shared between women's and men's teams and aiming to make the club more socially inclusive with regular events to promote mixing between teams (Jeanes et al., 2020). While this made some spaces more welcoming to women – those designed specifically for women's netball – it did little to change the culture of the club that was imbued with perceptions and behaviours reflecting a gender order underpinned by hegemonic masculinity. Even as the club went to great lengths to give women and girls greater representation in decision-making roles, they were unable to stop the men from taking up social space and sometimes acting in ways that made women feel unwelcome (Jeanes et al., 2020).

This can also happen in the virtual world on doping forums, as noted in the previous section. Besides simply taking up the virtual space with posts, quantitatively, men may flood exchanges with their own views and voices also substantive. In doing so, masculinity and the male body is centred in discussions, and set as the norm, at the expense of women's own experiences, views and expertise. We observed this in relation to doping in several ways on the 'Women and Steroids' forum on *ThinkSteroids* (Henning & Andreasson, 2019). *First*, some men behaved in aggressive ways towards women in some of the forum threads, including commenting on their bodies or making sexually suggestive statements. While some women would engage and push back against this kind of social behaviour, it also came through that there were women members who decided to leave the site because of it. One longtime member noted in a thread that she wanted the men to stop so that women would remain on the site (Henning &

Andreasson, 2019, p. 14). This not only acknowledged the problem of men taking over the 'Women and Steroids' discussions and making women uncomfortable to the point that they stopped posting, but it also underscored how men's voices tended to dominate discussions to the detriment of women. As a result, women may have been less likely to contribute to discussions or to share their own experiences for fear of this kind of treatment from men. This then had the knock-on effect of there being fewer experiences and first-hand accounts being shared, which may prevent the development of a woman-centred ethno-pharmacological culture and store of knowledge from being established (see Sverkersson et al., 2020).

Second, and directly related to the first, men often gave advice to women seeking information about dosing, side effects or other doping-related issues. As experiences with AAS and other IPEDs can vary significantly between individuals and certainly between sexes, this was sometimes not what women were looking for on the forums. Some expressed that they wanted more information or advice from other women who had used substances they were currently using or considering using. Others intentionally posted their own experiences or use logs so that other women could find them more easily. However, even when these preferences were stated, men would still contribute their own advice. Again, these posts then filled this social space, making the relatively few accounts by women harder to find in the mass of threads and posts. Despite much of the advice offered by men being well intentioned and even useful, it was still filtered through the male voice, experience and gaze. This had the effect of centring men's voices and positioning them as the experts or, at least, as the avenue through which knowledge was shared. Women, then, were positioned as novices reliant on men for directing their use rather than agents who could bring their own expertise and successfully coach other women. Advice and information was also usually based on the assumption that women all had roughly the same goals and body ideals as men, meaning women were being advised on how to conform their bodies to meet hegemonic expectations, usually positioning them in accordance with hetero-normative expectations and notions of emphasized femininity. As we will discuss, this was not always the case.

Third, men also spoke on behalf of women. This commonly involved men relating doping experiences and side effects experienced by a female partner. One surprising exchange on a thread about AAS and menstruation included only posts from men, all of whom lacked any first-hand experience. There was no reflection by the men in the discussion that they were debating a phenomenon amongst themselves without any direct input from women. They were reliant on their own observations and what their partners (or other women) disclosed to them, which may be incomplete. Men seemed unaware that their knowledge of women's experiences may be flawed or misunderstood. Instead there was a sense of entitlement about sharing and discussing these second-hand experiences due to their proximity to women who had their own experiences with these drugs and menstruation. By sharing women's experiences for them rather than them speaking for themselves – reasons for which we cannot be certain – men's voices filled the virtual-social space and caused women and their experiences and knowledge to be backgrounded in the process. Even though men were relating information ostensibly based in women's experiences, women's voices were absent in many conversations involving their experiences. This erasure, especially in discussions about and on behalf of women, keeps men as the default sources of knowledge about doping and doped bodies. Not only were they dominating conversations and relegating women's voices, they were also shaping the narrative around women's experiences. What men focus on may not be what women would focus on, and their perception of women's goals or motivations might differ from a woman's own.

Socio-Sexual Dominance

The third aspect of cultural manspreading in doping culture is related to questions of sexuality and intimate relationships. Virility and muscles are often linked in both the popular imaginary and in the expectations and imaginations of men who use AAS or other IPEDs. Research has found that individuals engage in IPED use, especially AAS, as a way of becoming more attractive according to broader cultural ideals (Underwood, 2017) and to impact gender power relations (Monaghan, 2001). Further, a study of Swedish bodybuilders who doped found that while steroid using men were aware that they may be perceived as being too muscular or even deviant, they still valued muscles and sexual potency as a foundational part of their muscular masculinity (Andreasson & Johansson, 2020). These highlight the relationship between doping, sexual prowess and power – and, of course, masculinity. Yet, there has been relatively little focus on the pleasurable aspects of use, with much focusing on the risks and potential harms (Mulrooney et al., 2019), despite this being a common topic of discussion within doping subculture. Even as women are becoming a visible user group, discussions of sexual interactions on doping forums are still centred around men, with little socio-sexual space in this subculture focusing on women/women's pleasure.

One way we see this play out is in terms of how men discuss sexual desires and interactions. As part of doping ethnopharmacological subcultures of online forums, men exchange information about the positive and virilizing side effects of doping substances. These exchanges often include sharing experiences about which substances or combinations of substances are most effective at increasing sex drive and/or how to prevent sexual dysfunction, such as so-called 'deca-dick,' a commonly reported side effect from use of the steroid Decaduranibol (Andreasson & Henning, 2021b; Andreasson & Johansson, 2021). While some men discuss their partners, even including difficulties in maintaining intimate relationships due to an outsized sex drive (Andreasson & Henning, 2021b), avoiding dysfunction is often seen as an important part of side-effect management among men on the forums. Being unable to perform sexually is sometimes set against having multiple sexual partners in order to fulfil their heightened desire for sex on the forums. In almost every case, the latter is viewed as the preferred state – being able to over-perform sexually is valued while inability is met with pity or even scorn. This underscores how doped bodies are understood:

muscles, hegemonic/aggressive masculinity and hypersexuality are linked in ways that overshadow women or alternative masculinities. This leaves little space for any articulation of these alternatives that may challenge this pattern, reinforcing the hegemonic norm within this subculture.

Some men paint vivid and hyper-sexualized pictures of how steroids and other IPEDs boost sexual ability, clearly highlighting the expectation that this is what doping bodies do. Fantasies centre almost completely on male desire and satisfaction that borders on pornographic fantasy. In some cases, men disregarded women's feelings and consent in their descriptions of feeling like a 'rapist' (Andreasson & Henning, 2021b, p. 66). Other men on the forums also agreed with this characterization and included their own similar feelings. Such misogynistic descriptions went unchallenged by other users, including by any women who may have read the threads. This allows this type of narrative of masculinity to spread and become normalized within doping subculture. This can be seen also in Andreasson and Johansson's (2021) work, in which the construction of subcultural and sexual spaces among Swedish male fitness dopers was studied. This study showed how men's heightened hunger for sex, symbolically, can be seen as indicators of a hardcore, mythological masculinity. The effects of IPEDs are argued to create desires that belong in a pornographic fantasy of a perfect male and potent (hetero)sexual ability. At the same time, the men in this study also expressed feelings of being a victim of their desires and lust. Nevertheless, and no matter how the use is understood, as men's fantasies dominate discussions of sex and relationships, narratives that centre other behaviours or women's desires are marginalized, if touched upon at all. In many ways, these discussions highlight how hegemonic masculinity permeates this subculture through men sharing and reinforcing hetero-sexist views of sexual and intimate relationships that position women as subordinate.

As these sections have shown, cultural manspreading within doping subculture is one mechanism through which hegemonic masculinity is stabilized and the gender order is maintained across different domains: physically, virtually, socially and sexually.

CLAIMING SPACE AND CHALLENGING HEGEMONY

The previous section largely revealed a historical continuity in terms of how muscular masculinities and doped bodies can serve to reinforce hegemonic patterns, through the mechanism of cultural manspreading. This is a cultural and dominant narrative and structure that is repeatedly reproduced in relation to the experiences of women in the realm of IPED use and gender. Though we can establish that hegemonic patterns tend to be reproduced in diverse ways, this does however not mean that such patterns remain unquestioned. In this section, we will therefore take a closer look at different ways such structures are challenged and resisted.

Making Space for Women – Ghettoizing the Female Experience?

One way of counteracting cultural manspreading that excludes or limits women's access to fitness and gym spaces has been to set aside women-only spaces or even establish women-only gyms. This recognizes and seeks to address the discomfort and intimidation some women might feel about exercising in male-dominated weight spaces (e.g. Salvatore & Marecek, 2010), allowing some to engage in weightlifting they may otherwise avoid. However, women-only spaces might reinforce the idea that common space is really men's space (Fisher et al., 2018). This may also establish or support a hierarchy within fitness spaces, where men performing a specific type of masculinity are at the centre and everyone else is tertiary. This risk *ghettoizing* women in these alternative spaces, where equipment may be lesser or focused on cardiovascular exercise intended to reduce size, further linking women with taking up less space (Bladh, 2020; Sassatelli, 2010). Relegating women in ways that convey they are secondary does little to change the environment and masculine subculture that prevents their participation in the first place (Fisher et al., 2018).

Women on *ThinkSteroids* were offered their own space in the form of a women-only forum called 'Women's Doping Experiences.' This was established by the site moderators following the publication of our article (Henning & Andreasson, 2019) highlighting how men were taking over the 'Women and Steroids' forum space, potentially limiting the available space women could occupy (Andreasson & Henning, 2021a). The new space offered women the opportunity to develop this virtual space in any way they chose. Though men could still see the threads and posts, they were not allowed to participate in discussions. Preventing men from verbally/socially spreading into the new forum gave women the opportunity to fill this virtual secluded space with their own threads and posts. This strategy does run the risk of potentially leading women to remain marginalized or only active in the space designated for them, which could both prevent them from becoming fully accepted within doping subculture and leave men and masculinity as the default occupants of such forums. Still, we argue that it is important to try to discern and interpret signs of ongoing socio-cultural changes and transformations of the gender balance in society. Therefore, the introduction of a women-only virtual space presents the chance to reframe what happens in terms of discussion and narrative on women's experiences, bodies and gendered understandings. Indeed, offering women an exclusive space can be read as a way to allow women to create a culture on their own terms, moving beyond hegemonic conceptualizations of muscular masculinities (Andreasson & Henning, 2021a). When people dare to challenge or even violate the gender order, the boundaries of the system suddenly become visible.

Women-Made Social and Sexual Spaces

As with physical space, social space can also be managed or regulated in ways that can allow or encourage women to participate. In 2020, when the moderators on *ThinkSteroids* introduced a women-only forum ('Women's Steroid Experiences'), they provided a social space that men could view but not participate in.

Though initially met with some discussion, the new forum was generally well received. Many of the thread topics mirror those from the 'Women and Steroids' forum and are similar to male-dominated forums (Andreasson & Johansson, 2016; Bilgrei, 2018), but here women are able to converse and discuss without men intervening. Like an artist starting from a blank canvas, this allows them to shape the forum in any way they see fit and discuss things in any way they choose. This freedom and their continued access to all the other forums on the site may help to disrupt the ghettoization of the social domain of women's IPED use (Sassatelli, 2010).

Although the forum is still new, findings from our follow-up piece (Andreasson & Henning, 2021a) show that there are some changes happening. Women began posting information and advice to and for other women, along with their own experiences of side effects and muscular gains. Not only did this make it easier for women to find information about other women's first-hand experiences, it also allowed women to position themselves and be regarded as doping experts. Rather than being overshadowed or drowned out by men, or manterrupted, women were able to assert their own knowledge and help guide other women's use. This de-centred men and hegemonic conceptualizations of masculinity in these discussions, allowing the focus to be on the female body and women's accounts of their side effects, motivations and goals. Centring the female form and biology promotes the development of a new ethno-pharmacological subculture based on accumulated 'sis-science' (Sverkersson et al., 2020) rather than a broscience culture (Bilgrei, 2018). This further normalizes women's doping and enables the type of peer-coaching of IPED use found in male-dominated ethnopharmacological cultures (Kotzé et al., 2020). This kind of coaching, inclusion by exclusion, also had implications for the way doping and doped bodies were discussed on the forum. Doping sis-science on *ThinkSteroids*, included both positive effects as well as some of the negative or masculinizing ones. As muscularity and doping were normalized, women in some cases supported one another to push beyond the notion of emphasized femininity and ideas about acceptable women's bodies. Women began to reframe the narrative around doping and doped bodies in a way that centred strength gains, muscle building and even pleasure. This began to break the links between (hegemonic) masculinity and doping, allowing women to set their own new goals and reimagine their ideal bodies.

As discussed in the previous section, scholars have paid little attention to pleasure as a reason for IPED use among men and there is even less research on women's doping and pleasure (see Andreasson & Henning, 2021a). This does not mean that women are uninterested in or refrain from sharing some of their own pleasurable experiences, especially sexual ones. Rather, men's sexual virility is often centred within this subculture, which makes women's sexuality seem to be incidental or even non-existent. Within the women-only forum space, women began discussing side effects of drugs in new ways. For example, where masculinizing side effects (e.g. deeper voice) were previously discussed as something to avoid, women began to rethink these changes as signals that they were making progress towards their muscle-building goals. Further, they moved from being wary of some changes to accepting that they increased pleasure (i.e. enlarged clitoris) and were therefore acceptable or even desirable as part of a doped femininity. Deeper voices became sexy voices and the enlarged clitoris was not a small male sex organ, but an enjoyable feminine change. By having space to share these pleasurable experiences and desires, women on this forum were able to challenge emphasized femininity and rewrite femininity according to their own bodies, feelings and understandings. Similarly, a study of women discussing doping on a Swedish language forum found that women did discuss side effects in terms of sexual satisfaction and desire (Sverkersson et al., 2020). The authors described this as a potensification of the doped body – narratives that connect desires to the body. Though less normalized than men's discussions, women did discuss their sexual appetites in ways that centred their own pleasure. This included describing taking the lead with partners and initiating sex, something often construed as a masculine behaviour. In both studies, women were able to claim some narrative space to present and share a woman-centred view of sexuality within this subculture.

These conversations and shifts seem to have been made possible, to some extent, through the exclusion of men from this forum. By allowing women to discuss, debate and share free from interruption by men – disrupting the cultural manspread – women were able to begin developing their own store of knowledge based on their own biology and experiences. This supports the formation of a women's doping community of practice (Eckert & McConnell-Ginet, 1992) around doping independent of – rather than only in relation to – a men's doping community. This new community may allow for more focus on, for example, harm reduction related to use or focusing on more positive and pleasurable aspects of IPED use.

CONCLUSION

One of our aims in this chapter was to show one of the mechanisms through which hegemonic masculinity is upheld and reinforced within doping subcultures, as well as potential ways of challenging these patterns. By considering the intersection of physical, virtual, social and sexual spaces, we can begin to see one such mechanism, which we have termed *cultural manspreading*. As a conceptual tool, cultural manspreading allows us to easily envision how the question of space and who dominates that space shapes how (sub)cultures are formed and maintained. The historic dominance of men within the public sphere underpinned their dominance of and entitlement to public spaces, including sport and fitness spaces. Even as women continue to enter and share space, the division is not always equitable. One way this occurs is by men simply taking up space. Space is a finite resource and when one group dominates, others are left with less space and forced to shrink or contract in order to fit into what remains. Hegemonic masculinity legitimizes these inequalities, resulting in women and their voices remaining marginalized. This dynamic between the marginalized and the empowered then shapes how spaces and the communities within them develop in terms of what is valued or normalized, which in turn underpin a (sub)culture. With regards to doping subcultures, space can be in terms of physical space (gyms or sports facilities), virtual space (online forums), social space (discussion and debate), or sexual space (fantasy and desire), among potential others. By focusing on the complex interplay between these different types of spaces we can see how these work together to uphold a system underpinned by hegemonic masculinity. In this way, men are not simply spreading across physical space; they are spreading culturally – setting and maintaining a specific type of masculinity as the standard. Manspreading, then, can indeed be understood as a reflection and reinforcement of the values, norms and gender expectations that define a (sub)culture – it acts as a mechanism through which hegemonic masculinity operates. In this way, *cultural manspreading* offers a way of looking beyond the politics of physical space to see how these hegemonic patterns are both stabilized and contested. The online environment provides a rich example of how we can see these dynamics play out and allows us to explore these mechanisms of power and discuss how hegemonic patterns are maintained and challenged in different sporting settings, in gym and fitness culture, and more broadly.

Doping subculture is steeped in a masculinity that prioritizes the male body that is muscular, massive, aggressive and virile. This is played out in gym spaces where women can be normatively excluded by men's unwelcoming behaviour, in sport spaces where men simply may be offered superior facilities and recognition, and in online forums where men are positioned as experts and sources of knowledge on doping. Though these hegemonic patterns of dominance endure, they are not without challenge. As we noted above, it is not as simple as men being the problem and women being the solution. Both men and women play into and challenge hegemonic patterns and gender dynamics and negotiations over various types of space are complex. In various ways, hegemony is challenged with differing degrees of success, in sport, fitness and in relation to doping. At times, women's presence in these spaces can in itself be a challenge to the default male position. Often, however, more is required for women to launch a legitimate and lasting challenge, such as policies that protect spaces for women. Although this can risk ghettoizing women and women's voices by cordoning them off into an adjacent space while maintaining men in the cultural centre (Sassatelli, 2010), they also offer possibilities for preventing men from spreading into and taking over. As our previous research found (Andreasson & Henning, 2021a), allowing women an exclusive space – physical or virtual – that they can shape in any way they choose – socially and sexually – can allow them to redefine gender and what it means to be a doped body. Women within such intersectional spaces are able to claim it and redefine those cultural norms, values and expectations according to their own lived realities, goals and desires. Preventing men from spreading into these spaces means women are uninterrupted and can centre female biology and women's expertise as the norm, allowing for the development of a woman-centred, or sis-science based, ethnopharmacological subculture.

KEY READINGS

(1) Andreasson, J., & Henning, A. (2022). Challenging hegemony through narrative: Centering women's experiences and establishing a sis-science culture through a women-only doping forum. *Communication & Sport*, 10(4), 708–729.

Understandings of image and performance enhancing drugs (IPEDs) and their use has largely been conceptualized through the lens of male hegemonic patterns, treating women's doping as a threat to the "natural" gender order. This article focuses on an exclusive, women-only online IPED forum. It stresses the importance of moving beyond hegemonic conceptualizations to understand the ongoing socio-cultural changes to the gender balance of IPED use and to center women's doping experience.

(2) Connell. R.W. (1995). *Masculinities*. Polity Press.

This is a foundational work in critical studies on men and masculinities. Though challenged, Connell's groundbreaking work on hegemonic masculinity, the nature and construction of masculine identities, and the position of men in the gender order, remains central in the scholarly debate on men and gender relations and in feminist literature.

(3) Felski, R. (1995). *The gender of modernity*. Harvard University Press.

Combining cultural history with cultural theory, Felski offers a challenge to conventional and often male-centered theories and understandings of modernity and modern society. This book provides lenses through which our understanding of history can be rethought and challenged.

(4) Havnes, I. A., Jørstad, M. L., Innerdal, I., & Bjørnebekk, A. (2021). Anabolic-androgenic steroid use among women – A qualitative study on experiences of masculinizing, gonadal and sexual effects. *The International journal on drug policy*, *95*, 102876. https://doi.org/10.1016/j.drugpo.2020.102876

This article explores how the development of masculinizing effects are experienced and processed by women with current or previous steroid use. The article concludes that women who use steroids are at risk of developing irreversible and unwanted effects from their use, which may negatively influence their self-esteem, social life, and sexual function.

(5) Jane, E. A. (2017). 'Dude... stop the spread': antagonism, agonism, and# manspreading on social media. *International Journal of Cultural Studies*, *20*(5), 459–475.

Feminist campaigns on social media platforms have recently targeted manspreading as a phenomenon. In this article, debates around manspreading are used to explore some key features of contemporary feminist activism occurring in the online environment.

REFERENCES

Andreasson, J. (2015). Reconceptualising the gender of fitness doping. Performing and negotiating masculinity through drug-use practices. *Social Sciences*, *4*, 546–562.

Andreasson, J., & Henning, A. (2021a). Challenging hegemony through narrative: Centering women's experiences and establishing a sis-science culture through a women-only doping forum. *Communication & Sport*. https://doi.org/10.1177/21674795211000657

Andreasson, J., & Henning, A. (2021b). *Performance cultures and doped bodies: Challenging categories, gender norms, and policy responses*. Common Ground Publishers.

Andreasson, J., & Johansson, T. (2014). The fitness revolution: Historical transformations in the global gym and fitness culture. *Sport Science Review*, *23*(3–4), 91–112.

Andreasson, J., & Johansson, T. (2016). Online doping: The new self-help culture of ethno-pharmacology. *Sport in Society: Cultures, Commerce, Media, Politics, 19*(7), 957–972. https://doi.org/10.1080/17430437.2015.1096246

Andreasson, J., & Johansson, T. (2020). *Fitness doping. Trajectories, gender, body ideals and health.* Palgrave Macmillan.

Andreasson, J., & Johansson, T. (2021). "Welcome to Planet Porno." Masculinity, sexuality and fitness doping. *Journal of Bodies, Sexualities and Masculinities, 2*(1), 9–30.

Archer, A., & Prange, M. (2019). 'Equal play, equal pay': Moral grounds for equal pay in football. *Journal of the Philosophy of Sport, 46*(3), 416–436.

BBC. (2015). 'Manspreading' added to online dictionary. *BBC.* https://www.bbc.co.uk/news/uk-34070483

Bilgrei, O. R. (2018). Broscience: Creating trust in online drug communities. *New Media & Society, 20*(8), 2712–2727. https://doi.org/10.1177/1461444817730331

Bladh, G. (2020). Thresholding emancipation: Bodies within the vicinities of gym and fitness. *Idrottsforum.org.*

Bunsell, T. (2013). *Strong and hard women. An ethnography of female bodybuilding.* Routledge.

Christiansen, A. V. (2020). *Gym culture, identity and performance-enhancing drugs: Tracing a typology of steroid use.* Routledge.

Christiansen, A. V., Vinther, A. S., & Liokaftos, D. (2017). Outline of a typology of men's use of anabolic androgenic steroids in fitness and strength training environments*. *Drugs: Education, Prevention and Policy, 24*(3), 295–305. https://doi.org/10.1080/09687637.2016.1231173

Coen, S. E., Rosenberg, M. W., & Davidson, J. (2018). 'It's gym, like gym not Jim': Exploring the role of place in the gendering of physical activity. *Social Science & Medicine, 196*, 29–36.

Connell, R. W. (1987). *Gender & power.* Polity.

Connell, R. W. (1995). *Masculinities.* Polity Press.

Connell, R. W., & Messerschmidt, J. (2005). Hegemonic masculinity: Rethinking the concept. *Gender & Society, 19*(6), 829–859. https://doi.org/10.1177/0891243205278639

Dunn, M., Mazanov, J., & Sitharthan, G. (2009). Predicting future anabolic-androgenic steroid use intentions with current substance use: Findings from an internet-based survey. *Clinical Journal of Sport Medicine, 19*(3), 222–227.

Dworkin, S. (2001). 'Holding back': Negotiating a glass ceiling on women's muscular strength. *Sociological Perspectives, 44*(3), 333–350. https://doi.org/10.1525/sop.2001.44.3.333

Dworkin, S., & Wachs, L. (2009). *Body panic. Gender, health, and the selling of fitness.* University Press.

Eckert, P., & McConnell-Ginet, S. (1992). Think practically and look locally: Language and gender as community-based practice. *Annual Review of Anthropology, 21*, 461–490.

Fair, J. D. (1999). *Muscletown USA: Bob Hoffman and the manly culture of York Barbell.* Penn State Press.

Fisher, M. J. R., Berbary, L. A., & Misener, K. E. (2018). Narratives of negotiation and trans-formation: Women's experiences within a mixed-gendered gym. *Leisure Sciences, 40*(6), 477–493.

Griffiths, S., Murray, S. B., Dunn, M., & Blashill, A. J. (2017). Anabolic steroid use among gay and bisexual men living in Australia and New Zealand: Associations with demographics, body dissatisfaction, eating disorder psychopathology, and quality of life. *Drug and Alcohol Dependence, 181*, 170–176.

Harvey, O., Keen, S., Parrish, M., & Van Teijlingen, E. (2019). Support for people who use anabolic androgenic steroids: A systematic scoping review into what they want and what they access. *BMC Public Health, 19*(1), 1024. https://doi.org/10.1186/s12889-019-7288-x

Haywood, C., Johansson, T., Hammar'en, N., Herz, M., & Ottemo, A. (Eds.). (2018). *The conundrum of masculinity: Hegemony, homosociality, homophobia and heteronormativity.* Routledge.

Hearn, J. (2004). From hegemonic masculinity to the hegemony of men. *Feminist Theory, 5*(1), 49–72. https://doi.org/10.1177/1464700104040813

Henning, A., & Andreasson, J. (2019). 'Yay, another lady starting a log!': Women's fitness doping and the gendered space of an online doping forum. *Communication & Sport, 9*(6), 988–1007.

Hoberman, J. (2005). *Testosterone dreams: Rejuvenation, aphrodisia, doping.* University of California Press.

Howson, R. (2006). *Challenging hegemonic masculinity*. Routledge.

Jane, E. A. (2017). 'Dude… stop the spread': Antagonism, agonism, and manspreading on social media. *International Journal of Cultural Studies*, *20*(5), 459–475.

Jeanes, R., Spaaij, R., Farquharson, K., McGrath, G., Magee, J., Lusher, D., & Gorman, S. (2020). Gender relations, gender equity, and community sports spaces. *Journal of Sport & Social Issues*, *45*(6), 545–567.

Jespersen, M. R. (2012). 'Definitely not for women': An online community's reflections on women's use of performance enhancing drugs. In J. Tolleneer, S. Sterckz, & P. Bonte (Eds.), *Athletic enhancement, human nature and ethics. Threats and opportunities of doping technologies* (pp. 201–218). Springer.

Kidd, B. (2013). Sports and masculinity. *Sport in Society*, *16*(4), 553–564.

Klein, A. (1993). *Little big men: Bodybuilding, subculture and gender construction*. State University of New York Press.

Kotze, J., Richardson, A., & Antonopoulos, G. A. (2020). Looking 'acceptably' feminine: A single case study of a female bodybuilder's use of steroids. *Performance Enhancement & Health*, *8*(2–3). e100174. https://doi.org/10.1016/j.peh.2020.100174

Kozinets, R. (2010). *Netnography: Doing ethnographic research online*. Sage.

McGrath, S., & Chananie-Hill, R. (2009). 'Big freaky-looking women': Normalizing gender transgression through bodybuilding. *Sociology of Sport Journal*, *26*(2), 235–254. https://doi.org/10.1123/ssj.26.2.235

Mocio, L. (2018). United States Soccer Federation, Inc. v. United States Women's National Soccer Team Players Association: When winning isn't everything: An examination into a world where female isn't deleted, but figures after a dollar sign are. *The Sports Lawyers Journal*, *25*, 249.

Monaghan, L. F. (2001). *Bodybuilding, drugs and risk: Health, risk and society*. Routledge.

Mulrooney, K. J., van de Ven, K., McVeigh, J., & Collins, R. (2019). Commentary: Steroid madness-has the dark side of anabolic-androgenic steroids (AAS) been over-stated? *Performance Enhancement & Health*, *6*(3–4). https://doi.org/10.1016/j.peh.2019.03.001

Pavlidis, A., & Connor, J. (2016). Men in a 'women only' sport? Contesting gender relations and sex integration in roller derby. *Sport in Society*, *19*(8–9), 1349–1362.

Salvatore, J., & Marecek, J. (2010). Gender in the gym: Evaluation concerns as barriers to women's weight lifting. *Sex Roles*, *63*(7), 556–567.

Sassatelli, R. (2010). *Fitness culture: Gyms and the commercialisation of discipline and fun*. Palgrave Macmillan.

Sverkersson, E., Andreasson, J., & Johansson, T. (2020). 'Sis Science' and Fitness Doping: Ethnopharmacology, Gender and Risk. *Social Sciences*, *9*(4), 55. https://doi.org/10.3390/socsci9040055

Tagg, B. (2016). Men's netball or gender-neutral netball? *International Review for the Sociology of Sport*, *51*(3), 314–331.

Tyler, M., & Cohen, L. (2010). Spaces that matter: Gender performativity and organizational space. *Organization Studies*, *31*(2), 175–198.

Underwood, M. (2017). Exploring the social lives of image and performance enhancing drugs: An online ethnography of the Zyzz fandom of recreational bodybuilders. *International Journal of Drug Policy*, *39*, 78–85. http://doi.org/10.1016/j.drugpo.2016.08.012

Yin, R. (2014). *Case study research: Design and methods*. Sage.

Zahnow, R., McVeigh, J., Bates, G., Hope, V., Kean, J., Campbell, J., & Smith, J. (2018). Identifying a typology of men who use anabolic androgenic steroids (AAS). *International Journal of Drug Policy*, *55*, 105–112. https://doi.org/10.1016/j.drugpo.2018.02.022

Chapter 11

BODYBUILDING, GENDER AND DRUGS

Charlotte Nicola Jane Mclean

ABSTRACT

This chapter presents an auto-ethnographic journey into the world of women's bodybuilding and the role performance-enhancing drugs play in the pursuit of muscularity in this growing, but hard-to-reach, subculture. The research addresses a paucity in the literature and paves the way for further research to inform public health initiatives for this population. Synthesizing journal entries, field observations and informal conversations recorded over the course of 18 months, this chapter provides insight into the rituals and practices present in bodybuilding culture. This embodied narrative explores the decision-making process surrounding anabolic androgenic steroid use in the context of competitive endeavour, including the impact that cultural norms, peer influence and personal narrative have on their uptake. It also sheds light on the experiences of being a woman in a man's world and the additional stigma women face when attempting to increase their muscularity. It also highlights the personal and professional challenges involved in auto-ethnographic endeavour.

Keywords: Anabolic androgenic steroids; bodybuilding; women; gender; auto-ethnography; cultural norms

INTRODUCTION

This chapter is based on my auto-ethnographic account exploring the lived experience of women who engage in the sport of bodybuilding. Traditionally a male domain, female participation in the sport has evolved since its introduction in the 1970s (Aspridis et al., 2014) as has the number of divisions within which

Doping in Sport and Fitness
Research in the Sociology of Sport, Volume 16, 215–238
Copyright © 2023 by Emerald Publishing Limited
All rights of reproduction in any form reserved
ISSN: 1476-2854/doi:10.1108/S1476-285420220000016012

one can compete. The hyper-muscular female bodybuilding class has now been joined by physique, figure, wellness and bikini. These classes range with respect to the required levels of muscularity and leanness from the most to the least respectively, with an emphasis on the preservation of femininity (Tajrobehkar, 2016). This, alongside the shift away from the thin ideal towards a lean athletic, fit, and strong female physique (Andreasson & Johansson, 2020; Benton & Karazsia, 2015), has led to an increase in the number of women seeking to engage in the sport (Aspridis et al., 2014). However, fitness is not always synonymous with health, and evidence suggests that the consumption of anabolic androgenic steroids (AAS) has substantially increased over the last several decades (Huang & Basaria, 2018). While prevalence is difficult to quantify, it is acknowledged that women's use exists although very little is known about this population (Kotzé et al., 2020).

My research focussed on what motivates female bodybuilders to use AAS, including competitive endeavour, the influence of peers and coaches, and attitudes towards AAS use within the bodybuilding community. In this chapter I present my auto-ethnographic story, analysing my personal experiences in relation to the subculture to create what I hope is an empathic understanding of the journey from novice bodybuilder to potential competitor and AAS user.

I achieved this through 18 months of participant observation in two hard core bodybuilding gyms, where I was immersed in bodybuilding culture and all its rituals and practices. This involved systematic weight training, adoption of specific dietary and supplementation protocols, attendance at competitive events, and engaging with coaches in an attempt to achieve a competitive physique. These experiences provided me with an insight into the lived experience of my peers, shedding light on the emotions and physical and mental states they encounter (Bunsell, 2010). In experiencing the corporal reality of becoming a female bodybuilder, I was the instrument of research, who *deploys the body as a tool of inquiry and a vector of knowledge* (Wacquant, 2004, p. vii).

This chapter draws on diary entries and field notes recorded over the course of my research as well as memories and experiences prior. I present these here as an emergent qualitative narrative bookended by a more analytic scholarly voice to extend understanding of the sport of bodybuilding, the cultural setting and the decision to use AAS (Wall, 2006). I also provide an insight into the challenges, dilemmas and personal issues I faced as a result of my auto-ethnographic practice.

The aim of this chapter is to provide the reader with an insider perspective on how female bodybuilders negotiate bodybuilding culture and how AAS use can play a role in achieving competitive success. In doing so, it highlights the decision-making process involved and the influences and motivations inherent in AAS uptake. The chapter will begin with an overview of the role of AAS use within bodybuilding culture followed by an explanation of women's bodybuilding and the threat it poses to gender norms. After a brief overview of my background, it goes on to discuss the physical challenges of the research, my engagement with cultural experts, and the decision-making process surrounding AAS use. Before reaching a conclusion it also highlights some of the emotional and methodo-logical challenges I faced.

AAS USE IN BODYBUILDING

The use of AAS and growth hormone to increase muscularity and improve body composition has been closely associated and increasingly normalized within the sport of bodybuilding (Liokaftos, 2018). Use is often endorsed by trusted figures whose knowledge of bodybuilding practice, including drug use, is extensive and authoritative. These are individuals who have achieved practical mastery of the sport, having realized a competitive worthy physique for themselves and others they have successfully coached. As a result, they enjoy an expert status amongst the community, as they have proved that they possess the necessary nutrition, training and in many cases drug use strategies to be successful in the sport. Their knowledge of AAS compounds, regimes and side effects is often termed ethno-pharmacological expertise, an indigenous knowledge that is aimed at maximizing benefit and reducing harm (Monaghan, 2001b).

Within bodybuilding using AAS is viewed as a normal and appropriate part of bodybuilding methodology, especially when an individual wishes to compete at professional level (Kotzé et al., 2020; Pappa & Kennedy, 2013; Wright et al., 2001). Indeed, AAS use is now so normalized in the sport that there are 'natural' bodybuilding federations catering specifically for those who do not wish to engage in AAS use. These federations however exist on the margins of main-stream 'normal' bodybuilding, attracting less attention and prestige.

The uptake of AAS by women has been attributed to the desire to increase strength and muscle mass, to improve appearance (Andreasson & Johansson, 2021; Ip et al., 2010), and for competitive endeavour (Grogan et al., 2006; Korkia et al., 1996). The desire to be competitive may in turn be influenced by encour-agement from male bodybuilders, who work alongside women as coaches, training partners or even romantic spouses (Chananie-Hill et al., 2012). Bunsell's ethnography (2010) describes how women bodybuilders often spend time researching and seeking advice from trusted peers in the pursuit of the desired physique. Although many of the women Bunsell talked with experienced side effects both positive and negative, they managed these by keeping drug dosages low and cycles short, while also avoiding highly androgenic compounds. For most the pleasure and desire of bodybuilding outweighed any negatives and none were willing to rethink their muscular pursuits (Bunsell, 2013).

A MAN'S WORLD

Women's involvement in the sport of bodybuilding has evolved since the incep-tion of the Ms Olympia women's bodybuilding class in 1980. During these early days, success was achieved through a thin and toned physique such as that of Rachel Mclish. However, as the sport progressed muscularity increased and by

1984, Corey Everson had set the new standard for muscularity, being nicknamed the 'Female Arnold Schwarzenegger', and going on to win the title a further six times before her retirement in 1989 (Bunsell, 2010).

Contemporary competitions offer a wider variety of class divisions, expanding over the years to incorporate bikini (2011), body fitness (or 'figure' as it is called on the professional stage [2002]), wellness (due to be introduced to the Olympia competition in 2021), physique (2013) (IFBB, 2021; Olympia, 2021b) and women's bodybuilding (2020). Class divisions are distinguished on a continuum of muscularity and leanness ranging from the hyper-muscular bodybuilding division to the slenderer bikini physiques, as well as in requirements for posing and attire (Campbell et al., 2021) summarized in Table 1.

Table 1. Adapted From the International Federation of Bodybuilding & Fitness (IFBB) Rules 2021.

Division	
Bikini	(1) The assessment, beginning with a general impression of the physique, should take into consideration the hair; the overall body development and shape; the presentation of a balanced, proportionally and symmetrically developed, complete physique; the condition of the skin and the skin tone; and the athlete's ability to present herself with confidence, poise and grace.
	(2) The physique should be assessed as to its level of overall body tone, achieved through athletic endeavors and diet. The body parts should have a nice and firm appearance with a decreased amount of body fat but may have a 'softer' and 'smoother' look than in bodyfitness. The physique should neither be excessively muscular nor excessively lean and should be free from muscle separation and/or striations. Physiques that are considered too muscular, too hard or too lean must be marked down. *The overall image displayed should demonstrate poise,* ***femininity*** *and self-confidence. This is especially true at all times when the competitor is performing I-walking in the finals, standing in the line-up and during the comparisons of the quarter turns.*
Body Fitness/ Figure	(1) The assessment, beginning with a general impression of the physique, should take into consideration the hair, the overall athletic development of the musculature; the presentation of a balanced, proportionally and symmetrically developed physique; the condition of the skin and the skin tone; and the athlete's ability to present herself with confidence, poise and grace.
	(2) The physique should be assessed as to its level of overall muscle tone, achieved through athletic endeavors and diet. The muscle groups should have a round and firm appearance with a small amount of body fat. The physique should neither be excessively muscular nor excessively lean and should be free from deep muscle separation and/or striations. Physiques that are considered either too muscular or too lean must be marked down. *The overall image displayed should demonstrate poise,* ***femininity*** *and self-confidence. This is especially true at all times when the competitor is standing in the line-up and during the comparisons of the quarter turns.*
Wellness	(1) The assessment should take the whole physique into account. The assessment, beginning with a general impression of the physique, should take into consideration the hair; the overall body development and shape; the presentation of a balanced and symmetrically developed, complete, athletic looking physique; the condition of the skin and the skin tone; and the

Table 1. *(Continued)*

Division	
	athlete's ability to present herself with confidence, poise and grace. Vertical body proportions should be correct; however, the horizontal proportions should display a slightly bigger body mass in the hips, buttocks and thighs area.
	(2) The physique should be assessed as to its level of overall body tone, achieved through athletic endeavors and diet. The body parts should have a nice and firm appearance with a decreased amount of body fat, similar to that displayed by bikini-fitness athletes. The physique should not be excessively muscular and should be free from muscle separation and/or striations. Physiques that are considered too muscular or too hard must be marked down. *The overall image displayed should demonstrate poise, **femininity** and self-confidence. This is especially true at all times when the competitor is performing I-walking in the finals, standing in the line-up and during the comparisons of the quarter turns.*
Physique	(1) The judge should first assess the overall female athletic appearance of the physique. This assessment should begin at the head and extend downwards, taking the whole physique into account. The assessment, beginning with the general impression of the physique, should take into consideration the hair and makeup; the overall athletic development of the musculature; the presentation of a balanced, symmetrically developed physique; the condition of the skin and the skin tone; and the athlete's ability to present onstage with confidence.
	(2) During the comparisons of the Mandatory Poses, the judge should first look at the primary muscle group being displayed. The judge should then survey the whole physique, starting from the head, and looking at every part of the physique in a downward sequence, beginning with general impressions, and looking for a *symmetrical balanced development of all the muscle groups and definition*. The downward survey should take in the head, neck, shoulders, chest, all of the arm muscles, front of the trunk for pectorals, pec-delt tie-in, abdominals, waist, thighs, legs, calves and feet. The same procedure for back pose will also take in the upper and lower trapezius, teres and infraspinatus, erector spinae, the gluteus group, the leg biceps group at the back of the thighs, calves, and feet. *A detailed assessment of the various muscle groups should be made during the comparisons, at which time the judge must compare muscle shape, density, and definition while still bearing in mind the competitor's overall balanced development and femininity*.
	(3) The physique should be assessed as to the level of overall muscle tone, achieved through athletic endeavors and diet. The muscle groups should have a round and firm appearance with a small amount of body fat. *The overall image displayed should demonstrate poise, **femininity** and self-confidence. This is especially true at all times when the competitor is standing in the line-up and during the comparisons of the quarter turns*
Women's Bodybuilding	Judges will score competitors according to the 'total package', which is a balance of size, symmetry and muscularity (IFBBPro, 2021). *NB: I could find very little in the way of published rules for the women's bodybuilding division. Whilst some federations consider women's physique as the pinnacle of women's bodybuilding, the IFBB pro league and the National Physique Committee (NPC) do have a listing for the women's bodybuilding division on their website (IFBBPro, 2021; NPC, 2021) and there also exists the Ms Olympia title. Although the IFBB professional league and the NPC both list posing and / or attire based information for competitors, there is very little pertaining to the judging criteria applied to the athletes physiques. The above is the only sentence that refers to how physiques will be evaluated.*

Source: Santonja (2021a, 2021b, 2021c, 2021d).

The exterior territories of the body represent a capital resource, a social symbol and a representation of the self in the modern world (Lelwica, 2017). Diet and exercise are the first line in the taming of an unruly body, and traditionally it is women who have been under pressure to achieve culturally prescribed body ideals. The once thin body ideal has recently developed into a leaner more muscular look, the achievement of which represent virtues such as self-control and hard work (Lelwica, 2017; Marshall et al., 2019). However, there exists a glass ceiling for women due to the gendered nature of muscle, such that hyper-muscular females are often stigmatized and seen as less intelligent, less educated, less socially popular, less attractive, and violating traditional gender norms when compared to the 'average woman' (Marshall et al., 2019; Worthen & Baker, 2016). Indeed, judgement from outsiders can be harsh, as noted by Shilling and Bunsell (2009), evoking attitudes of aesthetic repulsion and suggestions that women interested in building muscle were psychologically deviant or deliberately attempting to offend others. Thus, violating gender norms set women body-builders aside as deviant, and this can be compounded with the use of AAS which further threaten the gender order through the 'unnatural' use of derivatives of the male hormone testosterone. This notion of double deviance can lead to a shroud of stigma and taboo, resulting in a veil of secrecy or the downplaying of use to everyone except trusted insiders. As a result, women engaged in bodybuilding and associated drug use must participate in much more corporeal management and will inevitably experience different body politics to their male counterparts (Bunsell, 2013).

Previous studies (Andreasson & Johansson, 2021; Campbell et al., 2021; Heywood, 1998; Kotzé et al., 2020; Lowe, 1998; Shilling & Bunsell, 2009; Sverkersson et al., 2020; Tajrobehkar, 2016) have highlighted the fine line women tread to uphold the necessary requirements of their class division whilst also preserving traditional gender distinctions via the feminine apologetic of makeup, hair, attire and in extreme cases breast augmentation to achieve the 'overall package' that the sport rewards. Note in table one the emphasis on femininity for each division, cited twice for the more muscular division of women's physique, yet specific statements with regards to the muscularity required for the International Federation of Bodybuilding and Fitness (IFBB) professional league bodybuilding division are conspicuous by their relative absence.

Women attending to feminizing practices must also attempt to eradicate or distract from the virilizing effects of AAS use. So while a traditional drug user's body might expose their addiction and mark them as a figure of self-pity or shame (Ettorre, 2007), the muscular physique of the female AAS user will, under certain circumstances, and within certain limits, be celebrated and rewarded. In body-building this is when the male gaze of the judging panel is satisfied that a competitor has successfully achieved the required muscularity and tone for their class without disturbing the natural gender order (McLean, 2020). For body-building the ideal competitive physique is one that delivers the 'overall package' which includes its ability to signal femininity to its audience.

The degree of muscularity that is valued by bodybuilding federations at any given time is also subject to change. For example, the 2005 '20% rule' which was announced by the IFBB, one of the most influential federations linked to the Olympia event, dictated that female bodybuilders across all divisions should decrease their muscularity by 20% (Bunsell, 2010). Another example is the Ms Olympia title, a class division above the women's physique which has been absent since 2014, only reinstated more recently in 2020 (Olympia, 2021a).

The sport also economically values male and female bodies differently. Women bodybuilders enjoy much less economic reward than their male counterparts when it comes to prize money. The Ms Olympia 2021 winner received $50,000 (Hall, 2021b), eight times less than Mr Olympia who netted $400,000 (Hall, 2021a). The competition itself mirrors this gap between the men's and women's events with the men's open bodybuilding being the last and therefore main event; certainly it is difficult to imagine a bodybuilding contest where the women's competition is the 'headline act' (Campbell et al., 2021).

Women engaging in the sport of bodybuilding must carefully negotiate the edge between masculinity and femininity (Worthen & Baker, 2016). Those who can successfully combine muscularity, femininity and sexuality will obtain the most power (Bolin, 2012; Heywood, 1998; Hunter, 2013; Tajrobehkar, 2016) and as a result attract the most resources, such as competitive titles, sponsorship and coaching opportunities. These are often the bikini and fitness classes which are more in line with current mainstream body ideals, but still devoid of adipose tissue and not marked by AAS use (Bunsell, 2013; Bunsell & Shilling, 2012). In this respect bodybuilding still works to keep women docile (Hunter, 2013) by engaging them in an ever-evolving body project, the limits (in terms of muscularity) of which are determined by male dominated bodybuilding federations who control which bodies are valued and rewarded (Bunsell, 2013; Heywood, 1998).

My physique goal was centred on muscularity in line with the 'bodyfitness' class. This was my personal goal for my petite frame, and I was interested to find that many of the women I spoke with had their own line when it came to the degree of muscularity they pursued, although this could be open to change over time. Comparison and judgement formed part of these narratives, usually focussed on the virilizing effects and loss of femininity with increasing muscularity and AAS use. This often led to an 'othering' of competitors and bodybuilding peers choosing to take this route. Even those competing in the physique division, that allows for more muscularity and dispenses with some of the feminine posing and attire, were still concerned with 'not taking it too far' (McLean, 2020). I also experienced a similar attitude amongst the male members of the gym I attended, as I wrote about in my field notes.

I have been following a physique competitor online for a while. I appreciate her body but it's not a muscularity I can aspire to, don't get me wrong I certainly wouldn't mind waking up like this tomorrow, sans the obvious virilising effects. However, I am aware this isn't possible, so I appreciate it rather than crave it like I do bodyfitness. I am interested in what some of the members of the gym think and so when I'm next engaged in some reception 'banter' I ask what they think of this competitor's physique. 'That's a bloke' says Barry, 'look at the square jaw, any bloke would be proud of those legs'. 'That's the gear isn't it', says Tom. Interestingly all the guys around the table seem to agree that it is unattractive. I ask them about bodyfitness to see if they will have a more favourable outlook, however Tom still sees it as masculine. 'It's like being a man, all muscly and hard, would you feel sexy like that?' he asks. I explain that it would be more of an achievement than anything else, he replies, 'You'd just be obsessed with your abs, wouldn't you?'

Barry tells me about a bodyfitness girl from the gym. 'She's always getting looks off other girls', he says and goes on to explain that she often reacts to them negatively, frequently leading to an altercation. 'You'd have to deal with this sort of reaction. People see female bodybuilders like a freak', he says.

I talk a bit about social media and how my ideal body has become aligned with that of a bodyfitness physique such that I won't be happy with anything less. Interestingly Barry explains that he doesn't like a six pack on a woman, he says it would be 'Like shagging a man, a woman should have a bit of belly'. They all agree that bikini is acceptable however, likening it to a porn star look and expressing the importance of breast augmentation, something that Barry has suggested would look good on me.

I come away with mixed feelings, on the one hand it is refreshing that as a woman in that environment it's not necessarily a negative that I don't possess the lean and muscular physique I desire. My need to achieve a certain physique to be accepted as a bodybuilder feels more urgent when attending bodybuilding shows or when I am with the more competitively oriented gym group. I realise that my view has to some extent been warped with regards to what is 'normal' or achievable. On the other hand, the main issue most of these men had with these women was the degree to which they challenged gender norms, and the sex appeal, or (in their opinion) lack of, that they possessed.

Whilst I got the impression most bodybuilders would keep their opinions to themselves, it still struck me as ironic that insiders were making the same value judgements towards their peers that they often experienced more openly from cultural outsiders. However, I was no exception, I recognized my own aversion to the virilizing effects of AAS, and it was one of the reasons why I was reluctant to use them. Indeed, a large proportion of my concern for using AAS was cosmetic as well as health related. Whilst relatively speaking building muscle as a woman within bodybuilding culture is more accepted, the culture and its members also strive to uphold gender norms.

Connell (1987) argued that gender identities arise by the denial or minimization of bodily characteristics shared by women and men, and through the performance of certain social practices that transform the body. These can be permanent physical changes like those that occur through the practice of bodybuilding and cosmetic augmentation, or temporary outcomes achieved through attire, makeup or the wearing of high heels. Women engaging in bodybuilding employ 'emphasised femininity', which Connell used to describe femininity that was 'oriented to accommodating the interests and desires of men' (Connell, 1987, p. 183). In the context of bodybuilding, gender differences are strategically manipulated by female bodybuilders in order to negotiate their femininity (Dilley et al., 2014) against the backdrop of their hyper-muscular body.

AUTO-ETHNOGRAPHY AND ITS CHALLENGES

Background: The Journey to Bodybuilding

My involvement in the sport of bodybuilding grew in my early 20s; before then I was blissfully indifferent to my diet and had an unproblematic relationship with food. Although I exercised to control my weight I was not wedded to the pursuit of a hyper-lean muscular physique. By chance, the gym nearest to my workplace was frequented by competitive bodybuilders. Set over two floors, it was a far cry from the aerobics sessions and commercial gym environments I was used to at that point. Packed tightly with a plethora of machines, dumbbells, plates and men, it was initially an intimidating environment; however, over time I began to become more integrated into the gym as a 'regular', and at the same time my attention was drawn to the few women who attended, especially those whose muscular lean bodies I had begun to covet. In the absence of social media, it was these women and the women in the pages of 'Muscle and Fitness Hers' that began to skew my focus towards the bodybuilding physique, and it would be from this point onwards that I would adopt this cultural ideal as my own, embracing a more focussed training and dietary strategy with the assistance of one of the professional male bodybuilders. It was at this point that I began to become familiar with the methodology of bodybuilding and it would capture my interest for decades to come. I felt drawn to its promise of complete control over my physical form and the sense of empowerment this provided. In a job I hated and in a relationship that was falling apart, bodybuilding offered me an opportunity not only to transform my physique but to take control of my life. Bodybuilding also replaced the heavy metal community, from whom I had become estranged, swapping head banging, piercing, tattooing, make up and clothes, for lifting weights, protein shakes, and, as I would learn later, image and performance enhancing drugs (IPEDs). I felt compelled to immerse myself in this culture and the community it offered, later even taking steps to make it my full-time career as a personal trainer and coach. I was filled with a sense of purpose, eager to adopt what felt like a magical process.

Although the transformative culture of bodybuilding offers a sense of salvation from a disobedient body, an escape from an unruly life and the integration in a new community and lifestyle, it also objectifies the body, such that it becomes like a possession, broken into its constituent parts (back, chest, shoulders, legs, etc.) that must be continually improved upon, where the cultural discourse asks competitors to 'bring a better package' to the stage with each competitive endeavour. Attempting to achieve the bodybuilding ideal can therefore lead to a lifelong body project that is required to maintain a competitive physique and retain one's position as a legitimate bodybuilder. In any given week I would weight train five or six times, arriving at the gym by 6 a.m. Lifting as heavy as possible within a repetition range of 8–12, I would perform multiple sets of several exercises targeting the major muscle groups to be trained that session. This might take an hour or more and may be accompanied by cardiovascular exercise either straight after or later that day. My routine over the week would be split up to ensure I trained all the major muscle groups at least once, whilst allowing for lagging areas to be hit twice.

Certainly I was personally very aware that both within bodybuilding culture and the fitness industry, a flawless lean and muscular physique communicates the prestige and authority of its owner (Lelwica, 2017). Thus, achieving this became increasingly important as despite having several academic and professional qualifications, I felt under pressure to achieve a physique that would be successful on the competitive stage. As I knew, this would elevate my credentials within the industry and I would more readily attract clients. This is because qualifications are not highly valued within the bodybuilding community without a physique to 'prove' such credentials and demonstrate an ability to put knowledge into practice. Like consumer culture, bodybuilding places a premium on youth, health, fitness and beauty, where appearance symbolizes inner discipline, invites moral evaluation and is a vehicle to express a particular attitude (Howson, 2007).

During the early days of entering the world of bodybuilding I was only vaguely aware of the role of IPEDs in the sport. I would occasionally hear conversations amongst the male competitive bodybuilders in the gym where I trained. However, despite seeking help from one of these gym members, AAS and any associated drugs were not mentioned explicitly. At the time I was supremely confident that simply adopting the training and dietary protocols prescribed to me would be enough to change my physique. However, I was uneducated and naive to the extremes of training and dietary manipulation necessary to achieve a muscular and lean competitive physique (Spendlove et al., 2015). I also associated this body with the maintenance of health, and therefore I would not have entertained the use of any IPEDs.

Doing Auto-Ethnography

Embarking on a research project within a community that was already close to my heart seemed ideal, especially as it meant I could spend more time within a gym environment engaging with members of the bodybuilding community. At the same time, it also reinvigorated my desire to achieve a bodybuilder's physique and engage more heavily with the rituals and practices of the community.

Initially I believed that training for a bodybuilding competition would further enhance my auto-ethnographic experience with a more fully immersive participant-observer role, whilst establishing me as a bodybuilder and fulfilling a long-held personal desire. However, this presented several challenges with respect to the preservation of my mental and physical health and involved far more emotional labour and risk than I could have predicted at the outset.

The Physical Challenge

Bodybuilders usually divide their time between competitive and off-season periods. Off-season training focuses on muscle hypertrophy in line with the athlete's chosen division, whilst competition preparation is aimed at reducing subcutaneous fat to enhance muscular definition in line with the levels of conditioning required for the stage (van der Ploeg et al., 2001). This competitive phase includes intense resistance exercise coupled with aerobic training and rigorous dieting in order to achieve a negative energy balance (Alwan et al., 2019). All of this work culminates in a 'peak week' prior to the competitive event that involves the manipulation of fluid, salt, water and carbohydrates in an attempt to reduce body water to enhance leanness and vascularity (Mitchell et al., 2017).

Prior to this research I had spent several years resistance training and had already attempted, albeit unsuccessfully, to diet down for competition. The intense training often took its toll, and I was no stranger to the physiotherapist. Thus, when I started training with one of the male bodybuilders, I was apprehensive, not wanting to aggravate old injuries but also keen to let him lead the session. Below is a diary excerpt that illustrates the physical toll these sessions sometimes took.

> I wake up in intense pain, I am used to delayed onset muscle soreness but this feels different and somewhat reminiscent of my chronic fatigue syndrome (CFS) pain (unexplained chronic muscle pain and weakness). I am scared, having suffered with CFS for a prolonged period in the past, some of it aggravated by previous contest preparation attempts, this is not a place I wish to revisit. Nor do I want to be faced with more physio bills to fix my broken body. In the dead of night I am ready to pull the plug, go it alone in the gym and do my own thing.

Despite these misgivings I carried on, having a training partner made me feel more integrated into the gym community, giving me renewed hope that this time I might successfully achieve the physique I desired.

> We start training and this is the first time I have worn my [gym branded] hoody since I bought it. I feel more a part of things with it on, as so many members wear them. I look in the mirror as I train, my lats are straining as I pull the weight towards me. I can feel myself becoming a bodybuilder, all the magic and promise of the training and diet are once again tangible. I can feel myself spurred on by my training relationship, and the comradery and ritual of gym life.

I was by now far more aware of the extremes of the sport and at the same time, I had become increasingly more exposed to the idea of IPED use, with AAS having been suggested to me on a few occasions as an option to help me build and then retain muscle whilst dieting. I was also aware of how normalized the use of AAS was within the sport, as part and parcel of the process of competition preparation. Was I naïve in thinking I could maintain my health and achieve the physique I desired without the use of AAS? I began to seriously entertain the idea that I should go 'all in' and adopt the drug protocols suggested. So, with this in the back of my mind, I approached coaches in both gyms to ask them to train me formally for a competition.

The Coach

The role of trusted others as a source of information is common in bodybuilding culture and is supported by the literature (Fussell, 1991; Monaghan, 2001a). As a result of this faith in those possessing ethno-pharmacological expertise, combined with the early denial of the efficacy of AAS by the scientific and medical community (Wood, 2008), many bodybuilders are reluctant to seek or heed advice from outsiders. As a result, to achieve success in the sport, individuals often seek out or are influenced by trusted insiders, and this frequently results in the formation of a coaching relationship.

This was certainly the case for me as well as many of the individuals I met during the course of my research, with some having more than one coaching relationship across their bodybuilding career (McLean, 2020). For this relationship to be successful, an individual must be able to 'trust the process' that the coach prescribes and adhere to the training, dietary and supplementation advice provided. Thus, the coach, often a male, is an important director in the bodybuilding process, assessing individuals' physiques regularly, guiding the process from week to week, motivating and supporting. As a result of their own success in the sport and experience with drug protocols, these individuals enjoy an elevated position within the culture, and are viewed as experts who can provide the formula required to achieve a successful stage physique. Trusting the process means trusting the coach, so if their protocol extends beyond nutrition and training strategies into AAS and other associated drug use, they can form a significant influence on uptake. Furthermore, in most instances, there is an unwritten rule that a client does not question a coach's methodology, as to do so not only undermines the important trust element of the relationship but can also be seen as bringing into doubt the coach's expertise. This trust afforded to a coach can also extend to the supply of the compounds and the implementation of other extreme practices associated with the sport such as dehydration strategies during peak week.

Both prior to and during my research, I had several experiences with coaches who promised to deliver results. At first, fresh to the process and naïve to its practices, I was able to adhere to the diet and training protocols they advised without question. However, despite my best efforts, my physique still failed to be lean enough to be competitive on stage. Nevertheless, I was still unable to let go of the idea of competing in a bodybuilding contest and my failure to achieve this goal had left me feeling shameful and inadequate. The inability to disengage despite these feelings were largely a result of my continued immersion in the culture, and the adoption of so much of the bodybuilding lifestyle. I was in the gym at the crack of dawn most days, I calculated every gram of protein, carbohydrate and fat I consumed, and I carried Tupperware with pre-prepared meals to meetings and events. I was living the life of a bodybuilder, just without the body to match. As a result, I often found myself starting a new coaching relationship to alleviate the situation, which meant there were many occasions where my body was evaluated. This process, often called 'checking in' and occurring regularly throughout the coaching process, especially during contest preparation, is a chance for the coach to appraise your physique and determine the appropriate course of action. For myself it sometimes involved walking though the gym dressed in a bikini, sending bikini pictures to an online (usually male) coach, or going to a hotel room to do the same, behaviours not normally acceptable for a married woman but in the context of bodybuilding culture perfectly legitimate. I documented one of these experiences in my field diary.

It's not the first time I've had to stand in a bikini for my body to be evaluated, my phone is filled with 'progress pictures' that have been sent to various online coaches over the years since I first started this journey. In person it is a little more confronting, and especially in the presence of a gym owner that I am less familiar with. As usual my legs are the 'problem' this is no surprise, but I feel exposed, and a bit humiliated this time. I fumble around for the words to express how hard I have tried to achieve the requisite body however I feel that much of this falls on deaf ears. At the end of the day any evaluation by a coach must be met with the attitude that they, a man, knows more about my body than myself. I am left feeling that familiar sense of failure, I have not trusted the process or engaged with it enough. 'What you need to do is hammer the cardio twice a day', says Barry, 'and don't weight train them [my legs] for now'. Barry seems to think I can spot reduce the fat in my legs, but I know from experience it will be the last place I will lose adipose tissue. 'Laura was up to 3 hrs a day of cardio before her show' he explains. I tell him I have been there and done this in the past with limited results. 'You'll just have to work harder' he replies. I leave feeling upset and despondent, tired of being less than and fatigued at the thought of having to engage in the same uphill struggle again.

Although the check in experience was often associated with a new beginning and therefore hope, it never failed to highlight the inadequacies of my body, which began to feel like an object that I had failed to augment in the appropriate manner due to my mismanagement of it, and my inability to fully engage with the process when it began to affect my health. However instead of disengaging with my physique goals I simply sought out another coach. This was because, despite my academic and professional training, I still believed there was an 'expert' out there that could provide me with a way of attaining a lean and muscular body without compromising my well-being. As a result, I continually handed myself over to a man within a community where knowledge is often bound to masculinity, and where some of that knowledge I knew to be questionable at best, and at worst, potentially harmful.

ANABOLIC ANDROGENIC STEROID USE: A TRICKY DECISION

With many 'natural' failed attempts at achieving the body fitness physique I desired, and with my body image suffering, I began to revisit the idea of AAS use. It was the one avenue that I had shied away from as it was not in line with my goal of achieving the physique I desired without risking my health or compromising my wish to achieve a certain body without pharmaceutical assistance. I was also concerned about the virilizing effects I might experience. Nevertheless, I came back to the idea time and time again, grappling back and forth with the decision. The journal entry below illustrates how after certain experiences in the field I would move closer to the idea of AAS use.

We have finished our training session and I am sipping my protein shake and simultaneously drinking tea while I chat to Barry. I am lamenting about my body again and discussing my goals and my temptation to step over the line into AAS use. I am beginning to get the impression that many of the bodies I covet in the bodybuilding world are enhanced. 'Well, that's what you've got to accept', says Barry, 'everyone is on gear, you should just go for it and not think about it too much'. I am aware that there are a few female National Amateur Bodybuilding Association (NABBA) competitors who train at the gym. 'What is the NABBA official line on steroids?' I ask. Barry laughs, 'No one is natural, it doesn't matter what federation or class division'. On the way home I mull over the conversation and my experiences in the culture so far, witnessing AAS use as routinely as the drinking of protein shakes. Maybe I am making a big deal of this I think, I mean as a woman and for my goals all I need to do is take a pill, perhaps I should just bite the bullet and give it a go. It is after all the one thing that has been suggested to me by past coaches as a valid route to success and part and parcel of their nutrition and training protocols. A route that many of the women I have spoken to have successfully taken, so why should I be any different?

Normalization can be thought of as the inclusion of stigmatized or deviant behaviour into everyday 'normal' life. AAS use in bodybuilding is an excellent example of this, as it is part of the discourse relating to training and diet, and it is often present in the coach and client relationship. However, AAS use is often hidden to those first entering the bodybuilding community, as there is a tacit understanding on the part of bodybuilders that it may jar with individuals whose goals are to train naturally. However, over time as more training practices are embodied, the option is almost always laid on the table by coaches or mentors. The stigma associated with doping by outsiders is quickly eroded as the individual becomes initiated into a community where AAS use is regarded as a legitimate means of achieving a competitive physique. What might first have been thought of as a deviant practice utilized by the few gradually becomes seen as part of heterodox bodybuilding practice.

Both prior to and during the research I was fascinated by how others negotiated and engaged with a decision to use AAS. Some embraced it as easily as the diet and training whilst I grappled with it time and time again. It often seemed to be not only my personal desire to achieve the physique without the artificial assistance of AAS but also my increasing inability to trust when it came to coach recommendations. As time went on, I became trapped in a cycle of indecision, as the following journal entry illustrates.

Consideration of another extended period of dieting and cardiovascular exercise to achieve the desired body, only to result in eventual failure, disappointment, and further disillusionment with the process, fills me with dread. Ultimately something within me now rebels against the process, perhaps some deep-seated self-preservation from further frustration, coupled with the diminished belief that it is an achievable goal for me. However, I am dissatisfied with the obvious solution of simply letting go. In short neither option settles my mind. I have tried many different strategies to force my body into submission, while some have been relatively successful, I recognise that more extreme levels of energy restriction and expenditure are required, rendering me at greater risk of losing lean body mass. There is of course one antidote to this, a solution presented to me on several occasions, most often by Daniel but more recently by Barry, the use of AAS, namely oxandrolone, trade name Anavar. Often implemented by women during competition preparation to assist in the preservation of muscle mass, to help negate the effects of a restrictive low-calorie diet and hours of cardiovascular exercise and taken in the offseason to facilitate improvement to 'bring a better package' to the stage. This oral steroid might be a solution to release me from the frustration and disappointment of my current corporeal inertia. I find being with people who view AAS use as 'no big deal' and just another part of the preparation process often reassures my worrying mind, leaving me feeling more open to use myself, excited by the possibility of significant changes in my physique. As despite all my dedication, the hours spent in the gym, the weighing and measuring of food, I do not feel like a true bodybuilder. I long to be on stage parading a lean and muscular body in front of a line of faceless judges. To belong and be endorsed by a gym 'team' cheering me on, wanting me to do well. Indeed, visualising such thoughts tempts me to pick up the phone and say, 'Yes sign me up!' if AAS is the one element I have been lacking then maybe it **is** worth it.

However, in the same instance I am held back by my reluctance to cross a line that will ultimately lead me to a regime of daily checks and measures, looking out for signs and symptoms of unwanted side effects and the resultant stress that this will elicit. I am incapable of placing absolute trust in any coach or preparation provided in the same way that others seem able. Maybe I am also scared of achieving success with a body that has been augmented not only by dedication and hard work but also by AAS. Am I setting myself up for long term use lest I return to my former inadequate body? Will I value the achievement of my ideal physique in the same way if I am assisted?

Sometimes I wish I could erase my memory so I can blindly trust the process and the drugs to get me to the holy grail, but I cannot. Maybe I am simply not prepared to 'do whatever it takes' to be a successful bodybuilder, something that others are more easily able to accept and embrace.

Hence each time I am tempted closer to the decision to use, I am catapulted back round to the start of the process firmly in the 'No' camp, and back to considering other strategies to achieve my goals, even though I have already exhausted many of them. My continued immersion in the community in real life and on social media allows daily viewing of lean and muscular physiques, transformations to stage-worthy bodies and with them trophies. This has left my own body image in tatters, such that a new encounter with a gym or coach has the potential to place me firmly back on this cycle of indecision.

Bodybuilders engaging in AAS use utilize several vocabularies of motive to justify and legitimize uptake under the guise of reasonable, informed and responsible use (Monaghan, 2002). This legitimization of use renders it acceptable and normal when constrained within these parameters and allows those engaging in it to retain authenticity of their achievements. This capacity was one I fundamentally lacked, in part due to my academic background and my inability to engage authentically with those narratives to convince myself to use.

This was in direct contrast to many of the women (and men) I spoke with who were not only able to engage in these justifications but also valued the body they achieved or would achieve with AAS added to the equation (McLean, 2020). I found this problematic for several reasons; firstly, as a result of my continued research, I was well aware of the risks associated with AAS uptake and the use of illicit preparations and secondly, I was still not prepared to compromise my health or risk virilizing side effects for the sake of a certain physique. Finally, I was aware that if I compromised myself to achieve my goal, I would either not value the body I attained in the same way as if I had achieved it 'naturally' or I would value it to such a degree that the use of AAS would become habitual. However, as I was unable let go of the idea of competing in a bodybuilding competition, and since I had already had several failed attempts at competition preparation, I became trapped in a cycle. My desperate desire to achieve a hyper-muscular physique tempted me back to AAS use repeatedly, while my wish to preserve wellness would prevent me from taking the final step. Another factor that set me aside from some of my peers was that despite my ethnographic study I was not entrenched in a bodybuilding gym or with a coach full time. Indeed, the most compelling encounters nudging me towards use were when I was with these communities for extended periods and when I attended bodybuilding competitions. Had I been continually surrounded by other competitors and bodybuilding peers, especially females, I may have felt more comfortable to make the decision. The perceived safety, normalization and close support may have been enough to quell my reservations.

MENTAL HEALTH CHALLENGES

The decision I faced with respect to AAS use was not the only stress on my mental well-being, as some of the other rituals involved in bodybuilding culture were also beginning to take their toll. There is a body of research that indicates that the internalization of societal ideals of appearance can be a risk factor for the onset of body image disturbance and eating issues (Thompson et al., 2012). For myself, the internalization of a competitive physique coupled with years of attempting to achieve it left me struggling with my body image and relationship with food. This is perhaps not surprising for someone so entrenched in a culture where appearance is the main criteria upon which one is judged. Indeed, there is persuasive evidence to suggest physique athletes may be vulnerable to disordered eating, eating disorders and body image dissatisfaction (Alwan et al., 2019; Andersen et al., 1998; Goldfield, 2009).

The diets I had followed for competition on the strength of a coach's advice were a mix of evidence-based and experienced-based recommendations, ranging from very prescriptive meal plans to the meticulous tracking of macronutrients. One commonality they shared was prolonged energy restriction to promote significant fat loss to achieve the levels of leanness required for competition. My most significant attempt was a 20-week preparation diet after which my legs were still not lean enough. This, coupled with several other failed attempts to achieve stage readiness, began to take its toll on my mental health as the extract below illustrates.

> I feel that my immersion with bodybuilding culture during this research process (but also over the many years prior) has begun to take its toll on my mental health. I do not think I have ever felt that this is as much of a problem as it is now. I feel my mind is plagued by thoughts of dieting, counting macros, and preparing food. I still look at my body every day and wish it was leaner and more muscular, each time finding myself seeking other solutions, and restarting yet another variation of a restrictive diet or training regime. I often feel stressed and overwhelmed by it and usually swing from highly controlled and 'on it' to completely off the wagon and feeling out of control with food. I guess I am totally exhausted and disillusioned with the 'process' [of bodybuilding contest preparation] that you are meant to 'trust'. However, I am not sure how to break free from this well-trodden path, and I envy my younger self who was able to make food choices without rules, stress, or regulation.

The poor relationship I developed with food and my body is one that has endured beyond my quest for a competitive physique; it still lingers like a 'hangover' from engaging so heavily in bodybuilding practice. Like AAS use, the extreme dietary practices that are necessary to achieve stage conditioning also present physical and mental health risk (Alwan et al., 2019). Whilst there are bodybuilding coaches who employ evidence-based nutritional methods, there are others promoting more restrictive and unproven strategies (Mitchell et al., 2017), such restrictive meals plans consisting of a finite list of 'allowable' foods, often under the guise of 'clean eating', a term that cannot be clearly defined (Norton & Baker, 2019), and thus may vary from coach to coach or between different gym micro-cultures.

The emotional and mental health risk that the qualitative research process might pose to the researcher is less well attended to during application for university ethical approval than those of the participants (Emerald & Carpenter, 2015; Hubbard et al., 2001), but as my encounters highlight they are important to consider. Even though these experiences are highly insightful from a research perspective, immersive methodologies such as auto-ethnography and participant observation carry greater risks for the researcher than surveys, focus groups or interviews.

METHODOLOGICAL CHALLENGES

Insider or Outsider?

Considering my biography and background, it could be easy to conclude that I am an insider in the world of bodybuilding. However, insider vs outsider status are not necessarily binary concepts, as adopting a singularity of 'insiderness' closes the door to multiple and conflicting narratives and identities (Shim, 2018). Instead, it is a dynamic continuum and I often found myself located between the two realms (Chavaz, 2008; Shim, 2018). I felt like an outsider because I had not achieved a physique that was worthy of the competitive stage. This was compounded by my decision not to use AAS as this meant that unlike many of my peers I had been unwilling to 'do whatever it takes'. I am not sure how significant this element would have been had I achieved success without pharmaceutical assistance. The advantage was that I was able to gain perspective on the decision-making process, allowing me to compare my perceptions with others who chose to use.

I felt like an insider with respect to my ability to proficiently weight train, my confidence in the gym, my physique goals and my ability to understand cultural terms and practices, all of which helped me to integrate myself into the community with ease. However, I often swung rapidly between insider and outsider status depending on the context and social situation. This was often most obvious when I was with the group where competing was the focus for the majority of the gym members. Here I felt like an insider whilst training but my body and my lack of competitive experience would leave me feeling very much an outsider at bodybuilding shows or whilst attending or observing competition preparation check-ins.

Bodybuilder or Researcher?

Whilst in the field, I found my identity fluctuated between researcher, aspiring bodybuilder or even 'one of the lads'. These personas grew in complexity as my relationships within the community developed, and as a result, the line between the personal and the professional grew cloudy. I was never simply a researcher in that setting, and such is the fluid and dynamic process of auto-ethnographic research (Richards, 2015). In the early days, I questioned my engagement with some of the more personal and sexualized conversations in the gym and worried about how to handle them. However, as a woman in a male-dominated environment, I wanted to be 'one of the lads' and engage with this gym 'banter'. As time passed, I became far more comfortable engaging in such conversations, often revealing personal information of my own. In the end I enjoyed it, and it became as routine as the AAS use I observed. Having been asked direct and personal questions, I also felt I could delve a bit further into my participants' lives, and their AAS use. This in turn led to some frank discussions that might not have occurred had I been unwilling to engage in sexualized and risky conversations in general.

As field work drew close, however, I began to become concerned as to how I would write authentically about the people whom I had begun to consider friends. I was aware of instances where during publication it had become evident that the expectations between ethnographers and their informants were mismatched (Bourgois, 2003; Scheper-Hughes, 2004; Venkatesh, 2008). Did my participants understand that everything I observed would inform my work? I had also witnessed first-hand bodybuilders' negative attitudes towards any media stories regarding AAS use even when they did attempt to present a balanced story. Essentially, I feared becoming ostracized from a community that I enjoyed being a part of.

CONCLUSIONS

The account I have presented here provides a powerful overview of the complex interplay of culture, sporting endeavour, body image, gender and perceptions of drug use in bodybuilding culture. I explain some of the experiences that drove me towards AAS use as well as describing some of the barriers that prevented me from taking it.

The pragmatic reasons cited for AAS uptake in this research support the existing literature, particularly those relating to the pursuit of competition and improvements to body image and physique (Andreasson & Johansson, 2021; Grogan et al., 2006; Ip et al., 2010; Korkia et al., 1996; Maycock & Howat, 2005). Of course, these reasons must be considered within the context of integration into the bodybuilding community within which there are several other key influencing factors such as the normalization of AAS use, the role of the coach and impact of peers. The uptake of AAS is part and parcel of the integration and adoption of the bodybuilding lifestyle and often a requirement to achieve a competitive physique, such that it is viewed as a positive deviance away from conventional norms (Coquet et al., 2018). A woman embarking on this route may choose to build a muscular and lean body through the necessary means, yet they are also required to preserve their femininity, a move which some authors argue results in a hyper-conformity by over identifying with what is 'acceptable femininity' (Kotzé et al., 2020) rather than a resistance of cultural norms through the accrual of muscularity. This potentially reproduces rather than transform what women's bodybuilding protests against in the first place (Hunter, 2013; Kotzé et al., 2020; Tajrobehkar, 2016). Secondly, the pursuit of hyper-muscularity alongside AAS use can render women doubly deviant (Bunsell, 2013) while their male counterpart is exonerated in his drug use or at least enjoys a much higher threshold before his use is viewed as problematic. Indeed, many women have a line which they chose not to cross, as to do so means stepping into 'freakdom', a line they judge other women harshly against (Hunter, 2013; Tajrobehkar, 2016).

The conclusion to my own auto-ethnographic experience was that in the end I was not able to fully embrace all the rituals and practices that bodybuilding demands. My prior and expanding knowledge on AAS use as well as my background in nutrition and exercise science made me unable to fully 'trust the process' and the coaches who steered it. I was also incapable of reconciling my prior association between a lean and muscular physique and the maintenance of health. Hence the intrinsic value I placed in an assisted body was less than one achieved 'naturally'. My risk averse personality, as well as my own prejudices towards the possible androgenic effects of use, also played a part. Unlike some of the women I met, I was not immersed in the culture on a daily basis, and I also enjoyed the influence of an academic environment allowing me to take a more analytical view of my options. This is not to say given different circumstances I would not have made different choices. I fully understood and envied my bodybuilding peers dedication to their pursuit, and their ability to engage with all its practices, because in the context of bodybuilding culture and methodology, the choice to use AAS can seem a perfectly reasonable and considered one to meet a desired goal.

What I was left with was a body image that was in tatters and a disordered relationship with food. Indeed some of the literature considering women involved in fitness sports have shown disordered eating practices can develop in relation to extrinsic motivation such as the desire to change outward appearance (Chaba et al., 2018). While body dissatisfaction in men has been linked to disordered eating and muscle dysmorphia (Griffiths et al., 2013), there is little in the way of literature regarding women's pursuit of the muscular ideal and the various dimensions of disordered eating and some authors have reported positive image and eating practices in female competitive bodybuilders (Guthrie et al., 1994). While the rule-driven behaviour that governs the pursuit of the thin ideal are in the opposite direction of the muscular ideal, research needs to focus on the rules that underlie disordered eating rather than the direction of the eating behaviour itself (Griffiths et al., 2013).

Of course my experiences are not wholly representative of bodybuilding culture, and thus any conclusions made must respect the particularity of the research (Hammersley & Atkinson, 2007). Every gym is unique, and there may be other groups of female AAS users that are not represented here. However, I hope this chapter contributes towards understanding bodybuilding culture and illuminates the gendered nature and complexity of AAS use in women's bodybuilding.

KEY READINGS

(1) Andreasson, J., & Johansson, T. (2021). Negotiating female fitness doping: gender, identity and transgressions. *Sport in Society*, *24*(3), 323–339.

A contemporary paper that highlights the relationship between bodybuilding and fitness, noting the increasing involvement of women within the fitness space, where muscularity is becoming more acceptable with the constraints of a 'normal' range of femininity. Using interviews and internet forum discussion this study highlights how female users' initiation of image and performance enhancing drug (IPED) use is largely connected to gym and fitness culture.

(2) Bunsell, T. (2013). *Strong and hard women: An ethnography of female bodybuilding*. Routledge.

One of the foremost ethnographies of female bodybuilding offering an insightful view into the lived experience of bodybuilding culture. It considers whether women's bodybuilding is transgressive and addresses the cultural uncertainties that exist around women, muscularity and strength.

(3) Coquet, R., Roussel, P., & Ohl, F. (2018). Understanding the paths to appearance- and performance-enhancing drug use in bodybuilding. *Frontiers in Psychology*, *9*.

This paper further explores the trajectory bodybuilders take towards the use of appearance and performance enhancing drugs (APEDs). Focussing on an analysis of bodybuilders' social configurations and lived social experiences, to contextualize their relation to APEDs.

(4) Goldfield, G. S. (2009). Body image, disordered eating and anabolic steroid use in female bodybuilders. *Eating Disorders*, *17*(3), 200–210.

This paper explores the relationship between bodybuilding, steroid use and psychological traits. It compares competitive female bodybuilders and recreational female weight-training controls on a broad scope of eating-related and general psychological characteristics.

(5) Monaghan, L. F. (2002). Vocabularies of motive for illicit steroid use among bodybuilders. *Social Science & Medicine*, *55*(5), 695–708.

Steroid users rarely need to account for their drug use when interacting with other members of the bodybuilding community, but how do they justify their motives outside of the setting? This paper provides an insight.

ACKNOWLEDGEMENTS

I would like to thank Dr Conan Leavey from the Public Health Institute at Liverpool John Moores University, for his continued moral and academic support and for taking the time to review this piece of work.

REFERENCES

Alwan, N., Moss, S. L., Elliott-Sale, K. J., Davies, I. G., & Enright, K. (2019). A narrative review on female physique athletes: The physiological and psychological implications of weight management practices. *International Journal of Sport Nutrition and Exercise Metabolism, 29*(6), 682. https://doi.org/10.1123/ijsnem.2019-0037

Andersen, R. E., Brownell, K. D., Morgan, G. D., & Bartlett, S. J. (1998). Weight loss, psychological, and nutritional patterns in competitive female bodybuilders. *Eating Disorders: The Journal of Treatment & Prevention, 6*(2), 159–168. http://search.ebscohost.com/login.aspx?direct=true&db=psyh&AN=1998-04841-005&site=eds-live

Andreasson, J., & Johansson, T. (2020). *Fitness doping: Trajectories, gender, bodies and health*. Palgrave Macmillan.

Andreasson, J., & Johansson, T. (2021). Negotiating female fitness doping: Gender, identity and transgressions. *Sport in Society, 24*(3), 323–339. https://doi.org/10.1080/17430437.2019.1672152

Aspridis, A., O'Halloran, P., & Liamputtong, P. (2014). Female bodybuilding: Perceived social and psychological effects of participating in the figure class. *Women in Sport & Physical Activity Journal, 22*(1), 24–29. https://doi.org/10.1123/wspaj.2014-0008

Benton, C., & Karazsia, B. T. (2015). The effect of thin and muscular images on women's body satisfaction. *Body Image, 13*, 22–27. https://doi.org/10.1016/j.bodyim.2014.11.001

Bolin, A. (2012). Buff bodies and the beast: Emphasized femininity, labor, and power relations among fitness, figure and women bodybuilding competitors 1985-2010. In A. Locks & N. Richardson (Eds.), *Critical readings in bodybuilding* (pp. 29–57). Routledge.

Bourgois, P. (2003). *In search of respect: Selling crack in El Barrio* (2nd ed.). Cambridge University Press.

Bunsell, T. (2010). *Building body identities: Exploring the world of female bodybuilding*. PhD thesis, University of Kent.

Bunsell, T. (2013). *Strong and hard women: An ethnography of female bodybuilding*. Routledge.

Bunsell, T., & Shilling, C. (2012). Outside and inside the gym: Exploring the identity of the female bodybuilder. In A. Locks & N. Richardson (Eds.), *Critical readings in bodybuilding* (pp. 58–72). Routledge.

Campbell, F., Haverda, T., & Bartkowski, J. P. (2021). Rival bodies: Negotiating gender and embodiment in women's bikini and figure competitions. *Social Sciences, 10*(2), 64. https://doi.org/10.3390/socsci10020064

Chaba, L., D'arripe-Longueville, F., Scoffier-Mériaux, S., & Lentillon-Kaestner, V. (2018). Investigation of eating and deviant behaviors in bodybuilders according to their competitive engagement. *Deviant Behavior*, 1–17. https://doi.org/10.1080/01639625.2018.1437652

Chananie-Hill, R. A., McGrath, S. A., & Stoll, J. (2012). Deviant or normal? Female bodybuilders' accounts of social reactions. *Deviant Behavior, 33*(10), 811–830. https://doi.org/10.1080/01639625.2011.647592

Chavaz, C. (2008). Conceptualising from the inside advantages complications and demands on insider positionality. *Qualitative Report, 13*(3), 474–494.

Connell, R. W. (1987). *Gender and power; Society, the person and sexual politics*. Polity.

Coquet, R., Roussel, P., & Ohl, F. (2018). Understanding the paths to appearance- and performance-enhancing drug use in bodybuilding. *Frontiers in Psychology, 9*. https://doi.org/10.3389/fpsyg.2018.01431

Dilley, R., Hockey, J., Robinson, V., & Sherlock, A. (2014). Occasions and non-occasions: Identity, femininity and high-heeled shoes. *European Journal of Women's Studies, 22*(2), 143–158. https://doi.org/10.1177/1350506814533952

Emerald, E., & Carpenter, L. (2015). Vulnerability and emotions in research. *Qualitative Inquiry, 21*(8), 741–750. https://doi.org/10.1177/1077800414566688

Ettorre, E. (2007). *Revisioning women and drug use: Gender, power and the body*. Palgrave Macmillan.

Fussell, S. W. (1991). *Muscle: Confessions of an unlikely bodybuilder*. Avon Books INC.

Goldfield, G. S. (2009). Body image, disordered eating and anabolic steroid use in female bodybuilders. *Eating Disorders, 17*(3), 200–210. https://doi.org/10.1080/10640260902848485

Griffiths, S., Murray, S. B., & Touyz, S. (2013). Drive for muscularity and muscularity-oriented disordered eating in men: The role of set shifting difficulties and weak central coherence. *Body Image*, *10*(4), 636–639. https://doi.org/10.1016/j.bodyim.2013.04.002

Grogan, S., Shepherd, S., Evans, R., Wright, S., & Hunter, G. (2006). Experiences of anabolic steroid use: In-depth interviews with men and women body builders. *Journal of Health Psychology*, *11*(6), 845–856. http://search.ebscohost.com/login.aspx?direct=true&db=rzh&AN=200932 1788&site=eds-live

Guthrie, S. R., Ferguson, C., & Grimmett, D. (1994). Elite women bodybuilders: Ironing out nutritional misconceptions. *The Sport Psychologist*, *8*(3), 271–286. http://search.ebscohost.com/login.aspx?direct=true&db=s3h&AN=20735161&site=eds-live

Hall, D. (2021a). 2021 Mr. Olympia men's open bodybuilding results and prize money: Big ramy wins the 2021 Mr. Olympia. https://fitnessvolt.com/2021-mrolympia-bodybuilding-results/. Accessed on December 10, 2021.

Hall, D. (2021b). 2021 Ms. Olympia results and prize money: Andrea Shaw wins the Ms. Olympia 2021 title. https://fitnessvolt.com/2021-msolympia-results/. Accessed on December 10, 2021.

Hammersley, M., & Atkinson, P. (2007). *Ethnography: Principals in practice* (3rd ed.). Routledge.

Heywood, L. (1998). *Bodymakers: A cultural anatomy of women's body building*. Rutgers University Press.

Howson, A. (2007). The body in consumer culture. In *The body in society: An introduction* (pp. 93–119). Polity Press.

Huang, G., & Basaria, S. (2018). Do anabolic-androgenic steroids have performance-enhancing effects in female athletes? *Molecular and Cellular Endocrinology*, *464*(C), 56–64. https://doi.org/10.1016/j.mce.2017.07.010

Hubbard, G., Backett-Milburn, K., & Kemmer, D. (2001). Working with emotion: Issues for the researcher in fieldwork and teamwork. *International Journal of Social Research Methodology*, *4*(2), 119–137. https://doi.org/10.1080/13645570116992

Hunter, S. A. (2013). *Not simply women's bodybuilding: Gender and the female competition categories*. Master of Arts thesis, Georgie State University.

IFBB. (2021). Our disciplines. https://ifbb.com/our-disciplines/. Accessed on May 10, 2021.

IFBBPro. (2021). International regional and pro qualifier rules. https://www.ifbbpro.com/international-regional-and-pro-qualifier-rules/. Accessed on December 10, 21.

Ip, E. J., Barnett, M. J., Tenerowicz, M. J., Kim, J. A., Wei, H., & Perry, P. J. (2010). Women and anabolic steroids: An analysis of a dozen users. *Clinical Journal of Sport Medicine*, *20*(6), 475–481. https://doi.org/10.1097/JSM.0b013e3181fb5370

Korkia, P., Lenehan, P., & McVeigh, J. (1996). Non-medical use of androgens among women. *The Journal of Performance Enhancing Drugs*, *1*(2), 71–76,

Kotzé, I., Richardson, A., & Antonopoulos, G. A. (2020). Looking 'acceptably' feminine: A single case study of a female bodybuilder's use of steroids. *Performance Enhancement & Health*, *8*(2–3), 100174. https://doi.org/10.1016/j.peh.2020.100174

Lelwica, M. M. (2017). *Shameful: Religion and the culture of physical improvement*. Bloomsbury.

Liokaftos, D. (2018). Defining and defending drug-free bodybuilding: A current perspective from organisations and their key figures. *International Journal of Drug Policy*, *60*, 47–55. https://doi.org/10.1016/j.drugpo.2018.07.012

Lowe, M. R. (1998). *Women of steel: Female bodybuilders and the struggle for self-definition*. NYU Press.

Marshall, K., Chamberlain, K., & Hodgetts, D. (2019). Female bodybuilders on instagram: Negotiating an empowered femininity. *Feminism & Psychology*, *29*(1), 96–119. https://doi.org/10.1177/0959353518808319

Maycock, B., & Howat, P. (2005). The barriers to illegal anabolic steroid use. *Drugs: Education, Prevention & Policy*, *12*(4), 317–325. http://search.ebscohost.com/login.aspx?direct=true&db=s3h&AN=17552491&site=eds-live

McLean, C. (2020). *Gains, juice and bikinis: An ethnographic exploration of women's use of anabolic-androgenic steriods and growth hormone in bodybuilding*. (Doctoral thesis). Liverpool John Moores University.

Mitchell, L., Hackett, D., Gifford, J., Estermann, F., & O'Connor, H. (2017). Do bodybuilders use evidence-based nutrition strategies to manipulate physique? *Sports, 5*(4), 76. https://doi.org/10.3390/sports5040076

Monaghan, L. (2001a). *Bodybuilding, drugs and risk.* Routledge.

Monaghan, L. F. (2001b). Looking good, feeling good: The embodied pleasures of vibrant physicality. *Sociology of Health & Illness, 23*(3), 330–356. http://search.ebscohost.com/login.aspx?direct=true&db=a9h&AN=4391817&site=eds-live

Monaghan, L. F. (2002). Vocabularies of motive for illicit steroid use among bodybuilders. *Social Science & Medicine, 55*(5), 695–708. http://doi.org/10.1016/S0277-9536(01)00195-2

Norton, L., & Baker, P. (2019). *Fat Loss Forever: How to lose fat and keep it off.* Biolayne. https://biolaynestore.com/collections/accessories/products/forever-fat-loss-how-to-lose-fat-and-keep-it-off. Accessed on March 20, 2019.

NPC. (2021). NPC bodybuilding division rules. https://www.ifbbpro.com/international-regional-and-pro-qualifier-rules/. Accessed on December 10, 2021.

Olympia, M. (2021a). 2021 qualified: Ms. Olympia. https://mrolympia.com/ms-olympia. Accessed on October 05, 2021.

Olympia, M. (2021b). 2021 qualified: Wellness. https://mrolympia.com/content/wellness-olympia. Accessed on October 05, 21.

Pappa, E., & Kennedy, E. (2013). 'It was my thought ... he made it a reality': Normalization and responsibility in athletes' accounts of performance-enhancing drug use. *International Review for the Sociology of Sport, 48*(3), 277–294. https://doi.org/10.1177/1012690212442116

van der Ploeg, G. E., Brooks, A. G., Withers, R. T., Dollman, J., Leaney, F., & Chatterton, B. E. (2001). Body composition changes in female bodybuilders during preparation for competition. *European Journal of Clinical Nutrition, 55*(4), 268–277. https://doi.org/10.1038/sj.ejcn.1601154

Richards, M. (2015). Turning back to the story of my life: An autoethnographic exploration of a researcher's identity during the PhD process. *Reflective Practice, 16*(6), 821–835. https://doi.org/10.1080/14623943.2015.1095731

Santonja, R. (2021a). IFBB Rules Section 6: Women's bodyfitness. IFBB. https://ifbb.com/rules/

Santonja, R. (2021b). IFBB Rules Section 7: Women's bikini fitness. IFBB. https://ifbb.com/rules/

Santonja, R. (2021c). IFBB Rules Section 8: Women's physique. IFBB. https://ifbb.com/rules/.

Santonja, R. (2021d). IFBB Rules Section 15: Women's wellness fitness. IFBB. https://ifbb.com/rules/

Scheper-Hughes, N. (2004). *Parts unknown: Undercover ethnography of the organs-trafficking underworld* (p. 29). SAGE Publications.

Shilling, C., & Bunsell, T. (2009). The female bodybuilder as a gender outlaw. *Qualitative Research in Sport and Exercise, 1*(2), 141–159. http://search.ebscohost.com/login.aspx?direct=true&db=s3h&AN=43429266&site=eds-live

Shim, J. (2018). Problematic autoethnographic research: Researchers failure in positioning. *Qualitative Report, 23*(1), 1–11.

Spendlove, J., Mitchell, L., Gifford, J., Hackett, D., Slater, G., Cobley, S., & O'Connor, H. (2015). Dietary intake of competitive bodybuilders. *Sports Medicine, 45*(7), 1041–1063. https://doi.org/10.1007/s40279-015-0329-4

Sverkersson, E., Andreasson, J., & Johansson, T. (2020). 'Sis science' and fitness doping: Ethnopharmacology, gender and risk. *Social Sciences, 9*(4), 55. https://doi.org/10.3390/socsci9040055

Tajrobehkar, B. (2016). Flirting with the judges: Bikini fitness competitors' negotiations of femininity in bodybuilding competitions. *Sociology of Sport Journal, 33*(4), 294–304. http://search.ebscohost.com/login.aspx?direct=true&db=s3h&AN=120773968&site=ehost-live

Thompson, J. K., Schaefer, L. M., & Menzel, J. E. (2012). Internalization of thin ideal and muscular ideal. In T. F. Cash (Ed.), *Encyclopedia of body image and human appearance* (pp. 499–504). Academic Press.

Venkatesh, S. A. (2008). *Gang leader for a day: A rogue sociologist takes to the streets.* Penguin Books.

Wacquant, L. (2004). *Body and soul: Notebooks of an apprentice boxer.* Oxford University ress.

Wall, S. (2006). An autoethnography on learning about autoethnography. *International Journal of Qualitative Methods, 5*(2), 146–160. https://doi.org/10.1177/160940690600500205

Wood, R. I. (2008). Review: Anabolic–androgenic steroid dependence? Insights from animals and humans. *Frontiers in Neuroendocrinology*, *29*, 490–506. https://doi.org/10.1016/j.yfrne.2007.12. 002

Worthen, M. G. F., & Baker, S. A. (2016). Pushing up on the glass ceiling of female muscularity: Women's bodybuilding as edgework. *Deviant Behavior*, *37*(5), 1–25. https://doi.org/10.1080/ 01639625.2015.1060741

Wright, S., Grogan, S., & Hunter, G. (2001). Body-builders' attitudes towards steroid use. *Drugs: Education, Prevention & Policy*, *8*(1), 91–95. https://doi.org/10.1080/09687630124157

Chapter 12

INTERSECTIONS OF GENDER, DOPING AND SPORT: THE SHARED IMPLICATIONS OF ANTI-DOPING AND SEX TESTING

Sarah Teetzel

ABSTRACT

This chapter focuses on what we know about the intersections of gender, doping and sport and addresses the history, complexities and nuances of how gender impacts perceptions of and research on doping in sport. After establishing briefly what the physiology, psychology, media studies and sociology literature demonstrates with respect to the intersection of doping and gender, this chapter addresses how and why gender was neglected in the creation of anti-doping policies. The lack of thought toward gender in the creation of the current anti-doping system, combined with the conflation of drug testing and sex testing issues by the International Olympic Committee's medical commission in the 1960s, has led to persistent gender stereotypes associated with anti-doping rule violations. As a result, unintended overlap between sex testing and drug testing continues, with implications for the eligibility of intersex and transgender athletes.

Keywords: Doping; gender; women; intersex; transgender; policy

INTRODUCTION

What do we know about how, when and why gender and doping intersect? While physiologists can explain how different banned performance enhancing drugs (PEDs) impact female and male bodies, psychologists can provide insight into

Doping in Sport and Fitness
Research in the Sociology of Sport, Volume 16, 239–252
Copyright © 2023 by Emerald Publishing Limited
All rights of reproduction in any form reserved
ISSN: 1476-2854/doi:10.1108/S1476-285420220000016013

differences in women and men's attitudes toward doping, and we can ascertain how media covers men and women who dope disparately, little has been written about gender and doping from a socio-historical perspective. Building on earlier research identifying how the gender binary maintained in sport disadvantages women athletes (e.g. Hall, 1996; Lenskyj, 1986), this chapter highlights how and why doping in sport remains a gendered practice, including the anti-doping movement's links to sex testing, also known as gender verification, of women athletes. The growing body of literature on fitness doping provides fascinating glimpses into the role of PEDs in recreational sports and the fitness industry; however, the emphasis of this chapter is on doping in sports that are signatories to WADA's World Anti-Doping Code, by athletes who are part of their national testing pools.

While there are notable exceptions (e.g. Burke, 2004; Henne, 2015; Magdalinski, 2009), much of the doping literature lacks analysis from a feminist perspective. Research on doping in sport continues to focus predominantly on quantitative studies regarding the prevalence of drug use, and usually among high-performance male athletes (Weaving & Teetzel, 2014). From these studies, it is well understood from a physiological perspective how banned PEDs impact female and male bodies differently, as well as the spectrum of health risks associated with PED use. For example, beyond the anabolic effects associated with doping, physicians can prescribe steroids for myriad reasons, including to stimulate appetite and muscle growth in patients afflicted with a variety of medical conditions. In some countries, however, healthy men and women can obtain a prescription for steroids from physicians for cosmetic purposes as well, including building muscle and reducing body fat. The risks inherent in using steroids for non-therapeutic purposes are well understood and consumers can work with healthcare professionals to make informed decisions. In addition to producing anabolic effects, prolonged use of high doses of testosterone produces androgenic effects, including body hair growth, acne, liver damage, high cholesterol, high blood pressure and changes to the left ventricle of the heart. For females, prolonged steroid use causes irregular menstrual cycles, deepened voices and enlargement of the clitoris (Graham et al., 2008). Descriptive sex differences of this nature are important to understand so that current and potential users can make informed choices, but sex differences do not tell us much about women athletes' lived experiences with doping, or how gender impacts the current anti-doping system in sport.

Beyond physiological observations, the psychology of doping literature addresses differences in men's and women's attitudes to doping. For example, a study of college athletes demonstrates that athletes' attitudes toward doping and drug testing differ by gender and suggests that gender specific drug education is warranted (Issari & Coombs, 1998). Even earlier studies found gender differences present in girls' and boys' attitudes toward the so-called 'gateway' drugs as early as the fourth and fifth grade (Katims & Zapata, 1993). Similar trends were noted in a study of sport science university students' use of and attitudes toward licit, illicit and doping substances (Lorente, 2003). Research on cosmetic doping in college-level athletes suggests that gender differences are present in athletes' motivations to consume supplements and drugs, with women more likely to use substances to decrease body fat and mass rather than build strength (e.g. Muller et al., 2009). Studies of this nature seek to understand why athletes and recreational sports populations use banned PEDs, with the goal of developing successful interventions to promote anti-doping attitudes and, correspondingly, foster anti-doping behaviours.

Like studies of athletes' attitudes toward doping, prevalence studies look for trends in who is using various PEDs to estimate the pervasiveness of doping in sport. As Miller et al. (2002) acknowledged two decades ago, 'contrary to popular assumption, adolescent anabolic-androgenic steroid use is not limited to serious male athletes' (p. 385). Their research highlighted that girls in grades 9 to 12 had an estimated 0.5%–2.9% prevalence of steroid use across their lifetime compared to the significantly higher estimate for boys of between 4% and 12%, but with body image as the prime motivator for most steroid users, not sport performance. For a variety of methodological reasons, it is surprisingly difficult to determine the prevalence of doping among women high-performance athletes with any certainty. Even the working group formed by the World Anti-Doping Agency (WADA) for the specific task of determining doping prevalence struggled to estimate the prevalence of doping in women's sports. The working group recommends that future doping prevalence studies account for gender whenever possible, as their group of experts was unable to draw meaningful conclusions from the 105 prevalence studies its members identified and reviewed. These doping experts convened by WADA determined that doping prevalence among all athletes is between 0 and 73%, highlighting that an insufficient number of studies sufficiently report doping prevalence by gender to pinpoint women's doping prevalence any more accurately than that very large range (Gleaves et al., 2021). This observation echoes earlier recognition that doping prevalence rates fluctuate between different groups, and that additional studies need to be conducted with specific populations (de Hon et al., 2015; Ntoumanis et al., 2014).

Anecdotal evidence highlights some of the difficulties involved in gaining insight into the extent of doping among high-performance athletes. As part of a 'blame and shame' form of doping deterrence, WADA requires national anti-doping agencies to maintain an online registry of sanctions imposed on athletes in their testing pools who have committed an anti-doping rule violation (ADRV). As an example, Canada's doping sanction registry lists 44 athletes and one coach with sanctions in effect, of which 43 of the banned athletes are men and only one is a woman (CCES, 2021). The sanction registries for both the United States Anti-Doping Agency (USADA) and United Kingdom Anti-Doping (UKAD) contain many more entries, but neither specifies the gender of the athletes included on the lists (UKAD, 2021; USADA, 2021). No widespread agreement in the prevalence of women who commit ADRVs can be gleaned from sanction registries, but a cursory examination suggests that women commit violations far less often than men.

From the physiology, psychology and prevalence of doping research, we know that sex and gender differences are present in how banned PED use impacts female bodies, what attitudes correspond to an increased risk of using banned

PEDs, and that while women commit doping violations less frequently than men, the extent of the difference is not clear. The increase in the number of women committing ADRVs in high-performance sport is surely connected to women's increased participation rates in sports requiring strength and the increased athletic opportunities available to girls and women. Drawing on the feminist sport literature, the remainder of this chapter connects the history of women, gender and doping in sport to analyze how stereotypes and heteronormative expectations attached to doping have allowed a misunderstanding of the overlap between sex testing and drug testing to continue, which has implications for the eligibility of intersex and transgender athletes. In doing so, this chapter highlights how and why doping in sport remains a gendered practice.

IMPACTFUL MOMENTS IN THE STUDY OF WOMEN, GENDER AND DOPING

Doping historians accept that steroids and other rudimentary PEDs were used by some athletes in the 'strength' sports by the 1952 Olympics, and drug use was prevalent in these events by the end of the 1960s (Beamish & Ritchie, 2006). Renowned male 'drug cheats' abound, and even people who do not follow sports at all can likely identify 'famous' male dopers like Ben Johnson and Lance Armstrong with ease. A plethora of male athletes including Jose Canseco, Alex Rodriguez, Floyd Landis and Alberto Contador have also served as the face of doping at the time they were 'caught' and 'punished', yet far fewer women athletes immediately come to mind when thinking of doping scandals in sport. Several momentous events in the history of doping in sport involve women, of which three are summarized here to highlight the roles that consent, musculature and race play in public reaction toward women and doping.

The first, the state-sponsored doping associated with the German Democratic Republic (but in effect in many countries between 1972 and 1989), resulted in considerable success in many women's sports and opened the public's eyes to the idea that doping was not just an issue in men's sport. Werner Franke and Brigitte Berendonk's translations of State Plan 14:25 highlight that most, if not all, athletes competing for East Germany in the strength and speed events were doped. The Stasi files reveal that several hundred physicians and sport scientist researched and administered unapproved experimental drugs to thousands of athletes. Additional files published in *Swimming World* magazine in December 1994 suggest all top East German swimmers were doping. German historian Giselher Spitzer reports that the Stasi files reveal over 10,000 East German athletes were given PEDs (Ungerleider, 2001). Testimonials from athletes confirm that officials and coaches administered the anabolic steroid Oral-Turinabol in tablet form to athletes as young as 10 years old without consent from their guardians or assent from the athletes, telling these children the pills were vitamins, with apparently no concern for the long-term health implications or development of the girls they were systemically doping (Franke & Berendonk, 1997).

A second scandal of note in the 1990s involved the use of the topical steroid dihydrotestosterone (DHT) by swimmers and track and field athletes in China. Many athletes' very muscular physiques led competitors and Western media sources to speculate that systemic doping was occurring, despite several Chinese coaches' claims that their athletes' strength and success came from rigorous training and consuming traditional Chinese herbal supplements (Plymire, 1999). After many athletes tested positive for DHT, investigators described an extensive doping network motivated by coaches' and clubs' desire to win prize money and endorsement contracts (Teetzel, 2011).

A third key moment involves American sprinter Marion Jones's doping plight. Jones, who won five medals at the Sydney 2000 Olympic Games, was a beloved American athlete, who throughout her career maintained that she completed cleanly. However, evidence of her doping emerged in a raid of Bay Area Laboratory Co-Operative (BALCO) founder Victor Conte's records, and in a televised interview following the BALCO scandal and trial, Conte told a 20/20 host that he provided Jones with banned substances (Sports Illustrated, 2006). Jones continued to deny ever doping, but records and testimonies suggested otherwise. She complied with the IOC's request to forfeit and return her five Olympic medals from the Sydney 2000 Olympics.

Like Florence 'Flo Jo' Griffith Joyner, Jones's attractive, likeable, feminine appearance initially protected her from overt speculation that her astonishing performances were fueled by banned PEDs. Griffith Joyner raised suspicions of doping given her extraordinary performances at the 1988 Olympics, the same games at which Ben Johnson was disqualified for doping and became the scapegoat for doping in sport (Moore, 2012). As reporter James Montague (2012) reflects, Griffith-Joyner's 10.49 second 100m sprint in Seoul 'encapsulated everything that would define Flo Jo for the rest of her life: speed, elegance, beauty, femininity, suspicion'. Critics contend that her retirement after the 1988 Olympic coincided with the introduction of random unannounced drug testing. Her 100m (10.49) and 200m (21.34) world records remain the fastest times ever run by a woman, with 2020 Olympic champion Elaine Thompson-Herah's gold medal victories 33 years later ranking #2 on the all-time list at 10.61 and 21.53 seconds, respectively (World Athletics, 2021).

Jones's popularity prior to her eventual conviction and confession, 'reveal how the success and glamour of an athlete influence the media and the consumers who 'bask in reflected glory' and close their eyes to the evidence of drug abuse' (Pfister & Gems, 2013, p. 137). Jones avoided media speculation about doping for years, despite her association with banned athletes and coaches, because of 'the imagery and dreams conveyed by her beauty and prowess' (p. 147) which was in stark contrast with the typical image of the doped female body stemming from the East German and Chinese doping scandals described above. Jones's physical appearance aligned with heteronormative feminine expectations; however, following her confession, public opinion turned drastically. As Delia D. Douglas (2014) demonstrates, Jones was the first woman to be sentenced to jail for lying about doping. In contrast, American cyclist Tammy Thomas's similar act of lying under oath in the BALCO trials resulted in only house arrest and probation, demonstrating that 'Jones's Black femaleness activated the anger and anxiety that, in turn, contributed to her legal and public shaming and humiliation' (Douglas, 2014, p. 6). These three moments in women's doping history suggest that racialized women's bodies, and extremely muscular bodies that challenge heteronormative standards of feminine beauty, tend to capture public interest and raise suspicions in ways that other bodies do not.

An intersectional lens, which recognizes that not only sexism but systemic racism and oppression impacts doping in sport, is useful. This is illustrated by the mild consequences white tennis star Maria Sharapova faced following her ADRV and doping sanction in 2016. Sharapova claimed she had been prescribed the drug meldonium for a medical reason for a decade starting in 2006, back when the drug was not included on WADA's prohibited substance list. Her ADRV for the continued use of the drug after it was banned by WADA did not result in similar shaming, vilification or humiliation that Jones and other women faced. Sharapova's ADRV initially garnered considerable media attention because of her very public profile and wide following, but her image was not damaged for long. She retained many of her sponsors and endorsements after completing her 15-month ban, and she retired from tennis in 2020 as the third highest paid woman in tennis ever, behind only Venus and Serena Williams (Badenhausen, 2020). The next section unpacks the differences in how the sport system and media can treat athletes based on their race, gender and bodies.

STEREOTYPES AND HETERONORMATIVE EXPECTATIONS ATTACHED TO DOPING

Jan Felshin's (1974) description of female apologetic behavior – the requirement for women to adhere to expectations of heteronormative femininity to participate successfully in sport – remains a conceptually useful lens through which to examine doping in sport today. Women competitors with androgynous appearances, or who reject obvious markers of the idealized feminine athlete, raise flags of suspicion (Pieper, 2016). There is a long history of women athletes avoiding heavy weightlifting or 'body movements that connote strength, violence, or much aggression' (Davis & Delano, 1992, p. 14). Athletes who refuse to adhere to female apologetic behaviours, that is who refuse to 'apologize' for their athletic talent by adhering to heteronormative femininity, continue to face increased scrutiny about both their sex and gender (Hardy, 2015). For more than four decades, scholars in the sociology and philosophy of sport have analyzed and challenged the naturalness of gender and heterosexual standards in sport (e.g. Fairchild, 1989; Hall, 2002; Lenskyj, 2003; Lock, 2003; Patton, 2001). Lock (2003) argues that doping bans function to promote a heteronormative gender order, and that public aversion to women doping stems from a wider dislike of women deemed 'ugly' because of their insufficient adherence to the requirements of female apologetic behaviour. As Jesper Andreasson and April Henning (2021) more recently observed, 'Understandings of image and performance enhancing drugs (IPEDs) and their use has largely been conceptualized through the lens of male hegemonic patterns, treating women's doping as a threat to the "natural" gender order' (p. 2).

Concern about women and doping stemmed primarily from fear of the resulting masculinizing side effects of many PEDs, rather than a concern for leveling the playing field or ensuring no woman had an unfair advantage. With doping, women's bodies often, but not always, undergo several striking physical changes; anabolic steroid use, for example, is associated with narrow hips, small breasts, increased musculature, severe acne, deepened voices and substantial amounts of facial and pubic hair. As a result, women who use anabolic steroids are criticized as looking and sounding like men. As Lock (2003) argues,

> Doping then is not the significant crime committed by female dopers; it is the failure to express heterosexual femininity. In popular sport discourse, I suggest that the hegemonic notion of doping is doping that has masculinizing effects of female athletes. Coherent with this, women who have not doped, but are not heterosexually feminine, are criticized in the same way as female dopers who are considered to have become more masculine. The offence then is primarily one of appearance; it is women who do not visibly express heterosexual femininity who are disgusting (p. 408).

Drawing on similar observations, Davis and Delano (1992) argued that anti-drug media campaigns tend to encourage readers and viewers to assume that bodies fit naturally into unambiguous categories of gender, and that steroids will disrupt this 'natural' gender dichotomization. The growth of women's body-building culture, and increases in doping by participants, challenges what now counts as acceptable and unacceptable forms of displaying femininity and masculinity in sport (Andreasson & Johansson, 2021; McGrath & Chananie-Hill, 2009; Roussel & Griffet, 2000).

As doping is still considered a form of cheating, lying and deceitful behaviour that directly conflicts with ideas surrounding appropriate feminine behaviour, women who dope continue to pose a serious problem for sport. Using banned drugs, substances or methods to excel at sport conflicts with the historical 'ideal' image of women as feminine, heterosexual, fair, honest and submissive. In contrast, male athletes taking anabolic steroids and experiencing similar physiological changes tend to be viewed as strong and powerful, not ugly and unnatural. Feminist philosopher Iris Marion Young's observations from over 40 years ago continue to ring true today. According to Young (1980), many people believe that if a woman succeeds at sport, she either demonstrates male characteristics and is not really a woman, or she is succeeding in an event that is not a real sport. As the next section highlights, many of the outdated gender stereotypes attached to female and male bodies persist in sport and are exacerbated by the conflation of drug testing and sex testing protocols in sport.

CONSEQUENCES OF CONFLATING DOPING, SEX TESTING AND GENDER POLICING

The historical and continued overlap in the International Olympic Committee (IOC)'s rationales for sex verification and drug testing, which emerged concurrently in the 1960s, contribute to the gendered nature of doping (Sailors et al., 2012). As the history of doping in sport demonstrates, the terms 'performance enhancing drugs' and 'doping' were not used with much frequency prior to the end of the 1950s in the sporting community as most sport governing bodies were unconcerned with censoring what substances or drugs were permissible for athletes to use. This changed following the well-publicized and well-analyzed deaths of cyclists Knud E. Jensen at the 1960 Olympic Games in Rome and Tommy Simpson during a stage of the Tour de France in 1967, both of which gathered substantial media attention when they occurred (Mignon, 2003). Because of the negative public reaction to the presumed drug-induced deaths of elite male athletes, IOC members began discussing what they could do to prevent similar situations in the future. One proposed solution was the creation of a medical commission to address the growing problem of doping in sport.

Archival documents contained in Canadian IOC member James Worrall's papers (available at the International Centre for Olympic Studies at Western University in London, Canada) show that the IOC sought to both promote fairness and protect athletes' health by regulating drug use at the Olympic Games. Worrall served as the president of the Canadian Olympic Committee from 1964 to 1968, and as an IOC member from 1967 to 1989, so had intimate knowledge of the work undertaken by the IOC and its newly created medical commission in the 1960s. The attitudes of key IOC members toward women in sport demonstrate the long history of merging the discourses surrounding sex testing and drug testing in sport, with both issues often being lumped together as issues of fairness (Sailors et al., 2012). While one might think that sex testing and drug testing are clearly different issues, undertaken with different intentions and underpinned by different arguments for their continued use in sport, their shared history suggests otherwise.

According to Olympic historian Wolf Lyberg's summary of the minutes of the IOC and IOC executive board meetings, a discussion of doping in sport by the IOC took place in 1960 at the 57th session of the IOC in San Francisco, USA, not long after Jensen's death. At this meeting, IOC President Avery Brundage declared, 'We need to look into doping', and echoed a similar call to action at the 59th session of the IOC in Athens, Greece, in 1961 (Lyberg, 1994). The need to do so led to the appointment of an IOC medical commission, which included male IOC members Sir Arthur Porritt (New Zealand), Dr Josef Gruss (Czechoslovakia), Ryotaru Azuma (Japan) and Ferreira Santos (Brazil). In 1962, at the 60th meeting of the executive board in Lausanne, Switzerland, the IOC medical commission agreed to study the issue of doping further by way of appointing a doping committee, which consisted of almost the same group of men appointed to the medical commission one year earlier (Lyberg, 1994). Lyberg's summaries do not mention any news or reports from the IOC's medical commission or the doping committee at the IOC or IOC executive board sessions again until Arthur Porritt presented a report in 1966 on doping at the 64th session of the IOC in Rome, Italy. This report echoes the report given at the 63rd session two years prior, stating: 'it is fully realized that the problem of doping can be met only by a long-term education policy stressing the physical and moral aspects of the subject' (IOC Doping Committee, 1967). It is here that the merger of the anti-doping and sex testing movements begins. Porritt reported the medical commission had identified three areas for further study: doping, sex testing and anabolic steroids. Members of the IOC medical commission agreed that these areas required attention to ensure fairness in sport.

The proliferation of women's events on the Olympic program, in the Cold War context, brought greater incentives for nations to win gold medals in women's events. Suspicions about women competitors' biological sex arose after athletes performed feats previously thought incapable by women or failed to embrace hegemonic femininity and the obvious feminine markers of the time (Beamish & Ritchie, 2005). For some successful athletes, such as sisters Tamara and Irina Press who represented the former Soviet Union, their great athletic talent led critics to contend that to perform at such a high level they must either be men or steroid users, fueling 'speculation about both steroid use and gender fraud' (Kraus, 2002, p. 2). Unfounded rumours of nations seeking men or intersex athletes to compete in women's events were also prevalent (Skirstad, 2000, p. 116).

To discourage gender fraud, the IOC's medical commission declared in 1967 that all women competing at the Olympics would require a sex test to verify they were women prior to competing (IOC, 1967). The following year, a member of the medical commission summarized in the report of the 1968 winter games that 'The IOC Medical Commission's activities at the Grenoble Games were carried out in two spheres: controlling the sex of women and controlling doping' (IOC Medical Commission, 1968, p. 1). In the same report, a member noted, 'It is inevitable that sooner or later, the representatives of the weaker sex should feel persecuted and ask that the feminine records be awarded to them' (p. 2). Athletes advocating for clean, doping-free sport and strong penalties for doping argue similar sentiments, but with far less paternalistic undertones. Fairness, the IOC medical commissions members believed, could be ensured through banning PEDs and verifying all competitors in the women's events had XX chromosomes.

The IOC's medical commission conducted sex tests on athletes officially between 1968 and 1999 (Pieper, 2016). Writing in the *Lancet*, Myron Genel and Arne Ljungqvist clarified that the IOC's decision to abandon 'gender verification', as they often called the process, in 1999 was not intended to end the sex testing era of sport, but instead to pass the responsibilities from the IOC to the international federations and Olympic host city organizing committees. As a bonus, they noted, this change would result in 'saving a lot of embarrassment – and money' (Genel & Ljungqvist, 2005, p. S41). Their statement suggests that the motivation for eliminating mandatory sex testing of all women at the Olympics was at least in part a financial consideration, rather than a human rights issue. Despite relieving itself of the responsibility for conducting sex testing, the IOC and its medical commission were left vulnerable to public scrutiny in the late 1990s following numerous events unfolding at the time, including the International Cycling Union and the Tour de France's doping scandals and bribery of IOC members by host city bid committees coming under public scrutiny. Mistrust and skepticism directed at the IOC, and its supposed fight against drugs in sport, reached the point where the IOC could no longer ignore the situation (Teetzel, 2004).

The IOC had to do something concrete immediately to demonstrate its commitment to addressing doping in sport (Jenkins, 2006). The result was the creation of WADA, and the transfer of responsibility for anti-doping from the IOC medical committee to the new agency. WADA's initial responsibilities included: (1) establishing a single list of banned substances; (2) coordinating standards of collecting random unannounced tests; (3) coordinating standards to collect and analyze samples; (4) advocating for unified drug sanctions and (5) promoting research (Wilson, 1999). A key goal was universality, to ensure athletes competing in different Olympic sports in different countries were held to the same doping standards and rules. None of these original initiatives directly address gender, specifically, or overtly acknowledge that motivations to commit ADRVs vary among athletes or that gender differences are present among men and women in sport.

The mingling of drug testing and sex testing protocols and rationales, which began with the IOC and its medical commission in the 1960s, continues today with questions about how intersex and transgender athletes can compete fairly in high-performance sport. Regulating testosterone has always played an enormous role in both sets of rules, and the current policies in force outlining eligibility requirements for transgender and athletes with differences in sexual development (DSD) continue to set maximum upper limits for endogenous testosterone for competitors seeking to compete in women's events. The moral acceptability of regulating endogenous testosterone production in women, particularly intersex athletes who identify as women and compete in women's sport, has led to human rights challenges by athletes who were told their natural testosterone levels were too high to compete in specific athletics events (Human Rights Watch, 2020; Karkazis & Carpenter, 2018). That testosterone provides performance enhancing benefits is not under doubt, but the extent to which endogenous testosterone levels provide athletes with an unfair advantage remains a highly contested issue in sport (Jordan-Young & Karkazis, 2019; Wells, 2020). From its formation, the IOC medical commission's attention to women was directed at sex testing to 'protect' the women's category from men and women with intersex traits, similar to the goal of protecting 'clean' athletes from those using banned PEDs. Neither the IOC's medical commission nor its doping committee appear to have expressed any concern about women athletes intentionally doping to improve their performances. Doping concerns, and the resulting rules and regulations to combat doping in sport, seem designed with men in mind to the neglect of women athletes.

CONCLUSION

Histories of doping and anti-doping in sport rarely recognize the stories of women who dope. As the research literature and WADA publications on women and gender in doping suggest, gender is rarely a focus of anti-doping research. That a WADA working group could not determine with any confidence the prevalence of women engaged in doping in high-performance sport highlights the lack of attention to women's doping in the research literature. The media has long perpetuated the idea that women are inferior and unnatural athletes, which impacts how women's doping is covered, portrayed and researched. In many traditional 'masculine' sports, women who excel are still considered 'mannish' if they sport overly muscular or androgynous physiques. For example, Plymire (1999) highlights former chief medical officer for the United States Olympic Committee Robert Voy's public statement that many female athletes do not look, in his opinion, sufficiently feminine: 'Anyone taking a look at these "women" would be hard pressed to remember in them the girl next door (unless you lived next to the New York Jets)' (p. 159). Further, because both drug testing and sex testing are concerned with athletes' testosterone levels, the eligibility of intersex and transgender athletes continues to be misconstrued in the media as doping and fairness issues. Women whose bodies do not reflect heteronormative feminine ideals continue to be heavily criticized and face suspicion that they are drug cheats.

Concerns about women doping do not seem to be rooted in health concerns, or even maintaining a level playing field, but instead seem preoccupied with policing what athletes should look like on the field and who should be permitted to compete in women's events. Moving forward, long-held assumptions in sport that strong, fast women are strong and fast as a result of doping or of 'gender fraud', not intensive training, must be challenged. The continued marginalization of women in sport, combined with the lack of consideration of women in the development of the anti-doping system, results in a lack of scholarly analysis of the intersections of women, gender and doping.

KEY READINGS

(1) Andreasson, J., & Johansson, T. (2021). Negotiating female fitness doping: Gender, identity and transgressions. *Sport in Society*, *24*(3), 323–339. https://doi.org/10.1080/17430437.2019.1672152

This article provides an excellent overview of women's experiences with doping in the fitness area. Andreasson and Johansson provide new insights into foundational issues associated with doping in the fitness industry.

(2) Beamish, R., & Ritchie, I. (2005). The spectre of steroids: Nazi propaganda, Cold War anxiety and patriarchal paternalism. *International Journal of the History of Sport*, *22*(5), 777–795.

For an in-depth analysis of how and why sports organizations began to care about steroid and hormone use in sport, Beamish and Ritchie's article provides a detailed and nuanced understanding of the history of doping in sport.

(3) Burke, M. (2004). What would happen if a 'woman' outpaced the winner of the gold medal in the 'men's' one hundred meters? Female sport, drugs and the transgressive cyborg body. *Philosophy in the Contemporary World*, *11*(1), 35–43.

In this thought-provoking article, Burke raises numerous issues about how we think about women's bodies and successes in sport.

(4) Henne, K. (2015). *Testing for athlete citizenship: Regulating doping and sex in sport.* Rutgers University Press.

Henne's book was the first to address both doping and sex testing in sport in a detailed and systematic way. Covering the history of and science behind rules designed to control athlete eligibility in sport, Henne's book is an accessible and fascinating introduction for readers interested in women's doping.

(5) Lock, R. A. (2003). The doping ban: Compulsory heterosexuality and lesbophobia. *International Review for the Sociology of Sport, 38*(4), 397–411.

Lock's work on doping and lesbophobia is foundational for understanding why women athletes continue to face stereotypes and double standards in sport.

REFERENCES

Andreasson, J., & Henning, A. (2021). Challenging hegemony through narrative: Centering women's experiences and establishing a sis-science culture through a women-only doping forum. *Communication & Sport.* https://doi.org/10.1177/21674795211000657

Andreasson, J., & Johansson, T. (2021). Negotiating female fitness doping: Gender, identity and transgressions. *Sport in Society, 24*(3), 323–339. https://doi.org/10.1080/17430437.2019.1672152

Badenhausen, K. (2020, February 20). Maria Sharapova retires from tennis with $325 million in career earnings. *Forbes.* https://www.forbes.com/sites/kurtbadenhausen/2020/02/26/maria-sharapova-retires-from-tennis-with-325-million-in-career-earnings/?sh=3a66c4b9f2cf

Beamish, R., & Ritchie, I. (2005). The spectre of steroids: Nazi propaganda, Cold War anxiety and patriarchal paternalism. *International Journal of the History of Sport, 22*(5), 777–795.

Beamish, R., & Ritchie, I. (2006). *Fastest, highest, strongest: A critique of high-performance sport.* Routledge.

Burke, M. (2004). What would happen if a 'woman' outpaced the winner of the gold medal in the 'men's' one hundred meters? Female sport, drugs and the transgressive cyborg body. *Philosophy in the Contemporary World, 11*(1), 35–43.

CCES (2021). Canadian sport sanction registry. https://cces.ca/canadian-sport-sanction-registry

Davis, L., & Delano, L. (1992). Fixing the boundaries of physical gender: Side effects of anti-drug campaigns in athletics. *Sociology of Sport Journal, 9*(1), 1–19.

de Hon, O., Kuipers, H., & van Bottenburg, M. (2015). Prevalence of doping use in elite sports: A review of numbers and methods. *Sports Medicine, 45*, 57–69.

Douglas, D. D. (2014). Forget me … not. Marion Jones and the politics of punishment. *Journal of Sport & Social Issues, 38*(1), 3–22.

Fairchild, D. L. (1989). Sport abjection: Steroids and the uglification of the athlete. *Journal of the Philosophy of Sport, 16*(1), 74–88.

Felshin, J. (1974). The triple option for women in sport. *Quest, 21*, 36–40.

Franke, W. W., & Berendonk, B. (1997). Hormonal doping and androgenisation of athletes: A secret program of the German Democratic Republic government. *Clinical Chemistry, 43*(7), 1262–1279.

Genel, M., & Ljungqvist, A. (2005). Gender verification of female athletes. *Lancet, 366*, S41.

Gleaves, J., Petróczi, A., Folkerts, D., de Hon, O., Macedo, E., Saugy, M., & Cryuff, M. (2021). Doping prevalence in competitive sport: Evidence synthesis with 'best practice' recommendations and reporting guidelines from the WADA working group on doping prevalence. *Sports Medicine, 51*, 1909–1934. https://doi-org.uml.idm.oclc.org/10.1007/s40279-021-01477-y

Graham, M. R., Davies, B., Grace, F. M., Kicman, A., & Baker, J. S. (2008) Anabolic steroid use: Patterns of use and detection of doping. *Sports Medicine, 38*(6), 505–525.

Hall, M. A. (1996). Feminism and sporting bodies. *Human Kinetics.*

Hall, M. A. (2002). *The girl and the game: A history of women's sport in Canada.* Broadview Press.

Hardy, E. (2015). The female apologetic within Canadian women's rugby: Athlete perceptions and media influences. *Sport in Society, 18*(2), 155–167.

Henne, K. (2015). *Testing for athlete citizenship: Regulating doping and sex in sport.* Rutgers University Press.

Human Rights Watch. (2020, December 4). *'They're chasing us away from sport': Human rights violations in sex testing of elite women athletes.* Human Rights Watch. https://www.hrw.org/report/2020/12/04/theyre-chasing-us-away-sport/human-rights-violations-sex-testing-elite-women

IOC. (1967). *Press Release Lausanne September 27, 1967.* Avery Brundage Collection, Reel 47, Box 86, Medical Committee Minutes and Reports January 25–26 1969, ICOS.

IOC Doping Committee. (1967). *Doping Committee Report,* 3 March 1966, Avery Brundage Collection, 1908–1975, Box 82, reel 45, ICOS.

IOC Medical Commission. (1968). *Medical Commission of the Olympic Games Reports: 1 Grenoble 2 Mexico.* James Worrall Collection, Box 25, Red Folder, ICOS.

Issari, P., & Coombs, R. (1998). Women, drug use, and drug testing: The case of the intercollegiate athletes. *Journal of Sport & Social Issues, 22*(2), 153–169.

Jenkins, C. A. (2006). *Establishing a World Anti-Doping Code: WADA's impact on the development of an international strategy for anti-doping in sport.* Master's Thesis, University of Windsor Electronic Theses and Dissertations. https://scholar.uwindsor.ca/etd/1959

Jordan-Young, R. M., & Karkazis, K. (2019). *Testosterone: An unauthorized biography.* Harvard University Press.

Karkazis, K., & Carpenter, M. (2018). Impossible choices: The inherent harms of regulating women's testosterone in sport. *Bioethical Inquiry, 15,* 579–587.

Katims, D. S., & Zapata, J. T. (1993). Gender differences in substance use among Mexican American school-age children. *Journal of School Health, 63*(9), 397–401.

Kraus, C. (2002). Sports: Transgender issues. *LGBTQ Archive.* http://www.glbtqarchive.com/arts/sports_transgender_issues_A.pdf

Lenskyj, H. (1986). *Out of bounds: Women, sport, and sexuality.* Women's Press.

Lenskyj, H. J. (2003). *Out on the field: Gender, sport and sexualities.* Women's Press.

Lock, R. A. (2003). The doping ban: Compulsory heterosexuality and lesbophobia. *International Review for the Sociology of Sport, 38*(4), 397–411.

Lorente, F. O. (2003). Substance use: Gender differences among French sport sciences students. *International Journal of Drug Policy, 14*(3), 269–272.

Lyberg, W. (1994). Minutes, 57th IOC Session, San Francisco – 1960. In W. Lyberg (Ed.), The IOC Sessions 1956–1988 volume II. IOC.

Magdalinski, T. (2009). *Sport, technology and the body: The nature of performance.* Routledge.

McGrath, S., & Chananie-Hill, R. (2009). 'Big freaky-looking women': Normalizing gender transgression through bodybuilding. *Sociology of Sport Journal, 26*(2), 235–254. https://doi.org/10.1123/ssj.26.2.235

Mignon, P. (2003). The Tour de France and the doping issue. *International Journal of the History of Sport, 20*(2), 227–245.

Miller, K. E., Barnes, G. M., Sabo, D., Melnick, M. J., & Farrell, M. P. (2002). A comparison of health risk behavior in adolescent users of anabolic androgenic steroids, by gender and athletes status. *Sociology of Sport Journal, 19*(4), 385–402.

Montague, J. (2012, August 10). Saving Flo Jo: Taking back a legacy. *CNN.* https://www.cnn.com/2012/08/10/sport/olympics-flo-jo-seoul/index.html

Moore, R. (2012). *The dirtiest race in history: Ben Johnson, Carl Lewis and the 1988 Olympic 100m final.* Bloomsbury.

Muller, S. M., Gorrow, T. R., & Schneider, S. R. (2009). Enhancing appearance and sports performance: Are female collegiate athletes behaving more like males? *Journal of American College Health, 57*(5), 513–520.

Ntoumanis, N., Ng, J. Y. Y., Barkoukis, V., & Backhouse, S. (2014). Personal and psychological predictors of doping use in physical activity settings: A meta-analysis. *Sports Medicine, 44,* 1603–1624.

Patton, C. (2001). Rock hard: Judging the female physique. *Journal of Sport & Social Issues, 25*(2), 118–140.

Pfister, G., & Gems, G. (2013). Fairy tales? Marion Jones, C. J. Hunter and the framing of doping in American newspapers. *Sport in Society, 18*(2), 136–154.

Pieper, L. P. (2016). *Sex testing: Gender policing in women's sports.* University of Chicago Press.

Plymire, D. C. (1999). Too much, too fast, too soon: Chinese women runners, accusations of steroid use, and the politics of American track and field. *Sociology of Sport Journal, 16*(2), 155–173.

Roussel, P., & Griffet, J. (2000). The path chosen by female bodybuilders: A tentative interpretation. *Sociology of Sport Journal, 17*(2), 130–135. https://doi.org/10.1123/ssj.17.2.130

Sailors, P. R., Teetzel, S., & Weaving, C. (2012). The complexities of sport, gender and drug testing. *The American Journal of Bioethics, 12*(7), 23–25.

Skirstad, B. (2000). Gender verification in competitive sport. In T. Tännsjö & C. Tamburrini (Eds.), *Values in sport: Elitism, nationalism, gender equality and the scientific manufacture of winners.* E&FN Spon.

Sports Illustrated. (2006, September 18). Fast women, foolish choices. *Sports Illustrated, 105*(11), 20.

Teetzel, S. (2004). The road to WADA. In K. Wamsley, R. K. Barney, & S. Martyn (Eds.), *Cultural relations old and new: The transitory Olympic ethos* (pp. 213–224). International Centre for Olympic Studies.

Teetzel, S. (2011). Steroid use. In M. Z. Strange & C. K. Oyster (Eds.), *Encyclopedia of women in today's world, volume 3* (pp. 1405–1406). Sage Reference.

UKAD. (2021). Sanctions ADRVs. https://www.ukad.org.uk/sanctions

Ungerleider, S. (2001). *Faust's gold: Inside the East German doping machine.* St. Martins Press.

USADA. (2021). *Sanctions.* https://www.usada.org/news/sanctions/

Weaving, C., & Teetzel, S. (2014). Getting jacked and burning fat: Examining doping and gender stereotypes in Canadian university sport. *Journal of Intercollegiate Sport, 7*(2), 198–217.

Wells, C. J. (2020). *On the resiliency of sex testing in sport.* PhD Dissertation, University of British Columbia.

Wilson, S. (1999, November 11). IOC establishes world drug agency. *Associated Press.* https://www.skimag.com/uncategorized/ioc-establishes-world-drug-agency/

World Athletics. (2021). World records. https://www.worldathletics.org/records/by-category/world-records

Young, I. M. (1980). Throwing like a girl: A phenomenology of feminine body comportment motility and spatiality. *Human Studies, 3*(2), 137–156.

CONCLUSION: DOPING: UNBOUND

April Henning and Jesper Andreasson

ABSTRACT

This chapter concludes the volume. This is done in two capacities. First, the contributing chapters within in each theme are brought together through a reflexive discussion on current debates on anti-doping approaches, health and risk, doping arenas and communities, and the gendering of doping. Second, the interrelationships between the themes are discussed, pointing to new research directions.

Keywords: Sport and fitness; anti-doping; health; risk; doping arenas; gender

Doping and IPED use have largely been discussed in narrow ways according to somewhat arbitrary lines drawn around and between contexts, categories and even groups of people. In many ways, doping divides and divisions have bound how doping has been researched, and even experienced. Rigid boundaries serve to maintain a partial picture of doping and IPED use, not only limiting our understanding but also obscuring the complexities of the issue. Though some may benefit from such stark divisions – such as anti-doping organizations who rely on a zero-tolerance, right-versus-wrong understanding of doping – we have endeavoured to look beyond such dividing lines. Here we build on our conceptualization of doping and IPED use as nesting dolls, in which one theme rests within or around each of the others. In the following sections, we take a look at each thematic layer in this volume to highlight the conversations happening between the authors. Following this, we offer a higher order summary and a look at where research in this area might go next.

ANTI-DOPING: SETTING THE TONE

Anti-doping blurs the lines between global policy (e.g. WADA) and more local policies (e.g. national laws). Though anti-doping policies can be separate in

Doping in Sport and Fitness
Research in the Sociology of Sport, Volume 16, 253–261
Copyright © 2023 by Emerald Publishing Limited
All rights of reproduction in any form reserved
ISSN: 1476-2854/doi:10.1108/S1476-285420220000016014

implementation and enforcement, they are often underpinned by similar motivations and understandings of doping and other IPED use. By definition,
anti-doping is in opposition to doping as both a practice undertaken by individuals, and as a phenomenon. To be against doping, one must also target
individuals who dope or engage in IPED use. Anti-doping policies are intended to
operationalize this perspective, often attempting to eradicate the phenomenon by
targeting various groups and individuals engaging in specific practices. In sport,
we see this through anti-doping policies that prohibit athletes from using certain
substances, enforce these rules through biological sample collection and testing
and punish rule violations with competition bans. Outside of sport, many
countries have passed national laws that regulate the sale, purchase, possession
and even use of IPEDs for whole populations. These can include criminal penalties for some substances (i.e. anabolic steroids in Sweden) or for some behaviours (i.e. importing anabolic steroids through the post in the UK). In gym and
fitness contexts, this individual-level focus has resulted in preventative measures
where muscular bodies are profiled and exiled. In sport we see ongoing discussions of athletes' responsibilities to avoid doping and the rights of athletes to
compete in doping-free sport. Receiving far less attention are the rights of athletes
who get caught up in the anti-doping system in one way or another and the
responsibilities of the anti-doping system to ensure that athlete rights are protected. For example, if an athlete does not receive anti-doping education and then
tests positive for a prohibited substance, the focus is rarely on the institutional
failure or that athletes are bound by a complex set of rules that can be difficult, to
say the least, for even medical professionals to understand and navigate.

In some ways, simply convincing athletes to not engage in any potentially
doping behaviour would solve the sports doping question. Indeed, anti-doping
rules are often accompanied by strategies to educate against or even attempt to
prevent doping. As Gatterer and Blank argued, these strategies have the potential
to be implemented in more effective ways and with more targeted messaging
relevant to an audience of athletes. Prevention may prove a way forward for
eradicating doping for some specific athlete groups. It is unlikely that all doping
would stop, even just in the sport context, as not all doping offences are related to
intentional use. Each year, athletes receive sanctions for positive tests resulting
from inadvertent or accidental use of a doping substance yet are treated the same
as athletes who fully intended their use. As such, sport anti-doping policies –
namely, the WADA Code – have implications for athletes' rights. As Dasgupta
argued, this can be related to the legal limitations of the Code and the relative
lack of access to non-sport legal recourse for athletes. It can also be the result of
the uneven application of rules across cases, as Lenskyj showed with examples
from the Court of Arbitration for Sport. Both chapters showed, in different ways,
how the Code, and hegemonic anti-doping policies more broadly, can be used in
ways that can be counter-productive to the goal of eradicating doping by targeting athletes with a blanket policy and justice system that cannot account for
specific circumstances. Such loopholes and blind spots can leave athletes
vulnerable to punishments that may not clearly align with an offence or allow

athletes who may be breaking rules to avoid punishment – neither of which seems to match the goals of fair play and doping-free sport.

Policies at any level can represent the largest, outer layer of the nesting doll that encompasses all the others. Anti-doping policies create environments in which IPED use will likely still occur and determine how those individuals will be treated legally, socially, and regarding their health. Yet, what all anti-doping policies have in common is that they reinforce anti-doping as a worldview. The result is that they position any individual who falls afoul of anti-doping rules as bad, such as being a sports cheat or by risking their health to use IPEDs for reaching body goals. They can also lead to suspicion of extraordinary performances or bodies that do not conform to traditional gender norms. Crucially, these policy environments can determine what is or is not possible in terms of access to health and medical care, both legally and socially. Where doping and IPEDs are approached punitively – such as in countries where use is criminalized or in sports where athletes can be banned from competing for years at a time – those who engage in these practices may be unable to ask for and receive support for use in ways that can reduce physical risks and protect health from negative outcomes. Policy environments may also have further effects, including limiting the research on how to potentially use substances in ways less likely to result in harm or even having IPEDs and treatment for those who use them left out of medical education. Our next section on *health and risks* picks up these themes.

HEALTH AND RISK: BRIDGING THE GAP?

Just inside the policy layer are considerations around health and risk. Notions of health and risk often underpin anti-doping policies, which also determine how these are addressed strategically. Policies, then, have the potential to create either a supportive or hostile environment for both practice and participants, as well as shape what services are or are not available to support those who engage in use. For example, prevention services may be available under a prohibitive approach, while harm reduction may be limited or even absent. This can directly impact users in terms of physical risks and has implications for service providers. Athletes may be reluctant to seek out support to manage or reduce negative side effects for fear of being banned from sport. Non-athlete IPED users may fear being arrested or even judged by clinicians, while medical practitioners may or may not be educated or willing to engage with IPED users, either due to a lack of knowledge or an unwillingness to support use.

In public discourse and in the scholarly debate, IPEDs and polydrug use have long been connected to questions of health and risk. In sport, for example, anti-doping approaches have been rationalized by policymakers as means of securing the health and prosperity of athletes, as well as protecting fair play. Seemingly, sport and athletes should be protected at all costs. In parallel, the gym and fitness industry has been revitalized in recent decades – perhaps even gentrified – by efforts to 'clean up' a culture with what is thought to be a questionable history. In this process, previous subcultural gym settings associated with extreme body ideals, steroids and risks have been replaced by a fitness culture where healthy-looking bodies are put on display, but where there are also amenities like social spaces and playrooms for children. Bodybuilders and steroid-fuelled bodies have been largely marginalized and culturally exiled in the process, seen as representations of unhealthy bodies and risky lifestyles.

Images of and cultural narratives about doping seemingly cut through the organizational, institutional and social dimensions of sport and fitness. Being social constructs, narratives of doping and IPEDs and any associated health risks also function discursively as moral compasses. The judgements of those unwilling or unable to comply with the narrative of harm have often been harsh and swift, regardless of whether certain drugs have been used for legitimate medical reasons, to get a competitive edge in sport, to achieve a certain look, or something else. Indeed, users have not only faced severe judgement for doping violations but have also been constructed as moral spectacles. The problem with discussions based on moral stances and convictions is that they tend to steer the course towards their preferred outcome, and at the same time contribute to extreme and even de-humanizing perspectives on the non-compliant; in this case, those engaging in use. The ability to dominate the narrative through organization, policy and more is power. But when rule enforcers also become what Becker (1963/2018) describes as *moral crusaders* and campaigns around a symbolic issue, such as doping, become institutionalized, there is always the risk of unintended consequences. Health can become risk, and support can become judgement. These processes tend to create more distance between perspectives rather than foster any alternative understanding.

Indeed, the gap between anti-doping stakeholders (organizations, policy-makers and others) on one side and users with hands-on experience who have a variety of motivations on the other has sometimes been abysmal. Controlling the doping narrative of harm also has meant that it has been sometimes taken for granted that doping is a public health issue. However, the impact of doping in society and in relation to public health issues has not been sufficiently addressed, nor have the anticipated and dose-related potential harms that may follow doping use, to determine if doping constitutes a public health issue. By introducing and debating criteria for what constitutes a public health issue, McVeigh, Bates and Yarwood contribute a way to systematize this discussion, not least by relocating it outside a context often steered by moral crusaders. This incentive has other clear benefits. It is vital for the 'broader brush' to set the scene and to analyse questions concerning doping, health and risks through a lens that allows us to see that users themselves operate in diverse contexts, sometimes simultaneously. Adding to this, we can also begin to debate health and risk in a more nuanced manner, taking into consideration that doping demographics are in motion and that the risks associated with use vary tremendously. This has further implications for how we can understand and look at healthcare providers' engagement with IPED users and vice versa, which is discussed by Dunn. The interaction between healthcare providers and users can also help us to zoom in on questions concerning health and risk when narrowing down the gap between institutional and user-oriented perspectives. This is further illustrated through Underwood's chapter on Trenbolone and its potential harms. The chapter not only highlights how (potential) harm needs to be understood in relation to the particularities of different IPEDs but also – as touched upon in the chapter before – how such knowledge is vital for healthcare providers to do their job in a respectful and informed manner. Underwood's chapter further illustrates how situated discussions on doping as a sport or fitness issue is largely outdated and that the narrative needs to be re-formulated. New arenas and user groups are emerging and many questions on how health and risks are debated and dealt with within these are yet to be answered.

DOPING SPACES AND GROUPS

Directly related to this are doping spaces/arenas and communities, our third layer. If community or services are unavailable in the local environment, individuals engaging in use may move to more supportive contexts where they are less likely to fall afoul of policies or face negative social consequences. Online forums and other digital platforms can help users share information and experiences with one another – including information related to harm reduction – in a less visible and sometimes anonymous way. Communities may also form as needs arise, despite a prohibitive context, including where particular body ideals, gender dynamics or identity goals exist.

As noted in the introduction, doping has most commonly been associated with elite competitive sport or bodybuilding. Seemingly cut into two pieces, much public awareness of, and the scholarly debate on, doping has been fuelled by these contextual rigidities and ignored other doping arenas. High-profile sports scandals of athletes found to be doping and commentary about freakishly built bodybuilding bodies, linking IPEDs with cutthroat competitions and hard-core bodybuilding milieus, have dominated. In either case, doping and people who use IPEDs are understood as marginal groups who operate outside the bounds of fair play, morality and often legality – as discussed in previous section. However, who uses IPEDs and where use behaviours are learned and supported have changed. New use communities are emerging – or being acknowledged within research – and connecting in new spaces, both online and offline. Some of these shifts may be due to a range of factors including changing body and gender ideals, internet-based routes of sale and acquisition, and the ability to connect and share experiences with others anonymously via web forums. The expansion of doping arenas beyond elite sport training camps and basement gyms also has implications for how we understand what doping and IPED use is and how it is debated, as well as for how substances are regulated.

The three chapters included in the theme *doping arenas and communities* each highlight aspects of these changing doping venues and user groups. Fincoeur and Rullo draw our attention to a group and setting largely overlooked by enhancement and doping researchers to this point: incarcerated individuals. As they show, despite steroids and other IPEDs making their way into prison settings, these substances are largely overlooked as a significant issue by researchers, prison personnel and even the inmates themselves relative to other recreational substances. These findings, in some ways, turn the sport-based idea of IPEDs as a problem on its head, as they are viewed as less risky than other substances in this arena. Prison is not the only venue in which IPEDs are discussed differently from sport and fitness. The sport and fitness divide has also backgrounded the significance of online communication, even though it is widely acknowledged that the internet has changed the routes of information and market exchange on doping. Online fitness forums facilitate digital spaces where IPED communities can form. As shown by Turnock and Townsend, these forums can shape use behaviours, in ways that makes the hegemonic divide between sport and fitness largely appear obsolete. Instead, this context can highlight how a broader group of recreational users, among others, engage in the practice and deal with questions concerning access, harm reduction, gender and more.

One user group that cuts through the sport and fitness divide is recreational athletes. Though the link between sport and doping seems quite clear, our understanding of doping at the recreational sport level has only begun. Even though the WADA Code now explicitly includes recreational athletes in much the same ways as elite athletes, the full impacts this could have on sport and athletes at these lower competitive levels is not yet clear. As Cox, McNamee and Bloodworth highlighted, fitting the Code onto this mass population of athletes brings new challenges to anti-doping among other things.

Taken together, these chapters show how narrowly focused research on doping and IPED use has been to date. Rather than being a sports problem or something that only marginalized bodybuilders would use, doping as a practice is expanding into new groups and leading to new user communities even where substances or their use is prohibited. Doping as a phenomenon is also expanding into spaces that enable use and sharing experiences among participants. These spaces may also act as sites for the sale and acquisition of IPEDs, further changing the shape of what doping looks like and who can access enhancing substances. This opening of new markets to new groups runs counter to policies seeking to eradicate or limit IPEDs. Both types of expansion also have implications for health and risks, as discussed in the previous section, as well as for how policymakers in sport and at the national level seek to prevent, prohibit, regulate or support use. Doping has many complex layers that, once explored, challenge the narrowly constructed narratives around IPED use. Focussing on previously overlooked groups and spaces allows us a fuller understanding of who engages in IPED use and where they do so. We return to this notion in our final thematic section on gender.

(RE-)GENDERING DOPING

Gender, the innermost layer of our four themes, acts as an always-present core to doping. As in many areas of life, gender is always at play. It structures and is structured by policies, socio-cultural norms of bodies and roles, health and medical knowledge and narratives, how and where users engage with substances and with one another – all in addition to the users' everyday life experiences. Though closely linked with men and masculinity, doping is not limited to a particular gender group. However, doping and social views of it impact individuals differently, often based on the intersection of a range of factors, including a person's sex, race, socio-economic status and occupation. The meaning and morality attached to IPED use for a straight, wealthy, white man is different from that by a homosexual, lower-class, non-white woman, which is different still from those of trans-men and -women.

In many ways, gender is at the heart of many debates about doping and IPED use. The immediate connection might be between men and anabolic steroids, but this belies the complex gender meanings and anxieties related to bodies, performance and substance use. One of the attractions of IPEDs is that they can enable individuals to shape or improve upon their bodies and performances. In sport, this might be in effort to win competitions by gaining strength, losing weight or improving endurance. Gym-goers might use similar substances to craft bodies that meet social standards of beauty or fitness. But it is this shape-shifting ability that causes controversy, especially where women are concerned. Traditional gender conceptions position women and men as opposites: where men are physically strong and powerful and women are physically weaker and subordinate. Though such stereotypes rarely hold in real life, such notions still underpin our ideas of ideal masculinity and femininity. These gendered meanings of doping have also continued to bleed into and inform the scholarly debate, stretching from how anti-doping incentives are implemented, to which user groups are researched or excluded.

Henning and Andreasson picked up on these ideas with the elaboration of their concept of *cultural manspreading*. Men are assumed to both require and be entitled to more physical and social space than women, particularly in sport and fitness, reflecting and reinforcing the idea that men are at the centre of these cultures. This also backgrounds women's voices, experiences and expertise. Women are marginalized in diverse ways: spatially, physically, socially, sexually, etc. They are also left to push back against men taking up more than their fair share of social, digital and physical space. This has implications for how women learn about and engage with IPEDs, as well as how they engage with one another. McLean explored some of these questions in her auto-ethnographic look at women, muscle-building and IPEDs. McLean's experiences highlight the importance of both gender and the social environment on the decisions to use or not use IPEDs as part of a gym routine. This chapter further contributes to an ongoing debate within feminist philosophy of science regarding researchers' immersion in their research, and its implications.

IPEDs, particularly when used by women, can help create bodies that challenge gender lines and norms, and show how deeply embedded these can be in culture and society. Women who achieve muscular bodies may be ridiculed for looking too masculine as testosterone and synthetic anabolic steroids can allow women to gain muscle mass and increase power. They may face questions about their character, as well as their sex and gender, if they present as too powerful, too competitive and too massive. Such bodies challenge the gender hierarchy, whether in fitness settings, in sport or elsewhere. These challenges have led to accusations of men masquerading as women for competitive advantage, leading to sport instituting sex testing. Teetzel examined this relationship between anti-doping and sex testing as modern sport has developed. As she showed, there have been recent questions and controversies around women athletes with differences in sex development (DSD) who tend to naturally produce higher levels of testosterone and trans-athletes have raised questions falling into the intersection of sex, gender and sport. In many ways, this shows how sport is attempting to simultaneously define sex, gender and unfair advantage while relying on our incomplete understanding of all three.

Gender is inextricably linked to doping and IPED use via athletes' bodies. Our understandings of what these substances can do alongside what we expect bodies of different sexes to do in terms of gender performance structure how such bodies are treated, regulated and ultimately judged – especially in terms of who is included or excluded – in sport, fitness and broader society. This picture is likely to grow in complexity as more people of all genders use various IPEDs for any number of reasons. Understanding the dynamics at play before moving to regulation may lead to a more effective, supportive and safer environment for those often overlooked in research and debate on this topic.

DOPING IN SPORT, FITNESS AND BEYOND

As above, we have illustrated the interdependencies of each thematic layer to show the complexities of doping and IPED use both in and out of sport and fitness contexts. The nesting doll imagery is useful for us as it helps us understand how each can be considered on their own but are inextricably related to each of the others. In this volume, our first outer theme (layer) focused on policy. Though a case could be made for any of our themes to be the one encompassing all the others, the policy environment has implications for each of the other themes. We put policy here to reflect how policies around doping and IPEDs create the environment in which use does or does not happen (Andreasson & Henning, 2021). In sport and society, prohibitive policies mean individuals have little or no ability to use or admit use in the open, nor to access some services and service providers who may support use and reduce risk. Such environments push use into the shadows and leave individuals vulnerable to a whole range of risks, depending on the particular context and their individual circumstances. Men and women, for example, face different kinds of risks. Beyond the physical, there are social, legal and even economic risks that can have uneven outcomes, including impacting men differently from women, young people differently from older, the wealthy differently from the poor and athletes differently from non-athletes. Policies can also guide public opinion on IPEDs and doping. Where doping is prohibited or criminalized, doping as a phenomenon is necessarily understood as bad or anti-social. However, doping as a practice – and therefore its participants – are often viewed in the same way. Doping becomes attached to certain physiques or performances, linking such deviant forms with negative moral connotations. This can be particularly damaging for individuals whose bodies already challenge social norms, including racialized norms of beauty and gender, as they may be viewed as morally dubious regardless of their IPED use status.

There are also ramifications for where and how individuals engage with substances and with one another. One clear example is the internet. The development of online spaces as doping spaces may be a response to the growing reach of anti-doping policies and laws. When harm reduction is not enabled elsewhere, or if access is limited by other factors, it may take place online. This is an efficient and potentially less risky way of engaging in this work, though it does come with its own set of risks. Information may not be reliable or accurate, there may be a lack of preventative work and the gendered dynamic of doping forums can all lead to negative outcomes for those engaging in these spaces. Further, use still happens in the offline world. No matter the online dynamic, there are still risks based around one's geographic and socio-cultural location.

The picture of the doping landscape presented here may seem overly complex, interconnected and riddled with shades of grey. It is certainly much more complex than the generally accepted two-dimensional, black-and-white, right-vs-wrong conception of doping and IPEDs. Though this may seem like an unsolvable problem, we see this as an opportunity to ask and answer broader questions related to doping and IPED use. By breaking down divisions between contexts, concepts and even research disciplines, we can see the relationships between all types of use, including of non-enhancing substances. Rather than focussing narrowly on elite sport or bodybuilding communities, there are ways to extrapolate lessons learned on one topic or in one context and apply them to others. There is further opportunity to cross or even break subject boundaries and consider the overlaps with topics such as recreational use, wellness, pleasure and many more. In short, the complexity of doping can be a strength if we are willing to understand it as more than a simple question of good or bad.

REFERENCES

Andreasson, J., & Henning, A. D. (2021). *Performance cultures and doped bodies: Challenging categories, gender norms and policy responses.* Common Ground.

Becker, H. S. (1963/2018). *Outsiders. Studies in the sociology of deviance.* Free Press.